The Food Is My Friend Diet

Sheldon —

Here's to new food friends & good health!

Best,
Ruth :)

The
Food
Is My
Friend
Diet

**The Ultimate 30-Day
Weight Loss Plan**

**Get Healthy, Conquer Emotional
Eating & Feel Energized**

Ruth Frechman, MA, RDN, CPT

Gales Publishing
Burbank, Calif.

Published by Gales Publishing, Burbank, California.

Library of Congress Cataloging-in-Publication Data

Frechman, Ruth.
The food is my friend diet: the ultimate 30-day weight loss plan.
Get healthy, conquer emotional eating & feel energized
/ Ruth Frechman
ISBN-13: 978-0-9845979-1-8

LCCN: 2010912275

Photography by Rick Redd
Editing by Robin Quinn
(who lost 35 pounds during the editing of this book!)
Copyediting by Flo Selfman
(who lost 11 pounds during the copyediting of this book!)
Cover Design and Layout by James Arneson
Illustrations by Memo Angeles

Books are available at quantity discounts for use in sales promotions, corporate wellness programs, or custom editions initiatives.

For additional information, please contact
GalesPublishing@gmail.com.
Printed in the United States of America
10 9 8 7 6 5 4 3 2 1

This book is dedicated to my wonderful sons, Rick and Jim, who are always there for me.

The Food Is My Friend Diet
Table of Contents

Foreword

*D*iet: a word that strikes fear into the heart of anyone carrying around a few (or more than a few) extra pounds. Most diet books are about deprivation—what you *can't* eat. This book is about what you *can* eat-and there's plenty. Ruth has impeccable credentials and has thoroughly researched everything she writes about, from government research to how to make your way through each section of a supermarket. The book is comprehensive, but the author cleverly breaks it down into doable daily sections, so the reader ingests small, easily digestible bites. It's all done with a positive attitude and a bit of humor. In addition to Ruth's straightforward teaching, you get to follow the progress of her sidekick Jackie Fabulous, and there's even space for you to record your own thoughts and notes. In short, if you didn't already know that food is your friend, you'll find out just how true that is when you go on *The Food Is My Friend Diet* journey.

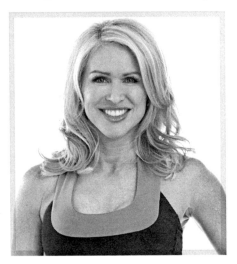

Chris Freytag is a nationally recognized health and fitness expert, blogger, author, and motivational speaker. She is a columnist for *Prevention* magazine, the fitness contributor for the NBC affiliate in Minneapolis, and ACE Board of Directors - Emeritus Member. www.gethealthyu.com.

*I*n a world full of misinformation with promises of "quick fixes," especially when it comes to fitness and nutrition, *The Food Is My Friend Diet* is truly a breath of fresh air. Ruth Frechman draws upon her years of experience helping people, both as a Registered Dietitian and as an ACE-certified Personal Trainer, to provide quality science-based nutritional information to empower readers to truly make lifestyle changes. Ruth takes the guesswork out of how to eat healthy and provides readers with the tools and tips they need to not only lose weight, but to keep it off long-term. She also pro-

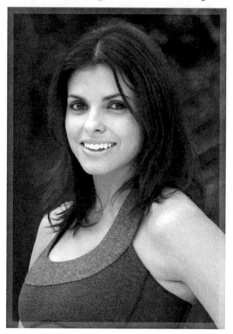

vides guidance on how to lead a more physically active lifestyle, a critical element for weight loss and maintenance, as well as strategies on how to truly change the way we think about food.

Jessica Matthews, MS, is a health and exercise science professor, keynote speaker, yoga educator, blogger, and writer for SHAPE.com. She is a senior advisor for the American Council on Exercise (ACE®). Jessica has been featured as a fitness expert on CNN and has been quoted in numerous publications. www.twitter.com/fitexpertjess.

Introduction

So You Want to Lose Weight

Whether you're new to the diet scene or a seasoned professional, welcome! We'll be spending some time together over the next 30 days.

This is not your typical "diet book." It's not a crazy diet to try for a while and then go back to your usual way of living. This is a "lifestyle book."

Are you always dieting? Are you trying to lose weight, but can't? Do you want to stop thinking about your weight and enjoy life? Sometimes it's the little things that bother us and prevent us from being who we want to be. Once and for all, this book will enable you to lose the excess weight and feel proud. Don't let weight stop you from doing what you want to do.

Why "The Food Is My Friend Diet"?

In helping people lose weight for over 20 years, I've realized that most of my clients, even children, are emotional eaters. When they first come to see me, food really *is* their friend. People and life let them down. Food doesn't, because it's always available. Over time, people learn to use unhealthy foods or excess amounts of food as an impersonal way of dealing with their problems. They eat instead of communicating thoughts, feelings, and desires to other people, sometimes not thoroughly resolving situations. Food helps them cope. This is how food becomes a "friend." However, eating too many unhealthy, high-calorie "food friends" will ultimately add excess weight.

The Food Is My Friend Diet is designed to help you make *new* "food friends." Soon you'll have more healthy "friends," like fruits, vegetables, and physical activity. You can still keep your old "friends," but you'll see them less often. I've also included an entire chapter (Day 4) to help you learn to curb your emotional eating and develop new ways of coping.

Your goal is to lose weight but, more important, to achieve a healthy lifestyle. My goal is to help you do it. With the help of new food friends, let's rid the world of the high blood pressure, high blood sugar, and high cholesterol caused from extra weight. It's a lofty goal; but if everyone tries a little bit, we'll make remarkable improvements to the world's health. If you don't have any health problems now, know that the likelihood of getting something becomes higher, statistically, as you get older. Whatever your reason, let's get started.

What's to Come

During the next 30 days, you'll discover new things about yourself and learn more about nutrition and physical activity. You're in charge, but I'll help you every step of the way. I will give you information and persuade you a little. You will slowly make changes to your lifestyle. If you don't succeed at first, don't give up. You can do whatever you want to do – in spite of the obstacles. Hopefully, you'll smile a little along the way. If you're having fun and enjoying yourself, it will be easier to change.

Meet Jackie Fabulous ... Here to Provide Inspiration and Comic Relief

As a weight loss program, *The Food Is My Friend Diet* works. Jackie has successfully lost eight pounds in 30 days. She is in the book to entertain you with her experiences and thoughts about this program. You'll see **JF:** and then her responses to my questions throughout the book, followed by lines for you to enter your own. Use Jackie as an inspiration. Maybe you'll relate. Maybe not. Be sure to have fun.

As I wrote the book, I wanted to keep the program as simple and painless as possible. You'll learn by doing. This is your personal journal. Keep my book with you. When you see the questions in italics, get ready to come up with some responses. Since I'm only with you in spirit, you can be honest with yourself. A lot of people tell their dietitian that all they eat is salmon and vegetables. It's okay to write down that you ate an entire bag of malted milk balls.

Since you can't lose 20 pounds in a week, and it takes time to change your habits, I suggest that you read one chapter a day and go through the book in 30 days. Each day, you'll learn nutrition information, think about why you want to lose weight, and set new goals. Know that some changes will be required. Sometimes people don't like to change their habits and you may find yourself being resistant at times. In those moments, it's important to remember why you're doing this. The 30 days will go by quickly. After the first 30 days, start over and keep repeating the program until your goals are a lifestyle.

Note: You may want to take a week for each of the chapters. You have the option of working at your own pace.

Know *This* About Weight Loss

There's no magic or quick fix when it comes to losing weight. Basically, you have to eat less than you're eating now and be more active to lose weight. There's no getting around "energy in" and "energy out." "Energy in" means the calories from carbohydrates, protein, fat, and alcohol. "Energy out" is your physical activity. If you can "pinch an inch," there's more "energy in" than "energy out." Adjustments will need to be made. Sometimes it will be easy. Sometimes it won't be so easy.

Follow my suggestions and, most likely, you will be successful. If you go back to your old, perhaps unhealthy habits, you'll gain the weight back. If you end up gaining some of the weight back, I'm confident that you will retain some of the healthy changes. Immediately get back on track and take off the extra weight. Keep practicing your new habits until they become second nature. Lose weight. Be healthy. And live longer!

Let's Move Forward Together

The Food Is My Friend Diet is based on the latest nutrition research and contains everything that you need to lose weight and achieve a healthy lifestyle. I've helped men, women, and children lose thousands, maybe even millions of pounds. When you feel good about yourself, you'll get more things done. It would be my pleasure to help you move beyond thinking about your weight and instead be on your way toward achieving your dreams.

Meet Jackie Fabulous!

Her best friends in the entire world were ice cream, chocolate bars, cake, and any cookie. Her biggest vice was definitely sweets, and Jackie turned to them when lonely, irritated, confused, or bored.

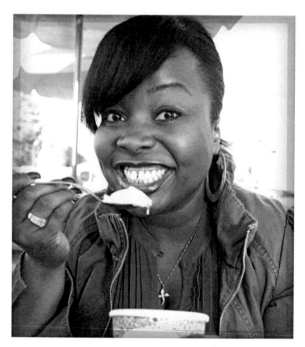

Day 1

Motivation, Motivation, Motivation

*M*otivation is the name of the game when it comes to losing weight. If you don't feel motivated, you're not even going to start. Without motivation, you're definitely not going to hang in there through the rough spots.

Tell yourself right now, "I want to do this … I'm ready to begin today."

Your Starting Point

Let's take a moment to assess your starting place.

How much weight do you want to lose? Be practical or be extravagant. Write down whatever you want.

JF: According to some chart I saw, at 5'4" my ideal weight should be 116 pounds. Since I want to be a healthy "woman" and not a nine-year-old girl, I will just settle for being around 135-140 pounds.

You: _____

_____

Have you tried to lose weight before? What are your comments about your past experiences?

JF: I recently lost 20 pounds through a very, very expensive and popular commercial weight-loss program. At the beginning, I considered staying obese just to save my money. No one should have to make that decision.

You: _____

_____

If you have extra weight, it's important to lose it. Excess weight causes health problems. The latest research says that body fat, especially around the stomach area, is *not* healthy. Fat causes hormones to be released, producing inflammation. The inflammation is a trigger for the start of various diseases, such as heart problems, diabetes, and even cancer. Scary stuff. In contrast, a lean body weight helps control blood pressure, cholesterol, and blood sugar. Good health should be your major reason for losing weight. *You may have other reasons, as well. More energy? Look better? Feel better?*

JF: Energy: I have an insane schedule that requires that I not fall asleep on stage or look drowsy when trying to make others laugh. I have 18-hour days and donuts are (sadly) what I've used for a short-term energy boost.

Look better: I love high heels and the lighter I am, the less painful they are for me.

Feel better: I occasionally have a few cocktails now to feel better but the negative effects of drinking heavily are for another type of book entirely.

The Emotion Factor

Now it's time to get in tune with your emotions. *How are you feeling right now about beginning this program?*

JF: Honestly? I hate change when it comes to food. To me, diets are evil and the only way I have ever lost weight was to stop eating all the foods that make me happy. I am excited about this program but I'm also jaded and scared. It's kind of like meeting another man who swears he's different from the rest.

You: _____

_____

Pictures speak louder than words. Draw a picture of how you feel.

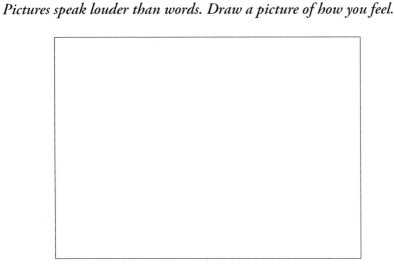

JF: The empty box shows exactly how I feel … empty inside. Which is why I turn to ice cream to fill the void.

When I ask my clients how they feel, some of them just say, "Fine." These people may not be tuned into their emotions. You may also be thinking that you're fine. But once you start considering how you feel about losing weight, you might find stuff going on under the surface. You may not have realized all of the different emotions that you're experiencing. In a similar way, without thinking about it, you may be eating comfort foods to distract yourself from your emotions.

This is where you're starting with the concept of food being your friend. But over the process of working with the book, you'll develop a healthier relationship with food. I believe that most excess weight in the world comes from learning to eat because of emotions. We learn these things early in life. Since every person is different, everyone eats for different emotional reasons. Many of the men, women, and children that I have counseled eat because they are bored or stressed. A lot of people are happy eaters and celebrate with food. Eating for emotions, along with giant portions, snacks galore, and lack of physical activity, can pack on many extra pounds over time.

Why Do *You* Want to Lose Weight?

Only YOU know the answer to this question. Before you start losing weight, you'll need to get your head "in the zone." The most successful losers are very motivated and determined. It's really important to take some time to think about *why* you want to lose weight. That way, you'll stay motivated and determined.

Here are some examples:

- ♦ I want to feel better and have more energy.
- ♦ I want to look better.
- ♦ I want to be healthier.
- ♦ I want to have more fun.
- ♦ I don't like people looking at me or making comments about my weight.
- ♦ I want to feel proud of myself.
- ♦ I want to wear cute, smaller clothes.
- ♦ I want a better job.
- ♦ I want to be able to exercise more.

Everyone says that they want "to look good and feel good." That's not enough motivation to make you lose weight and keep losing. Looking good is okay, but be more specific.

Here are a few more specific reasons why people want to lose weight:

- ♦ I don't want to take blood pressure or cholesterol medication.
- ♦ I don't like my thighs rubbing together when I walk.
- ♦ I don't want to get diabetes like my parents and lose a foot like my dad.
- ♦ Doctor's orders. Lose weight or live a shorter, less healthy life.
- ♦ I don't want to be short of breath when I climb the stairs.
- ♦ I want to fit into roller coaster seats.
- ♦ I want to lose the roll of fat around my stomach so I can get my belly button pierced.

If your reasons for losing weight are personal, and maybe seem a little crazy to others, you'll be more successful. Make an emotional connection. Then when you're tempted to eat more than you need, or you find yourself eating when you're not hungry, remember your reasons for losing. *What's in it for you?*

Again, why do *you* want to take off some pounds? I think that a person's motivations are the MOST IMPORTANT aspect of losing weight. Your reasons will help you stay strong when you're tempted to go off track.

Make a list of reasons for losing weight.

JF: Okay, this list might need its own supplement, but here it goes …

- I don't want to weigh more than the men I date. When your preference is men who are six feet tall and you're still heavier than they are, at some point something's got to give.
- I live in California and literally break out in hives when I hear the words "pool party."
- I want to be hot(ter). I am an attractive woman, but I want to be a "makes cars crash into stop signs," "makes women hate her," and "can fit into provocative outfits" type of hot.
- In the interest of time, I will just say to improve upon an already great life and not be limited because of any insecurity about my body.

You: _____

_____

*R*uth's **Rule:** *A person's motivations are the MOST IMPORTANT aspect of losing weight.*

Do You Care?

Remember … when you don't care, you aren't even going to try. So if you stop caring, you will quit this program. That's why people yo-yo diet. They get motivated for a while and then stop caring. After a while, they start caring again and look for a new gimmick or the latest fad diet to get motivated.

To stick with losing weight, the desire needs to keep coming *from you*. From deep inside. It *has* to be a driving force. Now is the time to think about it. You better start caring or it will catch up to you.

Take a minute to look in the mirror. What do you see? How would you describe your body? How do you feel about your body? What do you like about your body? Is there anything that you don't like about your body? Happy with it? Comfortable? Powerful? Depressed? Don't care?

Let it out.

JF: I seem to only get real mortified with my body in the dressing rooms in clothing stores. It is almost as if I am like "Who switched cute Jackie with this overweight mom of seven?" I love my skin and large boobs but hate my arms, back, and thighs (is that everything?). I just want to see what I would look like if my weight matched my small frame.

You: _____

_____

It's *your* body. Large or small. It's important to take care of your body. We only get one, and it needs to last a lifetime.

Did You Know?

This may surprise you, but there are likely to also be reasons why you *don't* want to lose the weight. These reasons may prevent you from dropping those pounds. To be successful, your reasons why you *want to* lose weight should be more powerful than the reasons why you don't.

Here are examples of reasons why people *don't* want to lose weight.

- I like to eat a lot of sweets.
- I eat lots of carbs (rice, bread, pasta).
- I eat too many high fat or fried foods.
- I drink too much alcohol.
- I love eating and eat too much. I live to eat!
- I can't stop myself from eating too much.
- I'm too stressed and need food for comfort and energy.
- I don't like to exercise.
- I don't have time to exercise.
- I don't want to change what I'm doing.

Why don't you want to lose weight? What stops you from losing weight?

JF: What stops me honestly is laziness. I am not usually lazy, because I fill my life with my love of entertaining people. But if that entertaining is followed by my getting up early to go to the gym, then I'd rather be fat and funny with an occasional nap.

You: _____

_____

Are your reasons for losing weight stronger than the reasons for not losing weight? Set goals for losing weight and eating healthy. It will help you stay motivated. It will make you accountable. Keep working on the goals over and over until they become habits.

However, there's no rush. Don't pressure yourself to lose 50 pounds in one month for a wedding. It's impossible. Have you noticed that it's very easy to gain weight but not so easy to lose weight? That's why, ideally, you don't want to gain any more.

Setting Weight Loss Goals ⌘

Your first goal might be to not gain any more weight. Make sure that your weight is stable. Then set a goal to lose ½-2 pounds a week or 2-8 pounds a month. The more you weigh, the more you can lose in the beginning. Realistically, it is difficult to consistently lose weight every single week. However, if you stick with it, your weight will slowly go down and keep going down until you reach your goal. Note that sometimes people gain a few pounds (rebellion) before they start losing weight.

If you lose weight slowly, you're less apt to gain it back. Sometimes it helps to give yourself a small reward for achieving short-term goals and a bigger reward for achieving larger goals. Be patient. Be persistent. Make slow, steady progress.

Commit with a Contract

Fill out the contract below so that you know exactly what you want to do, why, how much, and in what time frame. You don't have to be perfect. You can always adjust it. It helps to make a commitment.

Personal Contract

I, <u>Jackie Fabulous</u> **Your name here:**_____, am a good person. I am unique and special. My goal is to be the best that I can be. I am taking control over my life.

I want to: (lose weight) (exercise more) (eat healthier) (control emotional eating) etc.

JF: Add to the quality of my life with more energy, more confidence, and to have all that exhibited in the hottest outfits and shoes I can afford.

You: _____

_____

I want to lose weight for these reasons:

JF: I want to be comfortable in my skin and maybe even develop some muscles so the strength I feel inside is evident on the outside.

You: _____

_____

My short-term weight loss goal is (pounds and time frame):

JF: Twenty pounds in a few months.

You: _____

_____

My long-term weight loss goal is (pounds and time frame):

JF: I want this book to be the catalyst to losing my goal amount of weight, which is about 60-70 pounds.

You: _____

_____

Signature:_____Date:_____
Jacqueline Jeanette Champagnie, aka Jackie Fabulous (See ... I used my real name so I must be serious this time!)

Tracking Your Progress

Losing weight is a process. It takes time. Many, many clients tell me the same thing. If they don't lose weight quickly, they get discouraged and give up. Instead, be grateful for any loss. After all, it's better than gaining. Don't give up! You're in control. Hopefully, no one is tying you down and making you eat chocolate cake. Now that's an excuse! Losing weight and being healthy is all about MODERATION and PERSISTENCE. Keep making small changes. Eventually, these small changes will make a big difference! Below are several ways to track your progress.

1. **Weigh yourself** today and then again on the last day of each week. Plot your weight on the chart in the back of the book. Weigh yourself on the same scale at the same time of the day in the same amount of clothes or no clothes. Your scale doesn't have to be extremely accurate. Every scale is different. You're looking for consistency. It's good to know that you're making progress. If you're not losing, then you are still eating too much. You may be eating healthier, but you still need to eat less to lose weight. Your body weight can fluctuate daily depending on water retention. Look at a true measure of your weight every month.

   Starting weight:_____ Jackie's starting weight: <u>196.5</u> pounds

2. **Measure yourself.** As you lose pounds, it's rewarding to see the inches go down. If you don't have a scale or weighing yourself makes you crazy, take your measurements. Measure your chest, waist, hips, and the middle of your thighs every week. You can also notice how clothes fit. When you lose weight, your clothes will become baggy.

   Chest:_____Waist:_____Hips:_____Thighs: _____

3. **Take a picture of yourself** now and every time you lose 5 pounds. Your face will look thinner after losing just 2-3 pounds. It's encouraging to see pictures of your body changing.

You have the rest of your life to work on your weight. And believe me, there will be plenty of distractions along the way. Keep trying.

The Basic Food Plan

There is no one single best way to lose weight because every person eats differently, has a different situation, and has a different biochemistry. You have to find what works best *for you*. Some people have to eat small, frequent meals, or they get light headed and shaky. Other people don't feel much hunger and can go without eating for longer periods of time. For these reasons, I've provided only a very general, brief plan – one that all of you can follow.

Phase One: For the first four weeks, eat very little or no processed foods that contain sugar as the main ingredient. Do not eat fried foods. Drink very little or no alcohol. In the beginning, not consuming these foods is easier for most people than only eating small amounts. Abstinence from such foods and beverages may help you get these cravings out of your system. Solid fats, added sugars, and alcohol are not essential nutrients. They provide unnecessary "energy in." Also, try to get some type of physical activity every day.

Phase Two: For the rest of your life, eat sweets in moderation. Avoid high-fat foods and drink moderate amounts of alcohol. No one is perfect. Stay on track most of the time. Eat healthy foods and consistently eat smaller amounts. This is a healthy lifestyle. It's not deprivation. It's moderation.

Checking In with Your Doctor ℭ℞

If you have health problems, talk to your doctor before starting any weight loss program.

As you read the chapters ahead, you'll find information, suggestions, and a few tricks on how to eat healthy. This will help you expand on the basic plan as you lose the weight. There will be no magic foods, no crazy fads, no miracle pills or special drinks. Just smart advice that works!

Go for It!

Food is your friend. In the past, food has helped you gain weight. Now the right amounts of the right foods will help you lose weight and be healthy. Eating healthy and being active is a necessity of life. You can keep your old "friends" but also make new "friends."

You are doing this for yourself. Your health. Your future. You deserve a healthy future.

Let's stop the obesity epidemic. Losing weight will give you more energy. You'll feel better, look younger, and live longer. Does that sound good to you?

Go for it! What do you have to lose? Your weight, of course.

𝒟ay I CHECK-IN ☑

𝓘 recommend that you remind yourself every day why you want to lose weight. Typically, as people give in to hunger or temptation, they forget about wanting to lose the weight or don't care anymore. Keep reminding yourself.

Why do you want to lose weight? Summarize the reasons you uncovered while working with Day 1.

JF: I want to wear bathing suits to work, weather permitting.

I want to be comfortable with the men I date and not feel as if we are both eligible for the same weight class if we were to enter a boxing match.

I want to be extremely hot. A threat to all women, especially myself.

You: _____

_____

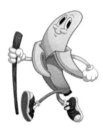

Day 2

Move It!

*I*f you were an Olympic swimmer or a Tour de France cyclist, you wouldn't need to lose weight. These individuals are regularly involved in a high amount of strenuous exercise. As a result, they're able to stay trim.

I believe that the most effective way to lose weight is to get more physical activity. Eating fruits and vegetables, whole grains, fat-free or low-fat dairy products, healthy fats, and lean protein will keep you healthy. But physical activity is necessary to be healthy, too. If you want to protect your health, and also have a goal of losing weight and keeping it off, physical activity will be important for you. As a bonus, weighing less and being physically fit will make you look younger.

What do you do for physical activity? How often?

JF: I started taking spin classes at my gym again. You know it has been a long time since you've been to your gym if you need a GPS to find it. Crazy, huh?

You: _____

_____

*R*uth's **Rule:** *The most effective way to lose weight is to get more physical activity.*

"Weighing" Your Options

There are **three ways to lose weight:**

1. Eat less and don't do any exercise.

2. Eat what you're eating but exercise more.

3. Eat a little bit less and exercise a little bit more.

The third way is the preferred option. While you're losing weight, you want to build muscle and lose fat. Physical activity, especially strength training, builds muscle. The more muscle you have, the faster your metabolism will be. When you have extra weight and it's muscle mass, you're better off. Muscle burns more calories than fat.

Also, to be healthy, you need a strong heart. Your heart is a muscle, just like an arm or leg muscle. Your heart pumps blood and carries oxygen throughout your body. You have to exercise to keep your heart strong, so that it can do its job.

If you say that you don't eat much and have extra weight, then you aren't getting enough physical activity. If you aren't active, your body doesn't need many calories. Way less than you think. Way, way fewer calories than you want.

A Lesson from the Past

Compare the life of a caveman, or even life in the early 1900s, to now. Today we sit in our cars to get to work. A lot of our jobs keep us sitting for hours. We pick up our food from a drive-thru window. We have someone else wash our car, mow our grass, clean our pool, and on and on and on. Our kids get a ride to school, don't get much or any physical education while they're there, and then sit in front of the TV or computer at home. Even our pets are becoming overweight. Our lives have become less active.

Not long ago, people had to get up to change the channels on the television. Car windows had to be rolled up and down by hand. People had to get up to answer the phone and climb out of the car to open the garage door. These activities burn calories. They add up, a little here and a little there. Life is good, and we got soft. Let's get back to the caveman days and be more active. We can't chase down a woolly mammoth for food, but we can go for a brisk walk after dinner.

According to the Centers for Disease Control and Prevention, 80% of Americans do not meet the recommended guidelines for aerobic and muscle-strengthening activities. Almost 30% are not active *at all.* Is it a surprise that over 70% of Americans are overweight? About 40% of those people are obese. Over one-third of our kids are carrying around extra weight. Do you see a correlation between excess body weight and the lack of physical activity?

You can lead people to a track, but you can't make 'em run.

If you're not physically active, why not?

JF: Why? Well, there are so many reasons (none of which are valid). For instance, I want to go to the gym in the morning because I hear that is the best time. However, that would mean 5 a.m. and I might rather die. Notice that I said "might," not "definitely" would rather die, maybe just be maimed.

You: _____

_____

What I Observed

Many people put on weight when they go on a cruise. When I planned a cruise vacation, I told myself that I would limit my portions. I was there to relax, not eat. Well … things change. The food was *so* delicious that I broke all my rules the first day. At meals, I ate until I was stuffed, and then I ate some more until I felt uncomfortable. I ate four desserts that day. At home, I rarely eat dessert. Soon it was time for Plan B. Starting on the second day, I refused to take the elevator, even if I felt exhausted. I walked up and down 13 flights of stairs all day long, and walked back and forth on the ship – plus I walked on land every day. At the end of the week, I started running up and down the stairs. Our body adjusts to exercise quickly. I weighed myself as soon as I got home and *voila!* My weight was *exactly the same.* Moral of the story? … *Physical activity saved me from gaining weight!*

I couldn't believe it! I ate at least *three times* the amount of food that I usually eat. Then it dawned on me. I can eat as much as I want *if* I get enough exercise. On the cruise, I was exercising at least *three times* as much as usual. Again, exercise (physical activity) is *the key* to losing weight or maintaining. If you absolutely cannot exercise, you MUST eat less to lose weight – no matter how little you think you eat.

I had another experience. One year during the holiday season, I was bombarded with delicious food gifts. Fancy chocolates, yummy cookies, and special cakes. I didn't want to eat them, but they really tasted delicious. They were worth eating. Well, it was a busier year than usual. More work. More parties. This meant less time for exercise. Guess what happened? I gained three pounds. *Aha! MORE eating and LESS physical activity results in weight gain.*

One year, I went to a party on New Year's Eve. A lot of the couples brought young kids. The adults sat around, ate food, and drank alcohol for hours. The kids didn't stop running around the entire night. Once in a while, they stopped for a bite to eat. I was exhausted looking at them burn calories. However, for the adults, the "energy in" was way more than the "energy out." If you don't balance eating with physical activity, you'll gain weight over time. Parties, holidays, and picnics shouldn't just be about eating. Celebrate, but include a walk, a game, a sport, or other types of physical activity in your plans. Do more than sit and eat.

A Simple Daily Energizing Exercise ❧

Stand up. While raising your hands up and over your head, inhale slowly and deeply. Exhale through your mouth and lower your arms. Do it again. Raise your hands over your head, breathe slow and deep. Fill your lungs with oxygen. Exhale through your mouth. Lower your arms. Feel the energy surging through your body. You're hot! Don't ever forget it. Remember to do this energizing exercise every day.

Ideas for Moving It!

How many times have you read that you should take the stairs instead of the elevator? Do you do it? It's just not catching on. Yet stairs are great for cardio, and they build wonderful leg muscles. So take the stairs, whenever you see them.

Here are other ideas for incorporating more physical activity into your daily life:

- Clean the house yourself – wash windows, vacuum, scrub the floor, etc.
- Do chores together as a family. (They will get done more quickly!)
- Wash the car yourself.
- Garden, growing flowers *and* vegetables.
- Mow the grass.
- Rake leaves.
- Trim trees.
- Play with the dog, the cat, the kids or the grandkids.
- Cut wood.
- Get together with friends for Exercise Boot Camp in the park.
- Pace while talking on the phone.
- Shovel snow.
- Park the car further away and walk.
- Fidget in your chair.
- Walk to the store, the post office, or school.
- Push a baby stroller. Start a new mom or dad stroller group.
- Hike around the mall as you shop.

Watching TV doesn't burn many calories. Find something active to do instead. When you do watch sports on television, think about the exercise the athletes are getting. They are burning *a lot* of calories. What are *you* doing? Just sitting. So think of some ways to move while watching the tube – place a treadmill nearby, buy some free weights, do some stretching, etc.

Any movement of your body burns calories. In a moment, we'll explore the many different types of formal exercise (jogging, tennis, golf, etc.) that are available. *But right now, can you think of some other ways to add more movement to the course of your day?*

JF: I started walking during half of my lunch break every day. If I go before eating lunch, it is a brisk walk. If it's after, I take a light stroll.

You: _____

_____

The Easiest Form of Exercise

Walking is the easiest, cheapest, and most convenient form of exercise. Walking one mile burns around 100 calories. If you walk one mile a day, seven days a week, for a year, you could lose around 10 pounds. Do you have an extra 15-20 minutes a day? What if you walked longer?

It's important to wear supportive shoes made for walking or running. Look where you're walking. You don't want to trip and fall, get hurt, and not be able to walk for three months. Find the best time for you. In the morning? After dinner?

Wearing a pedometer is eye-opening and fun. About 2,000 steps is one mile. People who aren't physically active walk around 2,000 steps a day. If you walk 2,000 steps, gradually increase the steps to 4,000 or 5,000. Write down the number of steps you take and keep increasing them until you get to 10,000 or more. Pedometers give an estimation of steps. They are not entirely accurate. If you walk on streets, clock the distance with a car.

What's Your Thing?

What can you do for exercise if walking isn't your thing? Match the physical activity with your personality. List some activities that sound good to you. *Is there something that you've always wanted to try?*

JF: I used to take martial arts and loved it! I felt like a fool walking around in a karate gi, but after class I had this sense of being able to beat anyone's butt. GREAT FEELING! Remembering that feeling reminds me of how well "moving" works, along with eating right.

You: _____

_____

Other possibilities include:

- Jogging or running
- Tennis
- Exercise DVD
- Lift weights
- Bowling
- Soccer
- Badminton
- Golf
- Biking
- Jumping rope
- Miniature golf
- Ping pong
- Throwing a Frisbee.
- Baseball/softball
- Hockey
- Rollerblading
- Dancing – ballroom, hip hop, salsa, line dance, ballet, hula, etc.
- Basketball
- Surfing
- Canoeing or rowing
- Handball
- Birdwatching
- Racquetball
- Hiking
- Fencing
- Trampoline
- Juggling
- Rock climbing
- Swimming
- Ice skating
- Volleyball
- Yoga and Tai Chi
- Skateboarding
- Boxing
- Exercise equipment – treadmill, stair stepper, stationary bike
- Martial arts
- Football
- Hula hoop
- Skiing – downhill or cross-country
- Hire a personal trainer.
- Join an exercise class.
- Sign up for a running or hiking club.
- Join an intramural sports league.
- Coach or referee a team.

What would you like to start doing? What are you willing to do more often?

JF: I will be looking into a boxing class as well as going to a park close to my house. I drive by the park all the time and wave at the people exercising. I plan to become one of them.

You: _____

_____

My mother always made me turn off the television and go outside. I'm glad she did. Being active has always been a part of my life. Whenever I could, I rode a bike to work. After work, I would swim in a fish hatchery with a 70-year-old friend. We had to keep moving every second or the fish would nibble our toes. Every once in a while, we would swim over an icy, cold spring. It felt great on hot, humid summer afternoons. Swimming in the pond surrounded by green weeping willow trees and looking at a bright blue sky and white puffy clouds is one of my fondest memories from my years in Wisconsin.

Categories of Exercise

There are three basic kinds of exercise. It's important to do all three. _Aerobic_ exercise (e.g., running, aerobics class) speeds up the heart rate and helps you lose weight faster. _Strength training_ builds muscle mass, which speeds up your metabolism. _Stretching_ helps you be limber.

Sit-ups (a form of strength training) weren't created to make you miserable in high school. There's nothing worse than back pain. Sit-ups do a lot to eliminate back problems. Make sit-ups a part of your life two to three times a week. As long as you're down there, do a few push-ups (another kind of strength training).

Stretching is especially important as people get older. Muscles get stiff. Stretching helps alleviate arthritis pain. Always warm up your muscles by walking in place for a few minutes before stretching, or you could pull something. Hold the stretch for 10-30 seconds. Don't bounce. If it hurts, stop. Stretch two to three times a week. Stretching every day is good, too.

Healthy Aging

As most people age, they have less muscle mass, which slows down their metabolism. To be healthy, you need to stay active. You also need to eat less to avoid gaining weight. By the time people are 65 years old, they have to eat 25% _less_ just to stay the _same_ weight.

No matter what your age, you should do some type of physical activity that you enjoy. Studies show that even people in their 80s and 90s benefit from strength training. Resistance bands are an easy and fun way to build muscles. Having strength from muscles is empowering. If you do strength training two to three times a week, you'll start to see and feel muscle in a few weeks. Before you know it, people will comment on your big "guns." Jack LaLanne should be an inspiration to all of us. There are 90-year-olds who swim and work out every day, and even participate in marathons.

Looking into the future, what would you like to be doing at 90?

JF: I want to be that hot, stylish 90-year-old who is in shape, blonde maybe, and just a firecracker of good health.

You: _____

_____

A Note on Burning Calories ೲ

Warning: Exercise doesn't burn as many calories as you think or want it to burn. Eating a donut means 45 minutes on the treadmill. Is the donut worth it? Since it's extremely difficult to accurately count food calories, it's also difficult to count calories that are burned in exercise, especially since every person's metabolism is different. Some people are blessed with a speedy metabolism. Others aren't so fortunate.

More on Benefits

Remember, physical activity could be the key to healthy aging and longevity.

Here are some more benefits of exercise:

♦ Stronger muscles, joints, bones, lungs, and heart
♦ More energy
♦ Lowers blood pressure and cholesterol levels

- Reduces osteoporosis
- Increases sensitivity to insulin – lowers blood sugar levels
- Decreases appetite
- Improves sleep
- Relieves stress
- Reduces depression and anxiety
- Burns calories resulting in weight loss
- Better flexibility
- Better balance
- More endurance
- Puts you in a good mood
- Reduces the risk of a heart attack, stroke, diabetes, and certain cancers
- Relieves arthritis pain
- Improves digestion
- Firms you up. Takes off inches
- Helps you be a role model for others
- Helps you live longer

What benefits would you like to accomplish from exercise?

JF: I want a higher level of energy more than anything else in my life!!! I also want muscles! A lot of them. Not the bodybuilder kind, but I love the way muscles look on women. I might even challenge a man to arm-wrestle ... a small man.

You: _____

_____

Staying Hydrated ൦൪

Always drink water before, during, and after physical activity to prevent dehydration. As a rule, your urine should be light or clear in color. If it's dark, you aren't drinking enough fluids. For workouts or strenuous activities lasting more than one hour, choose a sports drink to replace electrolytes. Always replace your sweat.

How Much Is Enough?

The Department of Health and Human Services releases Physical Activity Guidelines for Americans. It is science-based information to help individuals age 6 and older improve their health and reduce chronic disease through physical activity.

The guidelines are aged-based:

Children and Adolescents (ages 6-17)

- 1 hour or more of physical activity a day. Most of the hour or more a day should be either moderate- or vigorous-intensity aerobic physical activity.
- Vigorous-intensity activity should be included at least three days a week.
- Muscle- and bone-strengthening activity should be included at least three days a week.

Adults (ages 18-64)

- 2½ hours of moderate-intensity activity a week, or
- 1¼ hours of vigorous-intensity aerobic physical activity a week, or
- An equivalent combination of moderate- and vigorous-intensity aerobic physical activity a week. Aerobic activity should be at least 10 minutes at a time, preferably spread throughout the week.
- Do muscle-strengthening activities that include all major muscle groups on two or more days a week.

For additional health benefits, increase physical activity:

- 5 hours of moderate-intensity aerobic physical activity a week, or
- 2½ hours of vigorous-intensity physical activity, or
- An equivalent combination of both.

Older Adults (65 and older)

- Follow the adult guidelines or be as physically active as your abilities allow. Avoid inactivity.
- If older adults are at risk of falling, do exercises that maintain or improve balance.

Pregnant and Postpartum Women

- Healthy women who don't already do vigorous-intensity physical activity should get at least 2½ hours of moderate-intensity physical activity a week (preferably spread throughout the week).
- Vigorous-intensity activity can be continued, if the pregnant women's condition remains unchanged and they talk to their health care provider about their physical activity throughout the pregnancy.

What Is Moderate and Vigorous Physical Activity?

For exercise to be *moderate*-intensity, there should be an increase in heart rate and breathing. You should sweat. An example would be brisk walking, yard work, or dancing. The heart and lungs get stronger with moderate activity. Strolling would not be considered moderate-intensity physical activity. *Vigorous*-intensity physical activity provides more health benefits. For exercise to be vigorous, heart rate and breathing increases even more. Your sweat may drip. An example would be jogging, chopping wood, or competitive basketball.

There are 1,440 minutes in a day. Thirty minutes is 2% of your day. *Can you spend 2% of your day doing something that will improve your health and make you feel better?*

JF: The question of can is not the issue. My problem in the past is if I have wanted to make time for exercise. I really want to now. I am 40 years old. Yeah, talk about motivation!

You: _____

Additional Ideas on Exercise

If my clients say they don't like exercise, we always find something that they are willing to do. A lot of people don't like to run. They say that they were traumatized in gym class from running laps. But at some point in their life, they did enjoy *something*. Usually it's dancing. Dancing is great exercise. It's fun, and it burns a lot of calories. Turn on some music and dance. Take a dance class. Go to a club.

Here are some other things to consider:

- **If all you do is walk your dog or cat around the block, crank it up a notch.** Leave your pet at home sometimes, and walk faster. Also, walking for exercise once a week or every other week isn't enough. Get into a routine and stick to it.
- **If you work away from home, take a walk during lunch.** It might be inside or outside, depending on your situation. If you don't like to walk alone, invite a co-worker. Then there's someone to keep you accountable and motivated.
- **If you come home from work and feel too tired to exercise, take a 15-30 minute nap.** Then go exercise. It will do you some good.
- **Do you have allergies?** Stay inside and do exercise DVDs. Find a mall that allows early morning walking.
- **Do you need to be around other people to get motivated?** Join a gym, a YMCA or a YWCA, or an exercise studio. Sign up for a class at a recreation center or a senior center.
- **Physical activity doesn't have to be an intense hour at the gym.** It can be 10 minutes here and 10 minutes there. Just do something to get started.
- **Do you want to make the world a better place and get physical activity at the same time?** Pick up litter. Help build a house for someone less fortunate. Clean house for an elderly or handicapped person.
- **Like a challenge? Sign up for a 5K walk.** Increase it the next time to a 10K walk/run. Work up to a marathon. If you would like to receive an award for physical activity, go to www.presidentschallenge.org.
- **If you have a bad back, bad knees, or some other physical problem that limits your physical activity, find something that you**

can do … swim, do chair exercise DVDs, work with resistance bands. Look for workable options.

+ **Pick two cities, get the distance, and walk the equivalent steps with your trusty pedometer.** Los Angeles to San Francisco is 344 miles or 688,000 steps. That would really impress your friends. One step at a time.

+ **If you have kids, you are their most important role model.** Children tend to do what their parents do. Kids also love attention. Nothing would make your kids happier than going to the park with you. Bring along an inexpensive plastic ball and play volleyball. It's a win-win for everyone.

+ **As you get stronger and gain more energy, gradually increase the time and intensity of your activity.** You'll be asking yourself, "Why wasn't I doing this before?" You'll feel better and have even more energy.

What's Your Next Move?

Sun.	Mon.	Tues.	Wed.	Thurs.	Fri.	Sat.
Treadmill 30 minutes Garden 30 minutes	Walk at lunch 30 minutes Stairs at work 15 minutes Shoot hoops 15 minutes	Wash car 30 minutes Wash floor 15 minutes Vacuum 15 minutes	Gym - cardio 30 minutes Weights 20 minutes Stretch 10 minutes	Walk briskly at mall 1 hour	Walk in neighbor-hood 30 minutes Bowl 30 minutes	Dance 1 hour

Here's your chance to put it all together and make a commitment. What are your physical activity goals for pleasure and/or chores? How often? What days? What time? Plan your physical activities and put them on your calendar. Treat it like a doctor's appointment.

JF: I will keep it simple and say that my gym will know me. The staff, patrons, and the homeless people in the area. I want to be a fixture at my gym. That way, it is expected and I can be made to feel incredibly guilty if I miss a day.

You: _____

_____

Eating healthy and physical activity go together as a team effort. Both are important for a healthy lifestyle. Once you start being active, your body will crave more.

My last words about exercise … be active until the end.

Physical activity is your new best friend.

*D*ay 2 CHECK-IN ☑

*T*o help you make changes, you'll set a new goal for yourself every day. I will suggest some ideas that relate to the topic of the day. Feel free to come up with your own goals. As you add new goals, keep working on the previous goals. If you don't achieve some goals, keep going back and continue working on them until they become habits. One new goal a day is a lot, but when you're motivated, you'll be surprised at how much you can achieve.

What is your goal for today?

Examples: (Carry water on your walk.) (One minute of sit-ups) (Walk one block.) (Walk one mile.) (Buy a pedometer.) (Take the stairs at work.) (Walk in place for 10 minutes.) (Sign up for a dance class.) (Do an exercise DVD.) (Vacuum once a week.) (Go to the gym after work three times a week.) (Walk for a half hour every night.)

JF: Walk one mile every day at lunchtime and go the gym after work. Stop laughing, Jackie; you can do it!

You: _____

_____

Day 3

What's a Person to Eat?

*W*hat do you eat? How much do you eat? What *should* you eat? How much *should* you eat?

The majority of my clients are confused about what to eat and how much of it. Contradicting information is everywhere. When it comes to nutrition, there's a lot of *misinformation*. I'm not surprised that people are confused. They don't know who or what to believe.

The latest food guide for the public is MyPlate, which is discussed in detail in this chapter. It is based on the best and most current nutrition information. MyPlate replaces MyPyramid from 2005. MyPyramid replaced the Food Guide Pyramid from 1992.

Where did MyPlate come from? How do you follow it?

How the Guidelines Developed

MyPlate information comes from the *DRIs (Dietary Reference Intakes)*. The DRIs are established by the Food and Nutrition Board (FNB) of the National Academy of Medicine (NAM). This organization contains the nation's top scientists who volunteer their time and give advice to the federal government.

All of America's nutrition policies and programs are based on the information from the DRIs. The DRIs are the recommended intake levels for *micronutrients* (vitamins and minerals) and *macronutrients* (protein, carbohydrate, fat), depending on age and sex, also pregnancy and lactation. All of us need the same nutrients but in different amounts. The Dietary Reference Intakes (DRIs) used to be called the *Recommended Dietary Allowances (RDAs)*, which are now a segment of the DRIs.

The first RDAs were released in 1941 during World War II. The Department of Defense wanted nutrient recommendations for WWII soldiers because many of them were malnourished from the Depression. The government wanted to keep soldiers and the general population healthy during the war. Today, these guidelines continue to eliminate nutritional deficiencies, and the nutrient amounts that are recommended also reduce the risk of chronic diseases.

The Food and Nutrition Board updates the DRIs if there are advances in nutrient research.

In addition to the DRIs, MyPlate is also based on the *Dietary Guidelines for Americans*. The U.S. Department of Health and Human Services (HHS) and the U.S. Department of Agriculture (USDA) together publish the *Dietary Guidelines for Americans (DGA)* for healthy people ages two and up. The Dietary Guidelines are based on recommendations from the Dietary Guidelines Advisory Committee (nutrition and health experts), public comments, and the DRIs. The guidelines provide information on a nutritious diet as well as physical activity that helps to maintain a desired weight, along with food safety tips. These guidelines are updated every five years. This book follows the 2015-2020 Dietary Guidelines for Americans.

The USDA was established in 1862, and it started making dietary recommendations in 1894 with a publication called *Farmers' Bulletin* by W.O. Atwater. This was even before the first vitamin, thiamin (B1), was discovered in 1911. In 1902, Atwater seemed to be nutrition-savvy.

"Unless care is exercised in selecting food, a diet may result which is one-sided or badly balanced – that is, one in which either protein or fuel ingredients (carbohydrate and fat) are provided in excess …. The evils of overeating may not be felt at once, but sooner or later they are sure to appear – perhaps in an excessive amount of fatty tissue, perhaps in general debility, perhaps in actual disease."

Watch out for the evils of overeating. It could happen to you.

In 1916, the USDA printed its first food guide, called *Food for Young Children* by Caroline Hunt, a nutritionist. The first food guide had five groups, which included (1) milk and meat, (2) cereals, (3) vegetables and fruit, (4) fats and fatty foods, and (5) sugars and sugary foods. Over the years, new food guides have been released periodically, as nutrition research expanded. Surprisingly, the recommendations haven't changed drastically over the years.

How the Guidelines Are Used

As noted above, the purpose of the current Dietary Guidelines is to reduce the risk of chronic disease and to promote health through food and physical activity. A poor diet and lack of physical activity puts people at risk for heart disease, hypertension, diabetes, osteoporosis, and certain cancers. The guidelines take into consideration all of the necessary nutrients and translates them into food patterns depending on age, sex, and activity levels. There are 12 food patterns ranging from 1,000 to 3,200 calories. The Dietary Guidelines are used for nutrition programs and federal nutrition policy. The focus of the DGA 2015-2020 is the eating patterns not the food groups and nutrients.

Information from the RDIs and the *Dietary Guidelines for Americans* is used to determine the *Nutrition Facts food label.*

It's important for Americans to follow the guidelines in order to meet nutrient requirements. Specifically, American diets need more potassium, dietary fiber, calcium, and vitamin D. We should eat more vegetables, fruits, whole grains, oils, seafood, and fat-free or low-fat dairy products. Americans are over-consuming saturated fats, added sugars, refined grains, sodium, and calories.

Enter MyPlate

MyPlate puts the *Dietary Guidelines for Americans* into practice. MyPlate is a familiar, simple-to-understand symbol. Every time you eat a meal, think about building a healthy plate. Focus on the fruits, vegetables, grains, protein foods, and dairy foods. There are no "servings" or "portions" mentioned. Instead, MyPlate uses household units. There are "1 ounce" equivalents and "1 cup" equivalents.

MyPlate improves the quality of your diet by helping you choose what foods to eat from each group and how much of each food. This allows you to meet your entire nutrient needs from food.

Following MyPlate helps people increase vitamins, minerals, fiber, and other nutrients. It also helps lower sodium, saturated fats, trans fats, and cholesterol, along with added sugars. The food patterns can help people lose weight or prevent weight gain. MyPlate also makes recommendations for physical activity. It helps adults and children make good choices to improve their health.

Take a look at the daily amount of food suggested from each food pattern according to the calorie level on the MyPlate Daily Checklist chart. The Calorie Needs on page 34 gives you an estimation of how many calories a person should consume depending on activity level.

The 1,800-Calorie Starting Point ☙

Following the 1,800-calorie plan is a good place for most people to start when they're trying to lose weight. If you're not losing weight on the 1,800-calorie plan, go down to 1,600 calories. The calorie plans are balanced and healthy. Once you find your calorie range, use it as a guide to eat healthy.

Ruth's **Rule:** *MyPlate provides the basic guidelines that you'll need to meet your nutrient requirements and stay healthy.*

MyPlate Daily Checklist

Calorie level	1,200	1,400	1,600	1,800	2,000	2,200
Fruits	1 cup	1 ½ cups	1 ½ cups	**1 ½ cups**	2 cups	2 cups
Vegetables	1 ½ cups	1 ½ cups	2 cups	**2 ½ cups**	2 ½ cups	3 cups
Dark-green vegetables	1 c/wk	1 c/wk	1 ½ c/wk	**1 ½ c/wk**	1 ½ c/wk	2 c/wk
Red and orange vegetables	3 c/wk	3 c/wk	4 c/wk	**5 ½ c/wk**	5 ½ c/wk	6 c/wk
Beans and peas	½ c/wk	½ c/wk	1 c/wk	**1 ½ c/wk**	1 ½ c/wk	2 c/wk
Starchy vegetables	3 ½ c/wk	3 ½ c/wk	4 c/wk	**5 c/wk**	5 c/wk	6 c/wk
Other vegetables	2 ½ c/wk	2 ½ c/wk	3 ½ c/wk	**4 c/wk**	4 c/wk	5 c/wk
Grains	4 oz-eq	5 oz-eq	5 oz-eq	**6 oz-eq**	6 oz-eq	7 oz-eq
Whole grains	2 oz-eq	2 ½ oz-eq	3 oz-eq	**3 oz-eq**	3 oz-eq	3 ½ oz-eq
Enriched grains	2 oz-eq	2 ½ oz-eq	2 oz-eq	**3 oz-eq**	3 oz-eq	3 ½ oz-eq
Protein foods	3 oz-eq	4 oz-eq	5 oz-eq	**5 oz-eq**	5 ½ oz-eq	6 oz-eq
Seafood	4 oz/wk	6 oz/wk	8 oz/wk	**8 oz/wk**	8 oz/wk	9 oz/wk
Meat, poultry, eggs	14 oz/wk	19 oz/wk	23 oz/wk	**23 oz/wk**	26 oz/wk	28 oz/wk
Nuts, seeds, soy products	2 oz/wk	3 oz/wk	4 oz/wk	**4 oz/wk**	5 oz/wk	5 oz/wk
Dairy	2 ½ cups	2 ½ cups	3 cups	**3 cups**	3 cups	3 cups
Oils	4 tsp	4 tsp	5 tsp	**5 tsp**	6 tsp	6 tsp
Extra calories	100	110	130	**170**	270	280

Food groups are shown as cups per week (c/wk), ounce equivalents (oz-eq), ounces per week (oz/wk), teaspoons (tsp)

Adapted from Appendix 3. Dietary Guidelines for Americans, 2015-2020

Estimated Calorie Needs		
Female		
	Sedentary	**Active**
19-30	1,800-2,000	2,400
31-50	1,800	2,200
51+	1,600	2,000-2,200
Male		
	Sedentary	**Active**
19-30	2,400-2,600	3,000
31-50	2,200-2,400	2,800-3,000
51+	2,000-2,200	2,400-2,800

Source: U.S. Department of Agriculture. ChooseMyPlate.gov Website. Washington, DC. Assessed January, 2016.

Sedentary means a lifestyle with only the physical activity of independent living.

Active means physical activity equal to walking more than 3 miles per day at 3 to 4 miles per hour, in addition to the activity of independent living.

Adapted from Appendix Two. Dietary Guidelines for Americans, 2015-2020

The Fruit Group

Let's take a closer look at the food groups in MyPlate. We'll start with the *Fruit Group*. Fruits are on the top left of MyPlate. This is my favorite group. I could live on nectarines. Fruits contain vitamins, minerals, fiber, and phytonutrients. The Fruit Group includes any fruit and 100% fruit juice. Choose fresh, frozen, cooked, canned (in juice or water), or dried fruit. MyPlate recommends making half of your plate fruits and vegetables.

List your favorite fruit.

JF: Strawberry ice cream. Anything that is fruit-flavored. Okay, mangoes. Not nearly the first thing to come to mind when I hear "fruit," but my diet is what I'm working on improving, remember?

You: _____

34

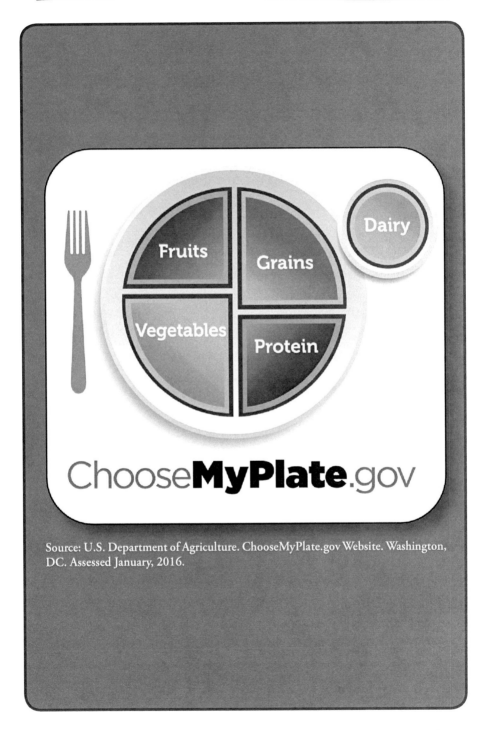

Source: U.S. Department of Agriculture. ChooseMyPlate.gov Website. Washington, DC. Assessed January, 2016.

Many fruit choices are available year-round. Eat a variety of fruits. Some of your options include:

- Apples
- Bananas
- Strawberries
- Blueberries
- Cherries
- Grapefruit
- Kiwi fruit
- Mangoes
- Watermelon

- Oranges
- Nectarines
- Fruit cocktail
- Peaches
- Prunes
- Apricots
- Plums
- Papaya
- Raisins

- Lemons
- Cantaloupe
- Pears
- Grapes
- Pineapple
- Raspberries
- Limes

Look for "100%" fruit juice (orange, apple, grape, grapefruit, pineapple, etc.). Limit juice to less than half of your fruit intake.

Depending on your age, sex, and activity level, **eat between 1½ to 2 cup equivalents of fruits a day**. In general, "1 cup" of fruit equals 1 cup of fruit, 1 cup of 100% fruit juice, or ½ cup of dried fruit. Here are some 1-cup equivalents:

- ½ large apple (3.25-inch diameter)
- 1 small apple (2.5-inch diameter)
- 1 large banana (8-9inch long)
- 32 seedless grapes
- 1 medium grapefruit (4-inch diameter)
- 1 large orange (3-inch diameter)
- 1 medium pear
- 3 medium or 2 large plums
- About 8 large strawberries
- 12 watermelon balls

Half of a large apple is 1 cup equivalent. So, one large apple would meet the 2 cups fruit requirement for a 2,000-calorie daily diet.

The Vegetable Group

Below Fruits is the *Vegetable Group*. Vegetables contain vitamins, minerals, fiber, and phytonutrients. Vegetables are important for your health. They can be eaten raw or cooked. Choose fresh, frozen, canned, or dehydrated vegetables. There are many choices. If you're watching your blood pressure, choose "no salt added" or "low sodium" canned vegetables.

MyPlate groups vegetables into five categories, and the vegetables in each category contain similar nutrients. The categories include dark green vegetables, red and orange vegetables, beans and peas, starchy vegetables, and other vegetables. The amount of vegetables needed every day depends on your age, sex, and physical activity level. However, here are some basic guidelines for 1,800 calories.

Eat 1 ½ cups of **dark green** vegetables a week:

- Broccoli
- Spinach
- Bok choy
- Romaine lettuce
- Collard greens
- Turnip greens
- Watercress
- Dark green leafy lettuce
- Kale
- Mustard greens
- Mesclun (salad greens mix including dandelion greens, mustard greens, and radicchio)

Eat 5 ½ cups of **red/orange vegetables** a week:

- Squash (acorn, butternut, Hubbard)
- Carrots
- Pumpkin (think outside the jack-o'-lantern)
- Sweet potatoes, yams
- Red peppers
- Tomatoes/tomato juice

Eat 1 ½ cups of **beans and peas** a week:

- Black beans
- Lentils
- Pinto beans
- Garbanzo beans (chickpeas)
- Soybeans
- Split peas
- White beans
- Navy beans
- Black-eyed peas
- Kidney beans

Note: Beans are the only food considered both a vegetable and a protein in MyPlate.

We're already eating enough starchy vegetables (probably because of French fries).

Choose 5 cups of **Starchy vegetables** a week:

- Corn
- Green peas
- Lima beans
- Potatoes
- Taro
- Plantains

The "other vegetables" contain various but important nutrients. Here are a few of the **other vegetables** (4 cups a week):

- Asparagus
- Beets
- Cabbage
- Mushrooms
- Zucchini
- Onions
- Eggplant
- Cucumbers
- Cauliflower
- Brussels sprouts
- Okra
- Avocado

In general, "1 cup" equivalent from the Vegetable Group equals:

- 1 cup raw or cooked vegetables
- 1 cup vegetable juice
- 2 cups raw leafy greens
- 2 medium carrots
- 3 spears broccoli (5 inches long)
- 1 large ear of corn (8-9 inches long)
- 1 cup whole or mashed cooked beans
- 2 large stalks celery
- 1 large pepper (3-3¾ inch)
- 1 large tomato (3 inch)
- 1 large baked sweet potato (2¼-inch or more diameter)
- 1 medium boiled or baked potato (2½-3-inch diameter)
- 20 medium to long strips French fries (2½-4-inch long) (contains added solid fat calories.)

In addition, 12 baby carrots equal 1 cup of vegetables. This is going to be easier than you think!

Vary Your Veggies ❧

Eat a variety of different vegetables. They are low in calories. I'm not sure that you can eat too many vegetables. I guess you could try.

In general, eat around 2½-cup equivalents of vegetables a day.

The Grain Group

The *Grain Group* is the top right on MyPlate. Grains are carbohydrates. Your body needs carbohydrate for energy to run up stairs. Grains are low in calories. Be particular about your grains. There are whole grains and refined grains.

MyPlate recommends making at least half your grains whole grains. Always look for the word "whole grain," "whole wheat," or "whole" on the ingredients. The amounts depend on age, sex, and level of physical activity.

Eat More of These Whole Grains ❧

Products made with whole wheat flour (whole grain bread, whole grain pasta, whole grain crackers, whole grain cereal, whole wheat tortillas, etc.)

- Oatmeal
- Whole cornmeal
- Popcorn
- Wild rice
- Brown rice
- Bulgur (cracked wheat)
- Whole rye
- Whole grain barley

Refined grains do not have the germ or the bran (fiber). These parts are removed in milling, and the grain is then enriched with some B vitamins and iron.

Refined grains are:

- Products made with white flour (white bread, crackers, pasta, flour tortillas, pretzels, cereals)
- White rice
- Cornbread
- Corn tortillas
- Couscous
- Grits
- Pita bread

MyPlate uses *ounce equivalents* for the recommended amounts of grains. The amount of ounce equivalents that you eat in a day depends on your age, sex, and activity level. In general, "1 ounce" equals 1 slice of bread, 1 cup of ready-to-eat cereal, ½ cup cooked rice, ½ cup cooked pasta, or ½ cup cooked cereal. The more active you are, the more you can eat. **The range for most adults is 5-10 ounce equivalents a day.** For 1,800 calories, aim for 6 ounces of grains a day.

Other "1 ounce" equivalents include:

- 5 whole wheat crackers
- 1 packet instant oatmeal
- 3 cups popcorn (good deal!)
- 1 mini bagel (1 large bagel equals 4 ounce equivalents)
- 7 squares of saltines
- ½ English muffin
- 1 small muffin (2 ½-inch diameter)
- 1 4½-inch pancake
- 1 6-inch flour tortilla
- 1 6-inch corn tortilla

Based on what you've read above, 1 cup of cooked rice is 2 ounce equivalents. Get it?

The Protein Foods Group

Protein Foods are below Grains on MyPlate. Foods that supply protein include *meat, poultry, seafood, dry beans and peas, eggs, processed soy products, nuts,* and *seeds*. Select lean or low-fat meat (at least 90% lean ground beef) and poultry. Avoid protein with unhealthy fats. Fish, nuts, and seeds contain healthy fats. Include at least 8 ounces of cooked seafood a week.

Here are some examples from each category:

Meats
- Beef, ham, lamb, pork, veal, game meats

Poultry
- Chicken, duck, goose, turkey

Eggs

Beans and peas

♦ Black beans, black-eyed peas, chickpeas (garbanzo beans), kidney beans, lentils, navy beans, pinto beans, soybeans, split peas, white beans, falafel, tofu, veggie burgers, tempeh, texturized vegetable protein

Nuts and seeds

♦ Almonds, cashews, peanuts, pecans, pistachios, walnuts, peanut butter, pumpkin seeds, sesame seeds, sunflower seeds

Fish

♦ Finfish (catfish, cod, halibut, herring, pollock, salmon, sea bass, snapper, trout, tuna)
♦ Shellfish (clams, crab, lobster, mussels, oysters, scallops, squid, shrimp, octopus)

Processed meats have added sodium. If you're watching sodium, check the sodium levels on the label for such foods as hot dogs, sausage, luncheon meats, and ham.

The recommended amounts of protein are in *ounce equivalents*. The amounts depend on age, sex, and level of physical activity. **Adults who get less than 30 minutes of moderate intensity physical activity only need between 5-6 ounce equivalents of protein a day.** When you consider portion sizes of protein these days, 5-6 ounces isn't much for the entire day.

Here are the "1 ounce" equivalents for protein according to My-Plate. 1 ounce equals:

♦ 1 ounce meat, poultry, or fish
♦ 1 egg
♦ ¼ cup tofu (about 2 ounces) or ¼ cooked dry beans
♦ 1 tablespoon peanut butter
♦ ½ ounce nuts or seeds
♦ 2 tablespoons hummus

Don't eat chicken or turkey skin. Beans are a wonderful, healthy choice. They are high in fiber, high in protein, and low in fat. Nuts are another healthy choice. Fish such as salmon, tuna, herring, and trout are good sources of omega-3 fatty acids and should be included in your meals.

The Dairy Group

The circle to the right of Grains is the *Dairy Group*. Milk, yogurt, and cheese are included in the Dairy Group because they are made from milk and retain their calcium content. Soymilk (calcium-fortified) is also included in the Dairy Group. Your body needs plenty of calcium for bones, muscles, nerves, teeth, and your heart. Dairy products also contain potassium, vitamin D, and protein.

MyPlate lists these "1 cup" equivalents for the Dairy Group (**it is recommended that you switch to fat-free and low-fat (1%) milk products for calcium and the least amount of fat**):

+ 1 cup milk
+ 1 cup calcium-fortified soymilk
+ ½ cup evaporated milk
+ 1 cup yogurt
+ 8 fluid ounces yogurt
+ 1½ ounces hard cheese (cheddar, Swiss, mozzarella, Parmesan)
+ 1/3 cup shredded cheese
+ 2 ounces processed cheese
+ 2 cups cottage cheese
+ ½ cup ricotta cheese
+ 1 cup pudding made with milk
+ 1 cup frozen yogurt
+ 1½ cups ice cream (1 scoop equals 1/3 cup milk)

Adults need 3 cup equivalents a day from the Dairy Group to meet nutrient requirements. Puddings, frozen yogurt, and ice cream contain extra calories from solid fats and added sugars. Don't overlook the Dairy Group. Are you getting enough?

Nearly 90% of my clients who come in for weight loss eat very little fruits, vegetables, and dairy foods that provide calcium. These are very important foods for your health.

Oils

Oils are not considered a food group. Oils are mentioned in MyPlate, because they provide essential nutrients that can't be made in the body. They have to come from food sources. Oils are also a major source of vitamin E.

Only small amounts of oils are needed. Fats and oils contain a lot of calories. One pat of butter contains almost the same amount of calories as one cup of vegetables. Think about how full you would be after eating one cup of vegetables. How full would you feel after eating a pat of butter? Watch out for salad dressings and fried foods. One tablespoon of oil contains 120 calories.

There are oils and solid fats. Oils are liquid at room temperature. Oils contain more monounsaturated and polyunsaturated fats than solid fats do.

Some common oils include:

- Olive oil
- Peanut oil
- Cottonseed oil
- Canola oil
- Safflower oil
- Corn oil
- Soybean oil
- Sunflower oil

Solid fats are solid at room temperature. Solid fats contain more saturated fat or trans fats, which raise cholesterol.

Solid fats:

- Shortening
- Stick margarine
- Butter
- Beef (tallow, suet), chicken fat, pork fat (lard)
- Milk fat
- Partially hydrogenated oil
- Coconut oil, palm oil, and palm kernel oil (liquid oil but high in saturated fats)

Limit solid fats and foods with unhealthy fat. The following foods contain solid fats:

- Cream
- Ice cream
- Prime rib roast
- Sour cream
- Bacon
- Croissant

- ♦ Whole milk
- ♦ Cheddar cheese
- ♦ Hamburger (80% lean)
- ♦ Pork sausage
- ♦ Cheese Danish
- ♦ Biscuit
- ♦ Pound cake

In the following foods, most of the calories come from oil, but it's healthy fat – olives, avocados, peanut butter, nuts, and seeds. My-Plate says to get most of your fat from monounsaturated and polyunsaturated fat; i.e., fish, nuts, and vegetable oils.

The daily allowance of oils depends on age, sex, and activity levels. The amounts are in teaspoons! There are 3 teaspoons in a tablespoon. **For adults who get less than 30 minutes of moderate physical activity a day the daily allowance of oils is 5-7 teaspoons.** For 1,800 calories, aim for 5 teaspoons of oils a day.

Here are the amounts of oil in some foods:

- ♦ 1 tablespoon oil (canola, corn, olive, sunflower) = 3 teaspoons oil
- ♦ 1 tablespoon margarine = 2½ teaspoons oil
- ♦ 2 tablespoons Italian dressing = 2 teaspoons oil
- ♦ 4 large ripe olives = ½ teaspoon oil (vegetable group)
- ♦ ½ medium avocado = 3 teaspoons oil (vegetable group)
- ♦ 2 tablespoons peanut butter = 4 teaspoons oil
- ♦ 1 ounce almonds = 3 teaspoons oil

Here are the amounts of solid fats in some foods:

- ♦ 1 tablespoon butter = 2½ teaspoons fat
- ♦ 1 tablespoon sour cream = ½ teaspoon fat
- ♦ 1 cup whole milk = 2 teaspoons fat
- ♦ 1½ ounces cheddar cheese = 3 teaspoons fat
- ♦ 3 ounces prime rib roast, lean and fat (1/8-inch trim) = 6 teaspoons fat
- ♦ 1 medium croissant = 3 teaspoons fat
- ♦ 1/6 of an 8-inch Chocolate cream pie = 5 teaspoons fat

As you can see, it's very easy to go over the recommended 5-7 teaspoons a day.

"Vitamin PA" (i.e., Physical Activity)

Remember the stairs on the left side of MyPyramid? Yes, there are stairs, not an elevator, for you to use for going to the top of the pyramid. Physical activity is essential for good health. Think of it as *"vitamin PA."*

MyPlate recommends following the Physical Activity Guidelines for Americans. Choose moderate (2 ½ hours per week) or vigorous (1 hour 15 minutes per week) intensity activities for health benefits. Light intensity activities that do not increase your heart rate do not count toward the recommended amounts of time.

Keep climbing MyPyramid's stairs high into the blue sky and bright sunshine of healthy living. The Egyptians climbed a lot of stairs building the pyramids. So can you.

How Does Your Diet Compare?

Some people eat healthfully. They just eat too much. Some people eat way too many sweets or high-fat foods. And some people eat way too many carbohydrates. Actually, I've found this last habit to be the case with most of my clients. People love carbs.

A Note to Vegetarians ℃ℛ

Vegetarians also need to follow the MyPlate recommendations to meet nutrient recommendations. It's important to eat a variety of foods and stay within the calorie limits. If you're a vegetarian, get enough protein, iron, zinc, calcium, and vitamin B12. Over the years, I've worked with many vegetarians for weight loss. When first coming to see me, many of them didn't eat vegetables. Vegetarians need to focus on eating foods with nutrients, not foods with a lot of sugar or refined grains.

Compare MyPlate's recommendations with what you're eating now. *Are you on track? Do you need to make some changes? Do you need to eat more fruits? More vegetables? More whole grains? Do you need to switch to fat-free or low-fat (1%) milk? Eat more lean protein? More seafood? Choose healthier fats? More physical activity?*

JF: I have recently switched from the glorious Danishes the size of my head to oatmeal for breakfast. More fiber has definitely curbed my appetite. At first, I tried plain old-fashioned oatmeal and realized a bowl of straw is no way to start the day. So I chose lower-sugar oatmeal with fruit.

You: _____

_____

Following MyPlate is the best way to eat healthy. *Did you notice that there's not a whole lot of room for sweets, fats, alcohol, and processed foods? Is eating excess amounts of processed foods more important to you than losing weight or being healthy?*

JF: Okay, is this a trick question? Because a couple of days ago my answer would have been: YES, DONUTS ARE MORE IMPORTANT THAN GOOD HEALTH. It's a matter of habit for me and understanding that loads of processed sugar feels great at first. But I imagine heroin does, too. It's a matter of conditioning. Once I condition myself to eat the proper foods, it will be easier.

Tracking What You Eat

It's time for the dreaded food journal. (You'll find a form to use on the next page.) Some people hate keeping a food journal, but it can be an effective tool for weight loss. Surveys show that people cheat and don't write everything down in their journals. However, you'll be the only one to see it. Whether you like it or not, it keeps you on track. You may not realize that you eat so much. Or you may not want to write down every bite, so it will help you consume less. If you don't already pay attention to what you're eating, it will be an eye-opening experience.

Keeping a food journal helps you identify patterns and problem areas. If you find it useful, continue writing down everything that you eat every day.

TIME	FOOD	AMOUNT	HUNGER LEVEL (1-5)	WHERE YOU EAT AND WITH WHOM	ACTIVITY	MINUTES SPENT EATING	FEELINGS

Food Journal

Take a look at each category:

- **Time:** When are you eating? Do you eat most of your calories after dinner? Find another activity during that time. Do you eat almost a whole meal in snacks because you are waiting for dinner and starving? *Eat earlier.*
- **Food:** Are you eating apples — or apple pie? There is a *big* difference in calories. Do you drink three glasses of wine with dinner? Alcohol calories add up.
- **Amount:** It's very important to measure food, at least in the beginning. Look at the food label for the calories. Are you eating a few cookies or the whole box?
- **Hunger Level (1-5):** Consider your hunger level: 1 is "starving"; 5 is "stuffed." It's important to only eat when you are *physically* hungry. Stop when you feel "just right."
- **Where you eat and with whom:** Do you automatically grab a bite every time you walk through the kitchen? Do you eat or drink when you're around certain people? Do some people insist that you eat?
- **Activity:** Do you eat while you're watching television or talking with friends? It's easy to eat until you are "full" or "stuffed" if you aren't paying attention. Do you nibble at your desk all day? Pick one place and only eat there.
- **Minutes spent eating:** Do you eat fast? Do you wolf down food and end up eating twice as much as you need?
- **Feelings:** A lot of my clients fill out the food journal and leave the feelings column blank. This is a key category for most people. Eating for comfort can become an unnoticed, learned behavior. Do you eat when you're bored, frustrated, or angry? Every time you put food into your mouth, ask yourself what you're feeling. You may discover something about yourself.

Try keeping a food journal for one week. I think you'll notice how helpful it is to see the foods you're eating listed on the page. This may inspire you to stick with your plan to lose weight. If you get busy, you can always fill in your journal later in the day.

Living the Guidelines

When scientists look at the people in the world who live the longest, there are a few common denominators. They eat a lot of fruits and vegetables. They are active. They may not go to the gym, but they garden and walk a lot. They are also happy and content with life. They don't know it, but they're following MyPlate guidelines, sprinkled with happiness.

According to the USDA, the number of people following the Dietary Guidelines is low. Yet the latest scientific evidence suggests that following the guidelines may reduce chronic disease. On the other hand, a poor diet, being sedentary, and remaining overweight or obese puts you at risk for chronic diseases. Do you want to be one of the more than 117 million Americans with chronic disease? You can choose how to live your life.

There are so many goodies and temptations, but you can do it. You'll do great. Say, "No thank you" to "The Cream Puff and Fried Cheese Diet." Get to know MyPlate foods. MyPlate is for you and for me. The website www.Choose**MyPlate**.gov provides more details and valuable information on eating healthy.

Eating the right amounts of healthy food is your new best friend.

$\mathcal{D}$ay 3 CHECK-IN ☑

What did you accomplish yesterday?

JF: I actually found the gym, went in, and got on some machines. My iPod battery went dead, and I still continued to work out rather than give up and go to Baskin-Robbins right next door. I also have been drinking a lot of water. I had to move the desk from my office into the bathroom; but this is about sacrifice, is it not?

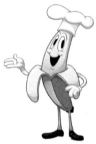

You: _____

_____

What is your goal for today?

(Study the MyPlate guidelines.) (Begin to follow the MyPlate guidelines.) (Keep a food journal.)

JF: To eat healthy every few hours and stay away from the vending machine.

You: _____

_____

Day 4

Food as a Friend

Who are your friends? Your spouse? High school buddies? Fraternity brothers or sorority sisters? The next door neighbor? A co-worker? A parent? Your kids? Your siblings? Do you have a best friend? List your closest friends below.

JF: Wow! This has turned into a therapy session. I don't have many friends. Almost none. I have one girlfriend who calls me daily to talk and check on me but she is allergic to driving to see me. I am single (cue feelings of pity). I have a sister 11 years younger than me. I am a comedian, actress and writer, so my co-workers are other performers.

You: _____

_____

Did you forget anyone? Your favorite aunt? A friend from the military?

JF: I spend most of my time alone. My audiences are the only groups of people I am around on a regular basis.

You: _____

_____

Who soothes and comforts you? Who puts a smile on your face? Who lets you be defiant? Who helps you forget and escape? Who is your loyal companion and unconditional best friend?

JF: I pray for comfort. I go to other comedy shows for comfort. I smile when I see other people happy. I enjoy putting people in a good mood. I am defiant when I'm told there is something I cannot do. I have no one to rely on but myself when I need to escape reality. My loyal companion and unconditional best friend is me.

You: _____

_____

Do you have any friends named Pizza? Pasta? Chocolate? French fries? Bread? Cheese? Candy bars? Ranch dressing? Beer? Ice cream? Chips?

JF: Okay, now the questions are digging deep. My favorite food is Italian and all things pasta. McDonald's French fries seem to be little gifts from Jesus to me. I once bought two loaves of monkey bread to give as gifts and I ate them both. Overindulging on ice cream during that special "lady time" of the month seems like a fight I would always lose. And chips? My favorite is Ruffles. THE GIGANTIC FAMILY-SIZE BAG! I feel like shedding a tear right now.

You: _____

_____

Do you have additional "food friends"? Are they from the sweet, fat, salt, protein, carbohydrate, or alcohol family? What are their names?

JF: My food friends are anything with multiple grams of sugar and carbs. I eat Snickers bars instead of healthy snacks. My friends' names are Pillsbury, Häagen-Dazs and M&Ms.

You: _____

_____

Emotional Eating

Some people use alcohol, drugs, work, or sleep to block out their problems. In my 20+ years of helping people lose weight, I've seen that there's usually an emotion or two behind the extra pounds. As I discussed earlier, people learn to use food to help themselves deal with life. (Some of us do this more than others.) Food becomes our friend. Everyone needs a friend sometime. We don't always realize when we're doing it. Day 4 will help you to recognize this habit and begin to change.

A six-year-old client once told me that she was an "emotional carb eater." I was stunned. At an early age, we learn that eating can make us feel better – or worse!

Emotional eaters are unique in that each person eats for *different emotional reasons*. Food can be a comfort. When everything's going wrong, macaroni and cheese makes everything right. Food can be an escape. When you can't deal with your kids, partner, or job, food is a good distraction. Temporarily, at least. People have their own special food friends to make them feel better.

Some people learn their behaviors from family members. If a parent used food to cope, this behavior could be passed down. Look at the last few generations. Every generation is getting a little heavier. Truthfully, we can't blame it all on genetics. Did you pick up eating habits from your family? Young children don't know anything different than what their family is doing. Unfortunately, the last few generations have more non-nutritious, high-calorie choices available and they're getting less exercise. Emotional eating, more food, and less physical activity equal more and more excess weight.

Did anyone ever try to cheer you up with a special food treat when you were feeling down? They just wanted you to be happy. Did your grandmother try to smother you in cookies when you went to see her? She was showing her love with food. Did your mother stuff you at mealtime so you'd be healthy?

JF: My mother and family didn't monitor what I ate. They would point out when I was gaining weight but never actually did anything to prevent further weight gain. I had a family that made very rich foods and served large portions. Actually, in many ways, it was a heavenly childhood. But after age 40, potatoes and chicken for breakfast has to stop.

You: _____

I had a client who loved to bake. Her daughters had a fresh bakery item waiting for them after school every day. Wouldn't that be great? What a wonderful way to show your love. However, if the girls didn't run five miles after their snack, extra weight could easily accumulate. Being conditioned to eat sweets every afternoon sets up unhealthy habits. Later in life, when the going gets rough, the girls could turn to bakery items or sweets to return to the safe and secure days of mom's home-baked love.

It's common for people to show their affection to others with food at holidays. Enter the food gifts. Food forms a bond between you and whoever gives you food. Who wouldn't love a person who gave you a pound of your favorite chewy, nutty chocolates?

Do you have a favorite food memory?

JF: Cakes, cakes, and more cakes!! Cake was a big deal for me growing up. Especially the kinds my mother made. I would be surprised when cake batter actually made it to the oven because I ate a lot of batter. Glorious, wonderful cake batter! The cakes were to celebrate good times.

You: _____

_____

People can easily give up on losing weight when staying in shape isn't important in their family. Some families use excess weight as a loyalty bond. When clients have health issues, it becomes easier for them to make dietary changes. The fear of taking medications, having health complications, and facing death is a motivator. Even when the food issues are deeply ingrained, as long as the person is willing, it is possible to take off weight. It just takes more time to reprogram your thinking.

Do you ever eat and not stop until you feel physically sick? Do you feel like you're out of control? Why? There's usually an emotion making you eat. Loneliness and depression could be whispering to you. Defiance or hopelessness could be shouting at you to keep eating.

JF: Depression is a concern for me. Actually, I have trouble figuring out if I'm depressed or ecstatically happy when I get to eat junk food.

I guess having to deal with most of life's challenges alone forces me to cope and sometimes it is easiest to cope at Coldstone Creamery. I am trying to use LA Fitness now to handle life's ups and downs.

You: _____

_____

When people are angry, a lot of them use food to calm down. Many clients have told me that they eat when they're angry. At first, I couldn't believe it. Why would anyone want to eat when they were angry? It is a learned behavior. As I found out, it can also be the power of suggestion. Over the years, I started grabbing something to eat when *I* became angry. It was great. Chocolate was always on my side. Chocolate is so creamy and soothing. Then I told myself, "Stop! You are *not hungry*. You are *angry*." It's easy to get into the habit of eating instead of dealing with an emotion. However, chewing gum and power walking are better ways to calm down.

I've seen a number of children overeat because they weren't getting enough attention from their parents. Children don't naturally know how to express themselves. Food becomes a substitution for their parents' time.

Emotional eating can get in the way of consistently eating fewer calories. You may know how to lose weight but find that you can't because of it. Or, once you lose the weight, it can come back and then some. I have seen it all *at least* a thousand times. So let's look at how you can work on this.

*R*uth's **Rule:** *When someone is overweight, there's usually an emotion or two behind the extra pounds.*

Identifying Your Emotional Triggers

It's time to get in touch with your emotions. Think of the times when you found yourself eating when you weren't hungry. Now circle the feelings you've had in those moments.

What Are You Feeling?	
Worried	Inadequate
Overwhelmed	Deprived
Lonely	Discouraged
Ridiculed	Hurt
Wound up	Stressed
Depressed	Happy
Angry	Controlled
Nervous	Self-destructive
Important	Apathetic
Frustrated	Rejected
Deserving	Relaxed
Tired	Bored
Fearful	Relieved

If you've been emotional eating for years, it may be difficult to change. This is why you have to have strong reasons for losing weight. Keep attacking the enemy. Don't let emotional eating win. Let's take a closer look at your opponent.

Does food listen to you when you're upset? Does food give you approval?

JF: Food allows me to close out the world and retreat. That's the problem.

You: _____

_____

Does food soothe you when you're angry?

JF: Yes, food definitely can be soothing at those times. It's when I get happy again that I realize that food is the enemy ... or at least the 2 pounds of chocolate that I ate when I was angry.

You: _____

_____

Does food help you to relax?

JF: Gigantic plates of homemade pasta have a surprisingly soothing effect on me.

You: _____

_____

Does food help you rebel? Give you freedom?

JF: Food allows me to escape to a very unhealthy place.

You: _____

_____

Does food make you feel safe and secure?

JF: Okay. Yes. Food has been my mom, dad, boyfriend, and enemy.

You: _____

_____

Does food give you something to do?

JF: The fridge provides more entertainment than the TV at times.

You: _____

_____

Do you use food as a reward? Do you go out for ice cream when your child scores a home run? When do you reward yourself or your family with food?

JF: When I feel I have eaten right for several days, I like to ruin it all and have the foods I love.

You: _____

_____

Do you eat instead of getting things done? Do you eat instead of dealing with problems?

JF: I have to work to make money to buy foods to eat. So I get things done while I eat.

You: _____

_____

I'm not saying that you can *never* celebrate with food ever again. That would make me the Food Police. Occasional food rewards are okay. Plan ahead. Be hungry. Make it part of the meal. Avoid excessive amounts. However, rewards do not have to be food. Going to the movies or the mall make good rewards.

Living to Eat vs. Eating to Live

Do you LIVE TO EAT or EAT TO LIVE? "Eat to live" means it's time for breakfast and you are hungry so you find something to eat. "Live to eat" means it's breakfast time, and you're already thinking about what's for lunch and dinner. When you "live to eat," eating is the highlight of your day.

Excess weight is usually not a big problem for "eat to live" people. They can take or leave food. Eating can even be seen as a chore. Some people are in the middle. If you're in the middle, cut back on sweets and fried foods and get moving.

If you "live to eat," food is important to you. The more delicious food is to you, the harder it is to eat less. Your world (time with family and friends) may be centered on food. I have found that these types of people have a more difficult time losing weight and maintaining. To make progress, you'll have to shift your focus away from food.

The Question of "How Much?"

Do you make your kids finish everything on their plates because there are starving kids somewhere in the world? That doesn't make sense. Instead, donate money to a humanitarian organization. Do you make your kids finish what's on their plates because that's what your parents did to you? This practice is still widespread and guarantees weight issues later.

Do you feel compelled or driven to eat all the food that's on your plate? Why?

JF: At times, yes. I feel guilty when I waste. I have to learn fettuccine Alfredo can be wasted.

You: _____

_____

To Each His or Her Own ℃℞

Attention parents and grandparents, new and old! Every person has to learn on their own how much to eat. Only the person who's eating knows when they've had enough. No one has to lick the plate clean. Stop emotional eating before it starts. Some people cannot waste a single bite of food. That's all right. Put less on your plate, or put the leftovers in the refrigerator for later. If you or your child gets hungry later, it's okay to have a small snack.

Binge Eating

Are you a "closet eater"? Do you only eat salad in front of people? If people only see you eating salads, then that must be all you eat. The extra weight must be from a slow metabolism. It couldn't be your fault. Or do you raid the kitchen when you're alone? What are you feeling? Be true to yourself. Eat with others so that you don't feel deprived and overeat later.

Do you binge eat (eating a whole lot of something at one time – cookies, chips, bread, ice cream, cheese)? What's going on emotionally?

JF: Overall, the answer is no. But a pint of ice cream is one complete serving to me. I don't know why people scoop it into a bowl. That makes no sense to me.

You: _____

_____

When and why is this happening? Overcoming binge eating can require the professional help of a psychologist, psychiatrist, or other mental health professional. It can be an unhealthy and dangerous eating behavior.

Additional Issues/Seeking Help

Often victims of sexual abuse use extra weight as a shield to keep people away. Traumatic experiences can cause extreme emotional eating. Some people had a time in their lives when they didn't have enough food. Now they make sure there's more than enough to eat. Some people use food to cope with a death in the family.

Do you feel like an empty shell with no reason to live? Take a break. Go outside. Feel the warmth of the sun on your face. Absorb its energy. Rejuvenate and be stronger than before. Contribute or belong to something to feel needed.

If you've had bad times in your life, seeing a mental health professional may be the only way to help yourself heal. If your issues are serious, it might be impossible to deal with the extra weight until the other issues are resolved.

Working on Your Emotional Eating

I truly believe that most overweight Americans are emotional eaters. The giant portions and lack of physical activity "feed the beast" and make the problem worse. The 80% of Americans who don't engage in enough physical activity aren't releasing their emotional pressure. They learn to suppress their needs and use food to cope instead of expressing themselves with words to deal with life.

We all have different personalities. We have different wants and needs. Some people are sensitive and very emotional. Accept and deal with the way you are and work with it. No matter what your problems, you will eat less *if* you communicate more. Do you have "willpower"? You will *if* you take control of your emotional life. Express your feelings instead of stuffing them down with food.

Think about the times when you can't stop eating. What's going on? Keep asking yourself, "Would I be eating if I wasn't (depressed, stressed, celebrating, angry, bored)? How do you stop yourself from overeating?

Let's role-play. You're bored, not hungry. You see a jar of hot fudge sauce in the refrigerator. Eating a hot fudge sundae sounds good to you right now. Talk to your friend, the sundae.

YOU: *Sundae, I'm bored. I worked at my boring job all day. I'm home. I had an early dinner. I have nothing to do but eat you.*

SUNDAE: *I am silky and delicious. But once you eat me, it's "a second on the lips and forever on the hips." I know that you're trying to lose a few pounds. After you eat me, you're going to be depressed. And you're still going to be bored.*

YOU: *Sundae, you're right. Anyway, a lot of sugar gives me a stomachache. I should go to the gym and work out. I might see some friends, and we could talk.*

SUNDAE: *That's sounds like a good plan. Do some cardio. Get your heart pumping. Talk with your friends. You won't be bored, and you won't feel like eating.*

YOU: *Thank you, Sundae. I almost ate for my emotions, not hunger. If I'm hungry, I will eat. If I'm not hungry, I won't eat.*

Bravo! That was easy. A sweet food friend helped you identify a trigger for emotional eating and brought you out of a dangerous situation. First of all, don't have the ice cream, hot fudge, and whipped cream in the kitchen. It can and *will* call to you. To get to the gym, remember why you want to lose weight. After you're done with your workout, you'll feel like a million bucks …

1. from the endorphins released from exercise.

2. for feeling proud of yourself for not eating and being on track for losing weight.

Not all situations are this easy. Stuff happens every day to trigger emotional eating. Fighting emotional eating can be a constant battle. Here's another example of emotional eating.

Your spouse always puts you down and makes you feel bad about yourself. Nothing you do is right or good enough. You feel rejected and self-destructive. You don't know what to do. You don't care about anything. Munching a big, juicy burger and greasy fries with lots of ketchup starts to fill the emptiness. It's a good escape. It seems like it's your only option. Food is a quick and easy comfort. The food begins to numb the pain, and it's making your stomach feel full and content. For now, you feel better. On the downside, your weight is steadily going up and so is your blood pressure from moments like this.

Six Easy Steps to Slowing Down Emotional Eating

1. **Recognize** that you are an emotional eater.
2. **Identify** the triggers. *Why* do you want to eat?
3. **Identify and feel** the emotion when you're triggered. Don't deny any emotion.
4. **Express** the feeling verbally or through writing to yourself, someone, or something. Start with "I feel …." Watch your desire to eat disappear.
5. **Let go** of the emotion. Move on. Holding in negative emotions can bring you down.
6. **Comfort** yourself. Tell yourself what you want to hear. Make yourself feel good. Start with "I need …." If possible, tell someone what you need. (See "Day 4 Check-In" for other ideas for comforting yourself.)

Try the six steps. This process works, and it's relatively easy.

Stop! Don't eat another emotional calorie. Ideally, talk to your spouse about how you feel. You never know what might happen. Change is possible *for everything*. However, if you feel you can't discuss this with your spouse right now, because you feel that this is the way it's always been and you know that nothing will ever change, start by connecting with your emotions. It may help you from turning to food for comfort.

For now, let's talk to a pretend friend. Tell your new friend (a pretend person), not your old friend (the burger), what's on your mind. Your desire to eat will begin to disappear. Since no one can read your mind, verbalize your feelings and start with the words, "I feel …." Every time you start a sentence with "You," stop because it will put the other person on the defensive. Go ahead and tell your friend how you feel.

"I feel depressed and worthless. I feel like nothing I do is good enough."

Good. You recognized that you were feeling depressed, and you expressed it.

Next, tell your friend what you need in order to comfort yourself. Tell your friend what you want to hear.

"I need my spouse to treat me with respect. I am a good person and don't deserve this."

Try telling your spouse how you feel and what you need. You may not be able to change your spouse's behavior, but expressing your feelings and your needs will make *you* feel better.

You can verbally express your feelings to yourself or another person. You can also write down how you feel or talk to a pet or a stuffed animal. They don't judge, and won't tell anyone. This is not in-depth therapy or a substitute for counseling. But it can help you slow down or stop your emotional eating.

Time to Practice

Now it's your turn to practice. Identifying and expressing emotions can be difficult and uncomfortable for people who aren't in tune with their feelings. It might take a while. You can't just say how you feel a few times and quit. It has to become a routine *every time* you find yourself emotional eating. No one will think you're a complainer or a wacko. They will understand you better.

Think of a situation when you eat for your emotions.

JF:

Situation: Dating a man who doesn't show how he feels about me

Express your feeling: I feel: Lonely and confused

What do you need to feel better? A friend to talk to and remind me of my worth

What are you going to do next time? Write out and journal my feelings. Go to the gym.

You:

*Situation:*_____

Express your feeling: I feel _____

_____

What do you need to feel better? _____

_____

What are you going to do next time? _____

_____

Your feelings are important. *Let them out.* I rarely keep any emotions inside. Strangers on the street know what I'm feeling. You may not get what you want or resolve the situation but that's okay. Putting it into words and expressing it relieves the pressure and dissolves the need to eat. Once you start noticing your emotions, it's surprising to see that minor annoyances can prompt emotional eating. Your mind can have a voracious appetite.

Think of Other Rewards Besides Food ଓ

What are some treats in your life that aren't food? What's fun and exciting to you? What will make you feel good and not think about food? How about taking a class, going on a hike, shopping for materials for a craft project, going to a scenic spot to watch the sunset?

JF: I love to read self-help everything. Also, I am trying to get into hiking. But I have a fear of mountain lions and being eaten.

You: _____

_____

A new client once swore to me that she never ate for her emotions. Two weeks later, she called to let me know that she moved. She had to let me know that she *eats for stress.* The client never thought that she ate for emotions until she started thinking about it.

Play "The Substitution Game"

What should you do if it's difficult to turn off the emotional eating switch? Instead of eating your usual comfort food, try substituting it with fruits or vegetables. At least it's healthy. For some reason, it's hard to eat an entire bag of apples. And you may lose interest after eating more than a few cups of beets. Not too many people are interested in eating five cups of oatmeal. On the other hand, have you noticed that it's possible to eat a family-size bag of chocolate-covered peanuts or an entire bag of potato chips? Isn't life interesting?

Give Yourself Time to Change

In the past, food may have been a good friend to you. But too much food can put on extra weight and make you feel worse. Get out of the habit of comforting yourself with food. Find a substitution for eating. Get busy and *do something*. Best of all ... release some endorphins by exercising!

Learning what and how much to eat is easy. Getting daily physical activity takes a little more effort. Not eating for your emotions is hard work. Honor your hunger and communicate your feelings. Feel the burden being released. *Be free.* Your waistline will thank you.

Expressing your feelings is your new best friend.

*D*ay 4 CHECK-IN ☑

What did you accomplish yesterday?

JF: I accomplished the art of mixing diet lemonade with Captain Morgan rum. Sorry if today was not an inspirational day.

You: _____

_____

What is your goal for today?

(Before you eat, ask yourself, "Am I hungry? What am I feeling?" Identify the emotion. Express the emotion. Set it free.) (Tell yourself or someone else what you need to feel better. "I need ....") (Be aware of the emotions that make you feel like eating – happiness, sadness, anger, boredom, stress.) (Become aware of how you use emotional eating – to comfort, cope, escape, sabotage, distract.) (Verbally express your emotions three times a day starting with "I feel ....) (Instead of eating for emotions, find a substitute activity – go for a walk, for example.) (Give someone a compliment. Make the world a better place a few words at a time.)

JF: Feel what I am feeling and not eat what I am feeling.

You: _____

_____

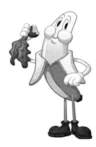

Day 5

The Power of Portion Sizing

*H*ow many times have you asked yourself, "Did I really eat the *whole* thing?" Being a fan of "no calorie left behind" spells trouble.

Portion sizes are out of control. This is an area where we really need to shift our thinking. Our plates, cups, and glasses are a lot bigger than they were 50 to 60 years ago. Restaurants are serving bigger portions on bigger plates. Warehouse stores are selling food in bulk. If you have a "clean your plate" policy and finish everything on your dish, you're in trouble. Some people never learn how to use hunger as a guide to determine how much to eat.

In some ways, eating is complicated. However, in other ways, it's simple. Think of it this way. A car needs gas to run. Similarly, your body needs food to run. If you put too much gas in the car's tank, it overflows. If you eat too much food and don't have enough physical activity to burn off the extra calories, food gets digested and turned into body fat. Unfortunately, we do not get any taller, just wider. Maybe if we were 10-12 feet tall, we wouldn't be so concerned about the extra weight.

Do you think that your portions are too big, too small, or just right?

JF: It really depends on what food it is, where I am eating, and what mood I'm in. If it is my own cooking and what I made is delicious, then I need someone to tell me that I can actually leave some for tomorrow.

You: _____

_____

A Closer Look at Your Portions

What's a portion? A portion is whatever you want it to be. The bigger the portion, the more calories it contains. Some people have no idea how much to eat. *What's a serving?* The Nutrition Facts food label uses servings. The label tells you how many calories and nutrients are in a particular serving. It's not telling you to eat a certain amount. Look at the number of servings in the package. One bottle could have three servings. Remember, MyPlate uses ounces and cup equivalents. Ounces and cups can be weighed and measured.

If a portion is gigantic and you eat fast, watch out! You will be eating a lot more calories than you need. The standard belief says that your brain takes 20 minutes to catch up with your stomach. For me, it's around 45 minutes. I often have to stop eating while I'm still hungry. If I keep eating, I will feel "stuffed" in 45 minutes.

Eat very slowly. You won't eat as much. Use behavior modification techniques to slow down. For instance, you can put down the fork after each bite. The trick that works best with my clients is to chew each bite 15 times. It gets you in the habit of slowing down.

If it's hard to break the habit of eating fast or you're in a hurry, put less on your plate than you think you want. When you're done, you're done. After a while, your brain will catch up to your stomach, and you'll feel "just right." If you find that you're still hungry, you can always eat more.

In Day 3, I recommended that you use a food journal. To work on how much you're eating, measure your food for at least a few days. Record your findings in the "Amount" column on the food journal sheet. After a day or two, you'll get an idea of how much you're eating and see where you can cut back.

Put down the fork and step away from the table. People usually have no idea that they eat more than they need. They just scoop food onto their plates. If it looks good, they scoop more. Our eyes are bigger than our stomachs. Clients are amazed to see a half cup of rice on a plate. It looks *so small*. A half cup of rice or pasta is only a few bites. It goes the other way, too. If you aren't eating many fruits and vegetables, getting a few more servings a day isn't that hard.

Measure your cups and glasses. How many fluid ounces do they hold? Be aware of *liquid calories*. They add up. Buy small bowls and plates. Use the salad plate for your lunch and dinner. It looks like you're getting more. You're probably getting just the right amount.

Take the Gradual Approach ℭ℞

If you usually eat four cups of pasta, go for three cups – not one cup. *Gradually* serve yourself smaller portions. Otherwise, you'll be too hungry. If your body has been used to eating more, it could rebel. You may get hungry an hour or two later and end up eating something unhealthy. Get used to eating two cups of pasta, then one cup or one-half cup.

Ways to Estimate Portions

After you're able to recognize the difference between a one-half cup, one cup, and two cups of pasta, you can start estimating. Estimating portions is a useful tool to use, especially in restaurants.

Here are some useful estimations:

+ **A baseball or a small clenched fist is about one cup.** Thinking about a baseball on your plate is a handy way to estimate amounts of rice and pasta. Go ahead and eat as many vegetables as you want. Large portions of vegetables are *not* a problem.
+ **A deck of cards is about the size and thickness of three ounces of meat or poultry.** The palm of a small adult hand can also be used to estimate three ounces. Fish can look like a checkbook. Three ounces is all the protein that you need at a meal.
+ **A tube of lipstick is good for one ounce of cheese.**

You can also use quarters, dominoes, thumbs and other body parts to estimate, but they can be too hard to remember. A baseball for one cup and a deck of cards for three ounces are often the most useful. Many times, you can think of one of these two tools and do the math (e.g., half a baseball equals ½ cup).

More Tips for Portion Sizing

The human body doesn't need much food to survive. Yet we've become accustomed to eating more and more. Then the bigger we are, the harder it is to be active. The activity levels become less, which causes the metabolism to slow down, which puts on even more weight. It becomes a downward spiral.

To help you avoid this scenario, here are additional ideas for working on your portions:

+ **A solution to overeating: downsize your portions.** If your mind is in the losing-weight mode, measuring your portions and only eating what's on your plate works. If you're eating for your emotions, you'll go back for more to satisfy your emotional hunger.

+ **Try eating three small meals a day with one or two little snacks.** Small, frequent meals can come in handy. Plus, everyone says that once they start eating smaller portions, they can't eat as much. It seems like the stomach "shrinks."

+ **Pick up some snacks packaged in bags of 100 calories.** However, be aware that if your mind is not in the losing-weight mode, you could eat all of the bags at one time. Don't be controlled by a bag. Just because it's 100 calories, don't feel like you have to finish it.

+ **Think of babies snacking on dry cereal. They take a piece and slowly nibble.** When they've had enough, they stop eating. They might only eat a few pieces. There are exceptions to the rule, of course. Some young children will keep eating. If children start gaining excessive amounts of weight, give them more fruits and vegetables – not high-calorie snack foods.

+ **Fresh or frozen packaged meals are good for people who need boundaries.** The portions are controlled. When it's gone, they're done. The prepackaged meals stop working when people get tired of eating the same food. Usually, people go back to eating their regular, big portions.

What About Counting Calories? ☙

I don't believe in counting every single calorie. I'm aware of calories but I don't like to count them. If you're miscounting by only 50 calories, it can throw the whole thing off. Who is to say whether an orange is 40 calories or 90 calories? If you eat an extra 50 calories a day, you will put on five pounds in a year. If you drink an extra can of soda every day, you will put on 15 pounds a year. Being off a little on each food doesn't work for counting calories. It's very common for clients to tell me that they only eat 1,000 calories a day and can't lose weight. The calories are probably underestimated. Follow MyPlate guidelines and fill in the blanks with a basic understanding of calories.

♦ **A relatively new and harmless gimmick for developing restraint is the "portion control" plate.** It has compartments for each food group. The plate reminds you to watch the protein and carbohydrate portions and to increase vegetables.

♦ **Meal replacements, such as shakes and bars, work for some people.** Drinking a shake from a can or eating a bar either for breakfast or lunch, with a normal dinner, limits portions and controls calories. These foods are convenient, and they can be consumed on the go. Read the label to see if there is enough protein and fiber. If they aren't enough calories for you, supplement the shake or bar with a string cheese or fruit.

Once you know *what* to eat and then *how much*, meals at home won't be the biggest problem. High-calorie snacks and eating at restaurants are bigger challenges.

Why Are You Eating?

It doesn't matter how big or how little the portion or serving, what matters is *how much you eat*. Besides your motivating reason for losing weight, *listening to your hunger cues is the second most important aspect of losing weight.* DON'T EAT IF YOU'RE NOT HUNGRY. What a revelation! How often do you eat and you're not hungry? Food is your friend. It's always there for you. Hungry or not.

Do you eat because food is there? What? When?

JF: I eat because I am hungry, happy, sad, confused, irritated, indifferent, nervous, confident, or excited. Actually, I have realized that I genuinely like food. The older I get and the more I try different foods, the more I realize that I AM IN A WORLD OF TROUBLE!

You: _____

_____

Do you eat if you see others eating even though you're not hungry? With whom? When?

JF: The only food that entices me when I see others enjoying it is alcohol. Wait, that's not food ... is it? Well, you get my point. If I'm in a festive atmosphere, I want to join in.

You: _____

_____

Do you eat if you're offered food? Can't say no? Where? Some friends and relatives are very persistent.

JF: I can turn down vegan and vegetarian meals because I don't believe that rocks, grass, sand, and twigs can pass for a casserole. But with any other food, I want to eat it if it looks yummy.

You: _____

_____

Do you eat just because it's mealtime?

JF: Actually, Jackie + eating all day = Happy Jackie.

You: _____

_____

These situations are very common for people with extra weight. Being aware of the triggers is half the battle.

"Full," "Stuffed," or "Just Right"?

Don't wait until you're starving to eat. If you do, you will automatically eat until you are "full" or "stuffed." You will be so hungry that you won't be able to stop eating. It becomes a shoveling motion. If you eat until you're "full" or "stuffed," you'll gain weight. Exception: You're exercising *a lot*.

Most of my overweight clients, young and old, eat until they are "full" or "stuffed," and they don't even realize it. Some people eat beyond "stuffed." Your goal is to eat when you're hungry, and stop when you feel "just right." Eating until you feel "just right" means that you still have a little more room left in your stomach but you feel satisfied. People from the island of Okinawa in Japan have a habit called hara hachi bu, which means eat until you are 80% full.

$\mathcal{R}$**uth's Rule:** *Eat when you're hungry. Stop when you feel "just right."*

Understanding Hunger

There are exceptions to the above rule. There is what I call *"tricky hunger."* You think that you're hungry but you really aren't. If you are gaining weight, know that you must not be allowing yourself to be hungry some of the time. There will be times when you'll have to ignore a little hunger. Some people may feel hungry all of the time. Maybe they're wired to constantly experience hunger and feel the need to eat. If that's the case, as long as you aren't going to pass out, go with a little hunger. Or snack on vegetables – *not* high calorie, processed foods.

Do you ever experience tricky hunger? You think you're hungry but you just ate an adequate amount of food an hour earlier?

JF: Yes, that happens to me a lot. I can have an amazing meal but within two hours I will open the fridge for food again. I tell people it's just to make sure the light in the fridge works, but it really is to see if there's anything I can put in my mouth quickly without looking like the greediest person in the world. That definitely is not hunger, but the beginnings of a problem. HELP!

You: _____

_____

Learn to recognize your hunger symptoms. Some people go from not being hungry to starving in 15 minutes. If you're suddenly starving, eat some fruit or drink a little juice to boost your blood sugar. After 15 minutes, you won't have that starving feeling which leads to overeating.

Some people tell me that they don't ever feel hungry. I think that if you wait long enough, you will notice a feeling of hunger. Get to know how your body reacts to being hungry. Some people get a headache. Some people get light-headed and shaky. Some stomachs growl like a lion. Recognize what hunger is like for you.

How does your body tell you that you're hungry?

JF: When I go hours without eating, I get very bad headaches. Also, I know that if three hours have passed, I should be eating something light so that the major meals are not made of enough food to feed a player from the Miami Dolphins.

You: _____

_____

uth's **Rule:** *Before you put food in your mouth, ask yourself: "Am I hungry?" If you do not feel hungry, don't eat. This is the key to not overeating and not gaining weight.*

Let's Give It a Try

Do you stop eating when you feel "just right," "full" or "stuffed" for breakfast, lunch, dinner and snacks? Track your habits below for two days and raise your awareness.

Breakfast: _____   Breakfast: _____
Lunch: _____   Lunch: _____
Dinner: _____   Dinner: _____

Snack: _____   Snack: _____
Snack: _____   Snack: _____

The Blindfold Test ○ঽ

The next time you eat, cut up your food and then put on a blindfold. Eat slowly. When you feel "just right," take off the blindfold. Is there food left on your plate?

Do you eat with your eyes or with your stomach?

JF: I eat with my eyes when it comes to the foods that I love – sweets, pastries, all desserts. I eat with my stomach in the mornings when I need food for energy. When I watch the Food Network, I eat with my eyes and stomach, ears, and heart because they make some yummy meals.

You: _____

_____

Protein at Each Meal

It's important to include a little protein at every meal. This has been beneficial for many of my clients. If you eat a big portion of carbo-hydrates, you may feel hungry again in an hour. Too many carbs make some people feel jittery. It has something to do with the rise in blood sugar, the release of insulin from the pancreas, and the result-ing blood sugar crash. It could happen after eating a bagel and juice, a bowl of cereal and juice, or a pastry and coffee with a lot sugar. It helps to eat a piece of low-fat cheese, some cottage cheese, or a hand-ful of nuts in the morning to maintain a steady blood sugar.

Other Things to Watch Out For

As you can see, Paul Bunyan's portions don't turn out to be a good thing in the long run. Start noticing the *portion sizes at restaurants* in terms of cups and ounces. One meal could be enough for two to three people. If you eat out, set aside a reasonable portion. Put the rest in a container and take it home. Say to yourself, "Wow! That steak is sixteen ounces. I only need five to six ounces for the entire day."

Be aware of *anything large*. A large coffee drink can be 500-600 calories. An extra large juice may be healthy but it could be 1,000 calories.

One Way to Avoid Disaster ℂℜ

Whatever you do, don't eat out of the bag or a carton. People often eat too many chips or too much ice cream because of this habit. It's a disaster waiting to happen. Put your snacks into small bags or buy snacks in little packages. If you buy a larger bag or container, make it a point to put a small amount in a bag or bowl. Don't go back for more.

Do you ever eat out of the bag or carton? What do you eat? Does it end up being more than you wanted to eat?

JF: Let's just say that I have never treated a pint of Häagen Dazs ice cream as a serving to be shared with others. I have always felt a pint of ice cream only needs a spoon, a napkin, and me.

You: _____

_____

Getting Bigger

The National Heart, Lung and Blood Institute, the National Institutes of Health, and the Department of Health and Human Services have a website www.nhlbi.nih.gov (search for portion distortion). It illustrates how portions have increased over the last 20 years.

A chocolate chip cookie used to be 55 calories. Now a large cookie can be 275 calories. A cookie is a cookie. You eat what's there. A cheeseburger used to be 333 calories. Now it might be 590 calories. A turkey sandwich on two pieces of bread used to be 320 calories. Today a 10-inch sub sandwich with lots of meat could be 820 calories.

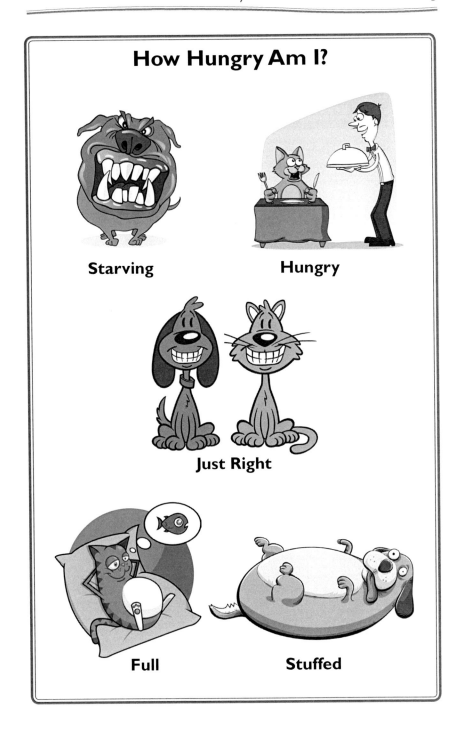

Popcorn at the movies used to be 270 calories. Today a tub of popcorn is 630 calories. A 1.5-ounce blueberry muffin used to be 210 calories. Today a 5-ounce muffin is 500 calories. A plate of spaghetti with 1 cup of pasta, sauce, and three small meatballs used to be 500 calories. Today a plate of spaghetti with 2 cups of pasta, sauce, and three large meatballs is 1,025 calories. The sizes of fountain soda are totally out of control. However, if you're young, the new huge portion sizes seem normal.

Portion Size the MyPlate Way ❦

Pay attention to your portions and compare them to the MyPlate amounts needed for your age, sex, and activity level. For 1,800 calories, it's 6 ounces of grains, 2½ cups of vegetables, 1½ cups of fruits, 3 cups of dairy, 5 ounces of protein foods, 5 teaspoons of oil, and 170 extra calories. Extra calories are bonus calories. Choose an extra 170 calories from any food group, including solid fats, added sugars, and alcohol.

Times have changed. We're eating more food. Don't be fooled by what's on your plate. It's probably more than you need. With the current portions, people will continue getting bigger.

With the way we're eating, is it any wonder that over 70% of Americans are overweight or obese? Is it possible to go back to the way it used to be 50 to 60 years ago? I think that we should try. If we eat the portion sizes from the sixties and use the nutrition knowledge from today, we could get the best of both worlds.

Listen to your hunger. Don't eat if you're not hungry. When you feel "just right," put your fork down.

A small amount of food is your new best friend.

$\mathscr{D}$ay 5 CHECK-IN ☑

What did you accomplish yesterday?

JF: I ate right all day. I had a show with all the free food I wanted. I wanted nachos but ordered shrimp instead. Free food is my vice, but I am learning.

You: _____

_____

What is your goal for today?

(Eat until you feel "just right.") (Measure portions.) (Estimate portions.) (Eat on a salad plate.) (Only eat if you're hungry.) (Notice other people's portions.) (Wear a blindfold while eating a meal as a portion-size test.)

JF: Eating five or six small meals when I am hungry in smaller portions that have a lot of fiber and protein, and doing this with the right attitude! I find that attitude is 95% of the battle. The other 5% is complete denial that I am changing my lifestyle.

You: _____

_____

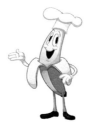

Day 6

Turn that Frown Upside Down!

"What's the use?" "I don't care." "I give up." "It won't do any good anyway." Does that sound like you? Do you need an attitude adjustment? If you keep telling yourself that you can't lose weight, how are you ever going to do it?

Many clients tell me that they can't lose weight. They walk through the door with negative attitudes and don't realize it. A negative attitude can drain you mentally, physically, and emotionally. Unrealistic fad diets and diet supplements impact the way people think about losing weight. People can feel like failures because they don't lose a lot of weight *fast*. I think they hear "lose five to ten pounds a week" too much.

Do you have a positive attitude? Or do you put yourself down about your ability to lose weight?

JF: I have an amazing attitude! It's the way the gym judges me and mocks me as I drive by that makes me angry. I hear the snickers of the mannequins of big-girl stores, despite my amazing attitude.

You: _____

_____

Choose a Positive Attitude

Losing weight is a mindset. Attitude is everything. You are the person in charge of your attitude. If you think positively, you'll have a better chance at succeeding. You can lose weight with a little perseverance and determination. It may take some time to get your mind ready to change, but that's okay. Forget about fear or obstacles (such as other people holding you back).

If you think you can, you can. Make the most of the day. Turn lemons into sugar-free lemonade. Make the best of a situation. Turn your "I can'ts" into "I cans."

A positive attitude means that you're willing to change and stick with it for more than a few months. This is *not* a diet. It's a lifestyle. Your cheery "can do" spirit will help you get through the challenges. Keep in mind that being positive doesn't necessarily mean being happy *all* of the time. Being positive means being confident and determined about losing the weight.

*R*uth's Rule: *Attitude is everything when it comes to weight loss.*

Turning a Negative into a Positive

See if you can catch yourself saying something negative, especially when there are goodies around and you want to eat them. What's more important to you? Losing weight? Or eating a loaf of garlic bread now, only to feel worse about yourself later?

People load their minds with negative thinking. Clients tell me that they haven't been able to lose weight because they like to eat dessert. How about eating some berries after dinner? Okay. That will work. Berries are sweet, satisfying, low in calories, and loaded with antioxidants. One time a client told me that she couldn't lose weight because she hated to exercise. But earlier in her life, she used to love cleaning. What do you know … she started cleaning her friends' houses. She got away from food and made some extra money, while losing weight. There are positive solutions to *every* problem.

Do you have unrealistic expectations? Have you ever quit because you only lost two pounds in a month? If you keep trying, that could be 24 pounds in a year.

Give yourself a pep talk on willpower. "I can buy a donut any time I want. The donut stores aren't going away. Today just isn't the right day. I will eat an apple and feel better."

One time a client stopped doing weights at the gym because he didn't like doing them for an hour. He thought that unless he did weights for one hour, it wasn't doing any good. I suggested that he drop by the gym for 30 minutes. He found that he got benefits and that this time frame was perfect.

Reframing a Possible Obstacle ℞

Consider how you might adjust (reframe) your attitude and behavior related to a recent visit from an out-of-town friend. Does the visit have to negatively affect your weight loss goals?

Negative attitude: *"I can't."*

I wanted to go to the gym but my friend from out of town called. We went out to eat and shared a big piece of chocolate cake after dinner. I blew it. "I can't" lose weight. "I can't" fit into my new jeans.

Positive attitude (reframe): ***"I can."***

*I hadn't seen my friend in a long time. It was good to get together. We had fun going out but I ate a little too much. **"I can"** go to the gym an extra day this week. **"I can"** bring my lunch to work four days this week instead of going out for lunch those days. **"I can"** and will wear my new jeans next month at the volunteer recognition party.*

What "I can't" situation do you notice in your life? (Food-, weight-, or exercise-related)

JF: I find that I can't have several good weeks in a row. If I have a good week of diet and exercise, I will celebrate the 3-pound loss with eating something that may very well set me back.

You: _____

_____

What "can" you do to make it happen?

JF: I can save up for liposuction or lap band surgery. Or I can be realistic and force myself to go to the gym. Then I can acknowledge how good I feel when I work out, bottle that feeling, and drink it every day when I feel like driving to the supermarket instead of walking. I just have a mental block keeping me from taking the 20-mile, I mean 2-mile walk.

You: _____

_____

Developing the Will to Lose Weight

Many years ago, someone told me that self-esteem is self-respect. I believe it. Be good to yourself. Do what's best for your body and your health. Respect yourself enough to say no to unhealthy eating and unhealthy behaviors.

Where there is a will, there's always a way! Focus on being a doer, not a downer. Gradually add things that you can do, like eating more fruit. If needed, focus on increasing exercise. With every accomplishment, you'll feel better about yourself. You'll be surprised at how much you can do.

Being negative is a way of thinking. Are you the one stopping your progress? This is *not* only related to losing weight. Being negative can affect your family, your job, and your relationships with others.

When you're determined, nothing stops you – not even a little hunger. One of my successful, young clients went from being round to being a stick. He had such great willpower that he said no to his own birthday cake.

Is your will to lose weight so strong that you'd say no to your own birthday cake?

JF: I have the kind of willpower that would keep me from allowing anyone else from having some of my birthday cake! I have treated birthday cake like a giant, God-given gift only for me.

You: _____

_____

That Person in the Mirror

When it comes to your body, you could probably list 20 things that you don't like. We are quick to put ourselves down. I used to ask my clients what they like about their bodies and also to name their best qualities. I stopped because it was too difficult for them. People don't think about the good stuff, and it's hard for them to express it to others. Start thinking about your good qualities to get the ball rolling for being positive.

Name three things that you like about your looks.

JF: I will actually enjoy this part!!! I love my face. I am a cutie pie!! I have nice legs/feet. Finally, I like my boobs.

You: _____

_____

We should feel good about our bodies, no matter what the size. It's unfortunate that weight discrimination is so prevalent, especially for women.

Name three of your admirable qualities or accomplishments.

JF: I gave up a career with financial stability to be in the entertainment business and have been successful thus far.

I am a big believer in karma and doing good for others and treating others with respect in order to get respect.

I have managed to stay single for a long time and didn't fall into the trap of settling for any type of man just so I can say I have somebody. I am proud of the woman I am and will be in the future.

You: _____

_____

Positive Affirmations for Weight Loss

Try saying these statements to yourself:

♦ I am ready to lose weight now.
♦ It doesn't matter how much I weigh. I am a good person.

- I don't have to be perfect.
- I am in control.
- Slowly, but surely. (Very important for not giving up!)
- I am doing the best I can.
- I could have done worse. (Isn't that the truth?)
- Everything will be okay.
- I know I can do it.
- Something good is going to happen to me.
- Today is going to be a great day.
- I feel good.
- I am relaxed and calm.
- I look and feel marvelous.

You can talk yourself into *anything*. It might as well be positive. Once you see the value in yourself, you can succeed at anything.

You Can Start with Small Steps ❧

If being positive isn't your thing, start small.
- Smile.
- Ask for help.
- Have faith and trust in yourself.
- NEVER GIVE UP!

Where Do You Want to Start?

Think about what you want to change about your attitude. Take that one small step. Believe that you will succeed. Could you handle the affirmation, "I'm going to lose three pounds a month"? Where can you start being positive? What would you like to do?

JF: I can look at each day as another day for success instead of another day of challenges I can't meet. I have a positive attitude with everything else, why not food?

You: _____

_____

If you're stressed, depressed, and feeling down, how important is the problem, considering the entire world? Don't dwell on negativity. Move on quickly. The sooner, the better.

More Positive Self-Talk

Give yourself frequent pep talks. Don't do anything unhealthy,–mentally or physically.

Here are more affirmations for you:

- If I lose three pounds a month, that's 36 pounds in a year.
- I would rather lose weight than eat a bag of chips.
- I feel great after I exercise.
- I want to fit into a bikini and look hot.
- I would rather exercise than eat chocolate.
- Other people can lose weight. I can, too.
- I have will power and self-control. I'm not a beast running wild through the forest.
- Who's in charge? Me or the donut?
- Food won't solve my problems.
- If I eat this double-bacon cheeseburger, I'll gain weight. I am trying to lose weight.
- I don't like ranch dressing on my food anymore. It makes me feel sluggish.
- If I keep trying, I will lose weight and achieve my goals.
- I don't want to be "obese" anymore. (BMI 30 and above; see Day 13.)
- I am a little hungry. It's okay. I know that I'm losing weight.

A Little Verbal Self-Defense

What should you say when a friend, co-worker, or family member tries to tempt you with unwanted food?

Try one of these lines:

- *No, thank you. I don't feel like eating. I'm full.*
- *I don't want candy. I am watching my blood sugar.*
- *I had lunch an hour ago. I'm not hungry.*
- *I don't want to go out to eat. I'm saving money for a vacation. How about going for a walk?*

Tricks of the Trade

When the going gets tough, here is a treasure chest of secret weapons to use. When one trick stops working, choose another one.

♦ You have reached the "just right" point but still want to keep eating. Grab a piece of sugarless gum to soothe the craving. You can also chew gum instead of nibbling and sampling food while you cook.

♦ Brush your teeth after dinner. Tell yourself, "Sorry. I brushed my teeth. I can't eat anything until morning." When I was in college, this was effective for me.

♦ Gulp down 1 cup of water before meals. It helps fill up your stomach.

♦ If you're used to eating dessert or something sweet after a meal, suck on a menthol cough drop. The menthol takes away the craving for sweet.

Smart Trick:
Target Your Problem Foods/Situations ଔ

Identify your problem foods, as well as the situations that can get you off track. Make some rules and stick to them. Keep adding more to your list, as needed.

• No sour cream. No cream cheese. No fried foods. No frosting.
• No eating in front of the TV or while reading. No eating after 7 p.m.
• No treats in the house. If it's not there, you can't eat it.
• Nothing sweet until noon.
• Only one treat a day.
• Fast food only one time a week.

♦ If you love to cook and make delicious food, it won't help your quest to lose weight. For a while, eat plain and simple.

♦ When you feel hungry, chew two to three *glucose tablets*. They're in the diabetes section at the drug store. Each tablet has 4 grams of dextrose, a fast-acting carbohydrate. When a diabetic's blood sugar is low, four tablets at a time are recommended to raise blood sugar. When I'm starving and it's not time to eat for another 30 minutes,

I find that the dextrose tablets raise my blood sugar quickly and take the edge off hunger. Then when it's time to eat, I don't eat everything in sight.

Are there other tricks that you would like to add?

JF: After reading "no sour cream," I'm not sure I have the emotional capacity to keep writing!! But here's another trick ... when I eat fruit, it keeps my hunger under control and keeps me from stealing other people's food when they're not looking.

You: _____

When You Get Off Track

If you mess up, forget about it. Get back on track right away. Keep moving forward and set small, achievable goals every minute, hour, day, week, or month. Be consistent, persistent, and patient. Think positive thoughts to get yourself re-started and to keep yourself going. Positive thoughts bring positive feelings, which cause positive behaviors and habits. Keep encouraging yourself on your progress. It makes sense that people with positive attitudes are happier and live longer. *Don't worry. Be happy.*

Visioning a Positive Future

This is your chance to look into the future. Close your eyes. Imagine that you have reached your perfect weight. How much do you weigh? What does your body look like? How do you feel? What are you doing?

JF: I am 135 pounds and, if it is possible, sexier than ever! I am not skinny, just incredibly fit and toned. And most important, happy with who I am inside and out.

You: _____

Excellent job. Keep going!

A positive attitude is your new best friend.

𝒟ay 6 CHECK-IN ☑

What did you accomplish yesterday?

JF: I went out with a girlfriend and shared one personal pizza. I so wanted my own. But after we ate, I was completely satisfied and happy that I had saved calories and money. It was her idea to split everything. My first reaction was to cut her in half (just kidding; you know what I mean).

You: _____

_____

What is your goal for today?

(When you wake up, give yourself a pep talk. Say, "I can, and I will, lose weight.") (Chew gum after meals.) (Visualize yourself losing weight.) (Give yourself an encouraging statement through-out the day.) (Stop eating in the car.) (Ask yourself, "Is there any-thing stopping me?" Then go for it.) (Tell yourself, "I'm never giving up!")

JF: Go to the gym!! Go to the gym! And did I say, "Go to the gym"? Right after I eat gym-friendly food.

You: _____

_____

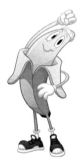

Day 7

The Check, Please ...

*W*hat happened to the good old days when your mother packed your lunch and a healthy dinner was sitting on the table at 6:00 p.m.? Times have changed. Rent and mortgages cost a lot of money. Mom has to work. And guess what? Mom is tired from working two jobs and driving an hour to get home, and doesn't feel like cooking. "Mom" could actually be anyone. The last thing anyone wants to think about is cooking. Not to mention doing the dishes and cleaning up.

It's no wonder that Americans are eating out now more than ever.

Looking at Your Patterns

Let's look at your eating patterns in restaurants.

How often do you eat out? What types of restaurants? What meals?

JF: I unfortunately eat out on a regular basis. When my schedule gets crazy, I don't exercise self-control and instead just grab what I can. I have shoveled down so much McDonald's since birth, I should get free French fries every time I drive past one of their restaurants.

You: _____

_____

Do you go to a drive-thru? Which ones? How often?

JF: Maybe I should ask for honorary stock in McDonald's instead of the free fries. The plain reality is that their food tastes good, it smells good. I think their fries are delicious, and the employees are usually very nice. Maybe if the McDonald's employees were a little meaner, I might break the habit. I'm not saying that I would stop going, but I would be less happy about each fry I ingest.

You: _____

_____

Do you pick up take-out food? From where? How often?

JF: All this being honest is making me uncomfortable and yes ... I usually go for Chinese takeout. I know to order steamed veggies, brown rice, and no sauce, but a bucket of greasy, sauced-up noodles has somehow always made it back to my house in the past.

You: _____

_____

There are many places to get something to eat. Food is everywhere.

Do you get something to eat or drink at any of these places? An espresso bar? A juice bar? A bakery? A grocery store? A food truck? A convenience store? A bookstore? An ice cream parlor? A liquor store? A deli? Movie theaters? Vending machines? What do you get?

JF: The answer to all these questions is yes. Ice cream parlor? If by this we mean Coldstone Creamery, then that would be a "heck, yeah, I go there." Wait, I shouldn't be so happy about that ... sorry. Liquor stores? To avoid being judged, I will choose to plead a fifth – I mean, the fifth.

You: _____

_____

When eating out, do you think about portion sizes or nutrients?

JF: I find that as I get older, "grabbing whatever" is not only a ticket to Tubby Town but it also increases the risk of heart disease, high blood pressure, etc. Wow! Could it be that at Day 7, I am finally catching on? Is JFab growing up?

You: _____

_____

Eating outside the home can be a major contributor to excess weight.

Why We're Eating Out More

Maybe you never experienced home-cooked meals so you're used to eating out. Every person has a different situation. People don't cook for a number of reasons:

- No time
- Too tired
- Too lazy
- Don't know how
- Don't want to cook

The alternatives to meal preparation are starving or eating out. It's easy for people to choose eating at a restaurant. Eating out has become a way of life. Take-out and drive-thru restaurants are quick and convenient. It's something to do. It's a place to meet friends or have a meeting. Kids are often by themselves so they may be picking up their own meals. Restaurants have many delicious and tempting items on the menu.

Buyer Beware

News alert. Restaurants are more interested in making a profit than lowering your cholesterol. Restaurants sell food that people want to buy. The food isn't always healthy. If the food is healthy and no wants it, they take it off the menu. Typically, people go to restaurants for food they don't get at home. Why go to a restaurant for oatmeal? Since over half of our food money is spent at restaurants, proceed with caution.

Know this about food served to you outside the home:

- Tends to be high in fat (butter, oil, dressings, sauces)
- Tends to be high in sugar (beverages, desserts)
- Tends to be high in refined carbohydrates (pasta, bread)
- Fruits and vegetables are usually lacking

- Can add *hundreds* of extra calories
- Many restaurants don't serve low-sodium or fat-free items, such as low-sodium soy sauce or fat-free sour cream.

Emotional Eating on the Run

If you're feeding wounded emotions, drive-thru restaurants are your secret friend. You can order whatever you want. No one sees you. No one knows what you're eating. Clients have told me that they pick up breakfast at one fast food place and move on to the next fast food place for a second breakfast, even a third. Emotions can be very hungry. Maybe you reward yourself with something comforting after a long, hard day. Food can be warm and satisfying. Are you a late-night eater? Restaurants are open 24 hours. When you're feeling vulnerable, vegetables aren't the first thing on your mind. Hot, salty, greasy fries usually fill the void better. Long ago, restaurants closed early, and grocery stores weren't open on Sundays. If you ran out of something, you had to go without and wait until Monday. This slowed down impulse eating.

Sweet, greasy, or salty foods are comfort foods to a lot of people. No one has ever told me that carrots are their comfort food. Do you eat at county fairs or amusement parks? You could spend a fortune on yummy comfort foods. Where are the vegetables?

A Closer Look

Eating is a social activity. Meeting at a restaurant is an excuse to get out of the house and see friends. It's much better than cooking your own food or preparing a meal for someone else.

Do you go to a movie, a play, a concert, or a sports event to eat unhealthy food and drinks? Try to separate eating from *the activity*.

Is eating out a trigger or excuse for you to eat or drink too much? Do you have special comfort foods that you like to order?

JF: There are so many instances as an entertainer where I can get drinks for free. THAT IS A PROBLEM! Not that I drink too much, but one fun cocktail can undo an entire day of eating right.

You: _____

Do you know what foods you should be choosing, but don't? When it comes to eating out, what's your biggest problem?

JF: I don't eat enough during the day to make eating out a non-issue. When it's time to eat while out, I am starving!

You: _____

Healthy Dining 101

It helps to remember the tools for portion sizing from Day 5. For _weight loss_, think "fat free" or "low fat," small meals, and no sweets. Limit alcohol. For _health_, think "low sodium," "healthy fats" and "high fiber" (fruits, vegetables, and whole grains).

When ordering, think about getting a small amount of protein, a portion of carbohydrate, and one or two fruits or vegetables. If your day needs calcium, add fat-free milk, low-fat milk or another calcium food. Eat less than you want. The hidden fat calories will kick in later.

No foods are forbidden. That's an invitation to eat them. A "bite" here and there is okay.

Here are some **foods to avoid:**

- Anything battered and fried – hash browns, fried chicken, French fries, onion rings, chicken nuggets, tempura, etc.
- Gravy
- Fried wontons, fried egg rolls, orange chicken, kung pao chicken, fried rice
- Refried beans made with lard
- Sour cream, cream cheese, mayonnaise, butter
- Sausage, pepperoni, bacon, salami, bologna, chorizo
- Creamy, white sauces – Alfredo, carbonara
- Cream soups, clam chowder
- Dishes with a lot of cheese
- Giant hot dogs, giant burgers, chicken wings

- Croissants, muffins, biscuits, pastries
- More than a few bites of a dessert or foods with a lot of added sugars
- Giant portions of *anything*
- More than one or two alcoholic beverages
- Liquid calories with no nutrients – soda, lemonade, punch
- Brunches and all-you-can-eat buffets

These tips for eating out are not new. Do you follow this advice? Why or why not?

JF: Consistency is my problem. That and a serious love/hate relationship with Krispy Kreme.

You: _____

_____

MyPlate and Eating Out

When eating out, keep following the MyPlate guidelines. Choose whole grains. Look for dishes with beans. Order fruit as the side. Look for ways to get more vegetables. Add fat-free or low-fat dairy foods to your meals. Limit steak or other protein portions. Know your calorie needs and check posted calorie counts at restaurants.

MyPlate suggests limiting the extra calories from saturated fats, added sugars, and salt. If you're trying to limit sodium, avoid salty foods – soy sauce, bacon, ham, canned soup. Watching sodium can be more difficult than watching the fat and sugar.

Portion Control at Restaurants

When it comes to eating out, portion sizing is probably the most important aspect. If a food is not healthy, a bite or two won't cause a weight gain. If it's a giant portion, you will most likely eat too much. Always order the smallest size. It will be plenty. Don't feel obligated to eat everything on your plate. Restaurant plates can be huge.

Look at the portion size of French fries at restaurants. The serving size is usually dependent on the size of the plate. There isn't a lot of consistency. People tend to eat what's in front of them. Do you ever see people dip their French fries in Ranch dressing? Talk about adding insult to injury. I would like to see raw carrot slices instead of fries as an option.

*R*uth's **Rule:** *Portion size is the most important consideration when eating out.*

Do's for Dining Out ℘

When eating out while losing weight, maintaining weight, or for good health, follow these simple guidelines – as often as possible.

- Enjoy baked, broiled, roasted, steamed, grilled, or poached foods.
- Always choose fat-free or low-fat, if available.
- Choose vegetables, fruits, beans, whole grains, lean protein, and fat-free and low-fat milk products.
- Ask for dressings and sauces on the side.
- Salsa, lemon, mustard, ketchup, and vinegar are good choices.
- For side dishes, order corn on the cob, baked beans, or coleslaw. Think *vegetables*.
- Select primavera or cacciatore dishes and marinara sauce.
- Order vegetable soup, wonton soup, black bean soup, minestrone soup.
- Trim the fat off meat. Don't eat chicken skin.
- Estimate portion sizes, decide how much to eat, and push the rest away.
- Stop eating when you feel "just right."
- Take home leftovers.
- Refrigerate within two hours.

Other Strategies

As you're seeing, there are ways to still enjoy a meal out while staying true to weight loss goals. Here are more tips to have on your side.

- **Order a low-fat appetizer for a meal or an a la carte item.** A salad and soup is enough for a meal at a restaurant. Try sharing a meal.
- **Look for ways to increase vegetables.** However, I'm not sure fried vegetables are better than no vegetables.
- **Don't be afraid to say "on the side."** Food smothered in sauces, gravy, and high-fat condiments can add hundreds of calories. If your order comes with a scoop of butter or sour cream, take it off the plate immediately.
- **Ask the server how the food is prepared.** A lot of times they know the type of oil/fat that is used to sauté foods.
- **Save your calories for the food. Don't drink them.** Choose water or unsweetened iced tea. Diet beverages are okay. Choose fat-free or low-fat milk. Lemonade has a lot of calories from sugar. It's soda without the bubbles.
- **Watch the bread.** One roll is not a problem. But if you know you'll eat a lot more, have the server take the bread basket away. Nonetheless, bread is filling and relatively low in calories. The bread calories are not as big a problem as the margarine, butter, or oil calories.
- **Be smart about omelets.** Watch the portion sizes. They can be enough for two people. Add a variety of vegetables instead of cheese or meat to the omelet. You're already getting enough protein from the eggs.
- **Alcohol can make or break a meal.** When you're losing weight, it would be better to skip the alcohol.
- **Slow down. You're not in an eating race.** It could save you some calories.

Know that if you frequently eat at restaurants, it's difficult to lose weight. In fact, it is difficult to *not* gain weight. You never know how many calories you're getting. Assume it's *a lot*.

Eating at Work

Do your meals come from a vending machine? Instead of a candy bar or a bag of chips and a soda, choose nuts, trail mix, whole grain granola bars, pretzels, dried fruit, and water. Vending machines are getting more creative and contain healthier choices. Look for protein, fiber, whole grains, and calcium choices.

Salads Can Be Deceiving ⊗

A salad can be filling to help you eat less, or it can be additional calories. How much dressing is on it? If a salad is big, it needs more dressing. A giant Chinese chicken salad or a giant Caesar salad can have a day's worth of calories. Always order the dressing on the side. Then dribble 1-2 tablespoons over the salad or dip your fork in the dressing and then on the salad. A salad should be more than iceberg lettuce and an unripe slice of tomato. Salads should have lots of vegetables, such as spinach, carrots, broccoli, peppers, etc.

Salad bars do not automatically mean healthy eating. There are many unhealthy choices at a salad bar. Choose a variety of colorful vegetables, not deli meats, bacon, or cheese. Pile on the vegetables and other plant foods. Beans are a great source of protein for salads. If you like a lot of salad dressing, choose a reduced-fat or fat-free dressing, or even salsa.

If you're at a conference or have an expense account and don't have to pay for meals, don't think that this is an opportunity to eat as much as you can. Pace yourself. It's okay to eat a small amount of different items to taste them. Leave some food on your plate.

Have an Emergency Food Stash ⊗

Stuck at work and can't get away? To avoid raiding the vending machines, keep emergency foods in a drawer: bean dip, peanut butter or tuna and crackers, instant oatmeal, heat-and-serve cans of soup, dried or canned fruit, beef jerky, cans of vegetable juice, nuts, and microwave popcorn.

Get Smart about Fast Food

I will say this about fast food. The portions are controlled, and you know the calorie and nutrient count. Knowledge is power. You still have to watch portions and fat. Avoid the temptation to order the larger choice and the combos to save money. It's more food than you need. Any restaurant food tends to be higher in fat and sodium than home-cooked food. You don't need the soda or the fries. Bring your own fruit or cut up vegetables. Forget the giant beef burger. A grilled chicken sandwich on a whole wheat bun may be a healthy option, but keep in mind the size. You don't need more than three ounces of meat or chicken. How big is the bun? Is it more than two pieces of bread? Forget the cheese. Get your calcium from a fat-free or low-fat dairy food. Forget the bacon. Since you can get the calorie counts at fast food restaurants, limit your calories to 500-700 calories a meal (depending on the number of snacks and your activity level).

Building a Healthier Sub Sandwich ❧

What could be unhealthy about a sub sandwich? For starters, a 10-inch bun is way more carbohydrates than you need. Even 6 inches is too much. Look at the size of the bun and compare it to one or two pieces of bread. Break off the rest and don't eat it. Choose a whole-grain bread. Watch the types of meat in the sandwich. Meats like salami and bologna contain a lot of saturated fat. You don't need chips or even baked chips with a sandwich. The bread is your carb. Bring along a fruit or cut-up vegetables. Add as many vegetables as you can to the sandwich. The meat or poultry is protein. Pass on the processed cheese.

If you order fast food, don't eat in the car. You could wolf down more than you need. Pull over and enjoy the meal in a park. Focus on the taste of the food. Many fast food restaurants are serving healthier choices. Scan the menu.

When you're eating take-out food, measure or estimate portion sizes. If you buy a rotisserie chicken, add your own vegetables or a salad and a whole-grain side dish. The portion size of the protein should look like a deck of cards.

Are you eating out with kids? Avoid the children's menu. It's usually high fat, high sodium, high sugar, low in nutrients, and low in fiber. Say no to chicken nuggets, fries, hot dogs, macaroni and cheese, and lemonade. Let them share your healthy choices.

Pepperoni pizza is the number one choice of pizza. Are you used to ordering pepperoni pizza because everyone automatically does? Maybe you really like the spicy, salty flavor? Well, pepperoni is a little circle of saturated fat that clogs the arteries. How about ordering a nice veggie pizza instead? Choose vegetable toppings on pizzas. Blot off any excess oil sitting on the cheese. Don't feel like you have to be macho and eat half a pizza to impress your friends.

Tips for Ethnic Cuisine

Every type of ethnic cuisine has healthy and not-so-healthy choices. Be aware of the fat content and the sodium.

Eating one or two baskets of tortilla chips at a Mexican restaurant can be a problem. Count out your chips in advance and load on the salsa. If you eat a lot of chips, a margarita, a big portion of the main course, AND the rice and beans, you'll leave stuffed. When you order a Mexican entree, the rice and beans aren't necessary. You're already getting the carb and the protein from the entree. If you want a light vegetarian meal, order rice, beans, and a vegetable or salad. Guacamole, *not* sour cream, is a healthy addition to Mexican food. As always, watch the portion sizes.

For Chinese food, it's easy to eat too much. It tastes so good. Do you fill up your plate with three or four different dishes and go back for more? Put everything on your plate that you're going to eat. Don't go back for seconds. Include a vegetable dish. Save the fried dishes for special occasions. If available, choose plain brown rice over white rice or fried rice. Assume that most Chinese dishes contain a lot of sodium.

What's for Dessert?

Do you love desserts? Just the dessert could have over 1,000 calories. Will eating a piece of cheesecake with chocolate sauce and whipped cream help you lose weight? Desserts and after-dinner coffee drinks add *a lot* of unnecessary calories.

Do you order dessert? Are you still hungry by then?

JF: I fall victim to the "Girls Night Out" trap where we order one or two desserts and decide to split them. This way, no one has to admit that they want their own.

You: _____

The FDA has an eating-out guide called "Whoa, Slow and Go." Here's their message. **Whoa:** Think about whether you should eat it or not. **Slow:** Okay. Eat it once in awhile. **Go:** Go for it. It's fine. Enjoy eating a moderate portion size. This is an easy concept to remember. Whoa! Slow! and Go!

*R*uth's Rule: *When you're maintaining weight, you can share a dessert with a few people. When you're losing weight, you can only afford a taste.*

A Basic M.O. for Restaurants

To lose weight, limit eating out as much as possible. When that's not possible, cut back on your portion sizes. Of course, you're not a robot programmed to only eat iceberg lettuce with lemon, beef broth, and boiled chicken. Just about any food can be ordered and consumed in small amounts, occasionally. How much fat is in chili cheese fries? Don't ask and don't tell your arteries.

Balance a high-calorie meal with a light-calorie meal and get physical activity. It's not that hard to eat an entire day's worth of calories in one restaurant meal. If you're unable to get any type of physical activity, only eat small amounts.

Home Sweet Home ଓ

As an alternative to eating out, there are numerous cookbooks and cooking shows offering ideas for quick, easy, and nutritious foods at home. It takes a little planning and a small attitude adjustment.

Trying new and different foods can be one of life's pleasures. It's okay to take delight in every bite, but avoid filling yourself up to the point of being stuffed. Eat really, really slowly, and savor the flavors.

Become a trend setter. After the server takes your order, ask for a salad plate. Put all of the food you're going to eat on the salad plate. Then put the rest of the meal in a container and take it home.

Eating can still be a social activity. Listen to your hunger. Talk more. Eat less.

Managing restaurant portions is your new best friend.

Week 1 Recap

This has been a week of big hitters. You thought about why you want to lose weight. Learned why physical activity is important. Reviewed what foods to eat and how much. Discovered that emotions can get in the way of losing weight. Reaffirmed the importance of being positive. Plus, you learned how to eat fewer calories when eating outside the home.

Congratulations!

Time to weigh in.

Weight:_____

𝒟ay 7 CHECK-IN ☑

What did you accomplish yesterday?

JF: Yesterday I turned down a free meal. Not big in the eyes of many, but to me this means that the world has tilted off its axis or that I am actually getting some self-control!

You: _____

_____

Eating out? What is your goal for today?

(Pack a lunch instead.) (No appetizer.) (No bread.) (Only drink water.) (Share a meal.) (No fried food.) (Salad dressing on the side.) (Smaller portions.) (Share dessert.) (Limit alcohol.) (No soda.) (Order a fat-free, sugar-free coffee.)

JF: My goal is to continue to eat well today. When I get hungry a little later, I will have a large glass of water and a low-fat string cheese. I feel that I should lose 10 pounds just by making the right decisions.

You: _____

_____

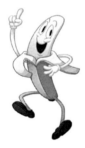

Day 8

Rise and Shine, Breakfast Time!

*G*ood morning! It's time for breakfast.

Do you eat breakfast? If you don't eat breakfast, why not?

JF: I do eat breakfast more often now. I have learned that eating breakfast means I am less likely to eat the office supplies at 11 a.m.

You: _____

_____

What do you eat? What about on weekends?

JF: I have oatmeal, with a packet of Equal or Splenda, of course. On weekends, I might eat eggs, turkey bacon, and low-fat yogurt.

You: _____

_____

Do you eat donuts or pastries for breakfast? On a regular basis or for special occasions?

JF: During that time of the month, I may feel obligated by the demons that take over my body to have sugary sweets for breakfast. I have no control over that side of me and the Jackie you know and love is not available for comment until the third week of the month. Sorry.

You: _____

_____

Many people tell me that they aren't hungry in the morning. Do you know why? It's because they ate too much at night. Either they ate too much for dinner, ate late, or ate snacks after dinner. Whatever the situation, it's crucial to get used to eating *less* the night before. Everyone should wake up with a hearty appetite.

Are you hungry when you wake up?

JF: I think to say I am hungry when waking up is a gross understatement. I would be more inclined to say I can be prone to cannibalism at that time of day. No one is safe.

You: _____

_____

Breakfast Games People Play

It's very common for people to skip breakfast. However, it's a good idea to eat small, frequent meals throughout the day to maintain steady blood sugar levels. If people don't eat breakfast, blood sugar levels could drop uncomfortably low by lunch time. People reach the "starving" level of hunger and then overeat.

Clients have told me that even though they only eat one meal a day (usually not breakfast), they can't lose weight. When they start eating three meals a day (including breakfast), they do lose weight. It seems hard to believe that you could eat more food in one meal than in three small meals. However, I have seen it many times.

Some people eat breakfast for the sake of eating breakfast. Many of my clients think that they have to eat breakfast, because it's the most important meal of the day, even though they aren't hungry. This is a problem. They wonder why they can't lose weight. The Golden Rule for losing weight: *Don't eat if you're not hungry.* If you're not hungry in the morning, you should *not* eat breakfast.

People worry about their children and often make them eat breakfast, again because it's the most important meal of the day. If children have excess weight, they could be snacking a lot, especially at night. They may not be hungry in the morning but their parents make them eat. Children have to learn to judge their own hunger and decide for themselves when to eat. Worried parents can pack a breakfast for their children to eat during nutrition break. Ultimately, parents should scale down dinners and limit after-dinner snacks so that the children will be hungry in the morning.

What Is Breakfast?

Breakfast means "breaking the fast." That means you eat because you're hungry after a long night of fasting.

A lot of people think of "breakfast" as bacon, eggs, toast, and hash browns at 7:00 a.m. But they aren't hungry and don't want to eat that much. So they say they don't eat breakfast.

If you grab a piece of cake or a candy bar at 10:30 a.m., that's breakfast. Eating any type of food in the morning is breakfast. It may not be the typical breakfast or be healthy, but still it's breakfast.

Some people who don't have time to eat breakfast grab a coffee drink in the morning. A coffee drink could contain 350-600 calories, depending on the size. That's breakfast. Consider the calories. The fat and sugar calories could equal the calories in a bowl of whole grain cereal with milk and juice, only with fewer nutrients.

Breakfast Strategies

If you don't have time to prepare breakfast in the morning, get it ready at night. It only takes a couple of minutes to spread some peanut butter on a piece of whole wheat bread. It takes 15 seconds to put a yogurt and a fruit in the front of the fridge.

Some people aren't hungry the minute they wake up. In that case, bring along something to eat and find a time to eat breakfast when you *are* hungry. It could be on the way to work, at work, or at school. When you get hungry, you will have it ready, and you won't be tempted to eat high-calorie, high-sugar, or high-fat foods. When you're hungry, sugary and fatty foods have a tendency to find you.

If you're at home, it's better to be on a schedule, and eat breakfast around the same time of day.

It doesn't matter what time you eat – 6 a.m. or 11 a.m. It's still your first meal of the day. Adapt the time to fit your hunger schedule. Whenever you start eating, space out the rest of your meals throughout the day.

Making a Healthy Breakfast

Now that you will be hungry and you've found a time to eat, what is a "healthy" breakfast?

A healthy breakfast contains protein, fruits, whole grains, or vegetables. Typically include foods from at least three food groups.

- **Protein** could be beans, nuts, eggs, lean meat, fish, fat-free or 1% milk, low-fat cheese, or yogurt.
- **Complex carbohydrate** could include whole grain breads and cereals, corn tortillas, or oatmeal.
- One hundred percent **juice** as well as fresh, frozen, dried, or canned **fruits and vegetables** are all good choices.
- It's okay to include **healthy fats.**
- Determine **portion sizes**, depending on age and activity level.

Foods like bacon, sausage, hash browns, processed cheese, donuts, pastries, croissants, biscuits with gravy, butter, cream, and whole milk contain a lot of saturated fat, trans fats, or cholesterol. They may be eaten in small amounts, occasionally. These foods contain a lot of unhealthy calories and can lead to excess weight, heart disease, diabetes, and cancer.

Such low-fat foods as fruits, vegetables, whole grains, low-fat dairy, and beans contain essential nutrients that protect health.

Breakfast at Restaurants

Do you go out for breakfast? Where? How often? What do you order?

JF: When I do order breakfast out, it is usually a low-fat muffin. Lately I learned that this is not at all low-calorie.

You: _____

_____

Going out for breakfast used to be a special treat to eat foods like omelets, French toast, or pancakes with strawberries and whipped cream. You ordered foods that you normally didn't make at home. Or you were on vacation and had to eat out. Today, there are many reasons for eating breakfast outside of the home. Meeting friends and family for breakfast has become a social event. It may be for business reasons. Your family may go out for breakfast after religious services. It might just be a good reason to get out of the house. Maybe you're in a hurry to go somewhere so you pick up a fast-food breakfast.

However, how many calories do you think are in one of those "specials" that include bacon, eggs, sausage, and hash browns, with toast dripping in butter? _A lot._ The unhealthy fat content is off the chart. How much sugar and fat is there in a giant portion of pancakes with strawberries and whipped cream? _A lot._ The calories from one breakfast could be enough for the entire table. How many eggs in an omelet? _More than you need._ Have you checked out the calories in fast food breakfasts? You might change your mind. The portion size may not be that big, but the large number of calories from fat and sugar is a lot. Many of these breakfast foods also contain large amounts of sodium. Fast food restaurants have calorie counts available. Do you need a 1,200 calorie breakfast? Lunch is a few hours away.

If you're going out for breakfast, follow the 1,800 calorie My-Plate guidelines to the best of your ability. Order what you would eat at home. It's not a special treat to eat breakfast in a restaurant anymore. If you're eating breakfast for social or business reasons, don't make the high calorie, unhealthy breakfast the focus. Be careful of the portions. Juice could contain 200 calories or more. The calories in the cream for your coffee, instead of your usual milk, add up. If you're on vacation and want to try something special, share it with the group.

A lot of people tell me that when they're on vacation, they don't care about their weight and eat whatever they want. Is it worth it to gain five pounds? Take-out restaurants have delicious and healthy breakfast items but the portions tend to be enormous. When eating out, it's okay to order cold cereal, oatmeal, or a low-fat muffin with fat-free milk. It's okay to order one egg, two pieces of whole wheat toast, and 100% juice.

Ruth's **Rule:** *Eating high-calorie restaurant breakfasts can be unhealthy and does not encourage weight loss.*

Ideas for Homemade Breakfasts

Here are some quick, easy, and healthy breakfast ideas to make at home:

- Whole-grain cold cereal topped with fruit and fat-free or 1% milk or soymilk
- Oatmeal with fruit and nuts and calcium-fortified orange juice
- Whole-wheat bagel with low-fat cheese and 100% fruit juice
- Toasted whole-grain waffle topped with fruit and yogurt
- Low-fat bran muffin and a fruit cup with milk or yogurt
- Peanut butter on whole-grain toast with juice or milk
- Fruit smoothie made with frozen or fresh fruit, protein powder, and milk, yogurt, or tofu
- Cheese quesadilla with salsa on a corn tortilla and juice
- A hard-boiled egg with fruit and milk
- Granola bar with fruit and string cheese
- Green pepper, onion, and salsa omelet with whole grain toast and juice
- Chocolate shake made with fat-free chocolate milk, peanut butter, and a banana
- Yogurt parfait with granola, nuts, and fruit
- Scrambled egg substitute with diced zucchini and onion, with whole wheat toast
- A fruit-filled breakfast bar and yogurt
- An egg, ham, or turkey on whole wheat bread or English muffin and juice
- Low-fat or fat-free cottage cheese and fruit
- Bean and low-fat cheese burrito and milk
- A slice of vegetable pizza and milk

♦ Multi-grain pancakes topped with pureed strawberries, and almond milk
♦ Hummus on a whole-grain pita bread with a few black olives and cucumber slices

These choices contain lots of important nutrients but not a lot of calories.

Other Healthy Options

Some people don't like typical breakfast foods. *No problem.* In the American culture, breakfast typically means cereal or eggs. Some people don't eat breakfast because they don't like cereal and eggs. Other cultures like to eat soup and salad or fish and rice in the morning. Eat foods that you like for breakfast. Is it healthy? Watch the portion size. Get the most nutrients for the least amount of calories. Pick lean proteins, complex carbohydrates, and healthy fats.

How do you feel eating *natural foods* versus processed foods? See how your body responds to oatmeal and fruit compared to a couple of donuts and fruit punch. When you stick with healthy foods, after a while donuts and pastries don't seem like food. They will seem like a big glob of white flour, sugar, and fat. Where are the nutrients?

A *bagel* with cream cheese is a popular breakfast. Bagels are mostly white flour. Cream cheese is fat. Not a lot of nutrients for the calories. Depending on the calories, one large bagel could be the equivalent of eating three to four pieces of bread. A small whole wheat bagel with peanut butter would be a healthy choice.

Weird Breakfasts ∞

What was the strangest breakfast you ever ate?

JF: Cold anything. Pizza, fried chicken, pasta. Anything cold from the night before that I may have had for dinner. I've had beer that I couldn't finish the night before. Your question didn't ask what "good things" I had for breakfast, just strange.

Waffles can be healthy. Buy whole grain waffles and top with pureed fruit. There are many healthy *pancake* recipes. Making a healthy breakfast on the weekend can be a fun family activity. If it turns out to be a larger meal than you thought, call it brunch. Skip lunch.

Some people can eat the same breakfast day after day for their entire life. Other people like variety and need to alternate what they eat. **Try to eat about the same amounts, varying the type of foods.**

The Low-Down on Cereal

Wondering what cereal to buy? *Read the label.* Above all, choose a *whole grain* cereal. Look for the word "whole" grain. Choose a cereal with 3-5 grams or more of fiber per serving. Since most people don't get enough fiber in their diet, cereal is a good option. Choosing a low-fat, low-sodium, and little or no added sugar cereal is preferable. Are artificial colors necessary? Is cereal supposed to be green and pink? If you're buying a cereal because of the added vitamins and minerals, finish the milk. The milk could wash the vitamins and minerals off the cereal. Besides, you need the calcium in the milk. Sweetened cereals are okay, as long as they are whole grain. A sweetened whole grain cereal contains fewer calories and is healthier than a donut.

What do you think about oatmeal? Do you eat it?

JF: Yes, I have grown to love it! But not the plain, natural kind that is the best for you. I would rather stay chubby. I have to eat the kind with flavor.

You: _____

_____

Oatmeal is low in fat, low in sugar, low in sodium, and high in fiber, especially soluble fiber. Oatmeal without the outer, inedible hull is called *groats*. What are *steel-cut oats*? Besides taking longer to cook, are they healthier? Steel-cut oatmeal is groats that are chopped into pieces. Old-fashioned rolled oatmeal is groats that have been rolled thin until they are flat. Quick oats are rolled thinner. Instant oats are rolled the thinnest. That's why instant oatmeal cooks the fastest. All variations of oats are whole grains and contain the same health benefits, just different widths. Flavored instant oatmeal can have more sodium and more sugar than old-fashioned oatmeal. If you're in a hurry, cooking oatmeal in the microwave is quick, and there's no pan to clean.

Some people eat breakfast foods for lunch or dinner. That's okay, too. Whole grain cereal with low-fat milk and topped with fruit is a light, healthy dinner.

And the Winner Is ... ೞ

Dietitian's choice for breakfast: oatmeal with fruit and nuts. It doesn't get any healthier. Oatmeal with blueberries and pecans is yummy. So is oatmeal with sliced bananas and walnuts. Add a sprinkle of cinnamon. Oatmeal doesn't need any added sugar, especially when you add fruit. Add a glass of milk.

The Size of Your Breakfast

How much breakfast should you eat? It depends on how much energy you need. Are you going surfing or sitting at home reading? What time is lunch? If you can eat a small snack midmorning, eat a small breakfast – but big enough so that you don't get to the point of starving and end up eating too much at the next meal.

If you're losing weight on MyPlate's 1,800-calorie food pattern, mix and match the food groups depending on your hunger. If you like counting calories, breakfast could be 350 calories; lunch and dinner 625 calories each, with two 100-calorie snacks.

Before Your Morning Workout ೞ

If you wake up and immediately exercise, drink a glass of juice or eat a fruit. Your body needs some carbohydrate for fuel. You'll have more energy to work out.

If you wanted to eat most of your calories early in the day, you could divide the food groups so that most of them are for breakfast and lunch. For 1,800 calories, breakfast and lunch would be 600 calories each and 400 calories for dinner, with two 100-calorie snacks.

Examine your hunger. If you feel "just right" at any time during the meal, stop eating. Don't feel like you have to finish eating all the food on your plate.

If you're not used to eating in the morning, a light breakfast would be a piece of whole wheat toast with peanut butter and orange juice.

Getting on Track

If you wake up hungry, you're probably eating fewer calories and losing weight. *That's good.* Get your body used to waking up hungry. Try eating a smaller dinner and no snacks after dinner. I wake up hungry. I tend to eat a big breakfast, a big lunch, and a small dinner. If I ate just a piece of toast and a glass of orange juice for breakfast, I would be starving in an hour.

I recommend eating breakfast. A healthy breakfast fuels your body with energy and provides important nutrients. Eating a bigger breakfast and lunch and then a smaller dinner makes sense. This is especially true if you need most of your energy for brain power and physical activity in the morning and afternoon. When you're losing weight, there is very little room for eating foods that don't contain nutrients.

*R*uth's Rule: *Eat a healthy breakfast daily to fuel your body with energy and nutrients.*

If you don't eat breakfast, are you willing to make a commitment to start?

JF: My issue is that some days I do and some days I don't. So, I do declare that from now on, me and breakfast go together.

You: _____

_____

What are some healthy foods that you would like to start eating for breakfast?

You: _____

_____

WEEKLY REMINDER ◆ ──────────

Your Reasons for Losing Weight

Every day, you should be reminding yourself why you want to lose weight. So you don't forget, you'll be writing your answers down in this book once a week.

Why do you want to lose weight? Have your reasons changed since you started reading this book?

JF: One of my reasons for wanting to lose weight has always been to become a healthier person. I also want to stretch myself, get out of my comfort zone, and overall just be able to be happier with what I see when I look in the mirror. Losing weight is an overall confidence-booster and a demonstration of what I am capable of when I don't take the easy route.

You: _____

_____

Day 8 CHECK-IN ☑

What did you accomplish yesterday?

JF: I ate breakfast but that's pretty much it. EVERY DAY CAN'T BE GREAT! Sorry, I didn't mean to get loud. Just feeling sad that I didn't accomplish more.

You: _____

_____

What is your goal for today?

(Eat breakfast.) (Eat a healthier breakfast.) (Eat a smaller breakfast.) (Eat less at night and wake up hungry.) (Buy oatmeal.) (Include protein with breakfast, such as beans, nuts, eggs, lean meat, fish, fat-free or 1% milk, or low-fat cheese and yogurt.) (Eat breakfast at home more.)

JF: I found a park near my house that I'm going to starting visiting. Maybe I'll find a husband there …. I mean, I'm going to the park to start a walking regimen to lose weight.

You: _____

_____

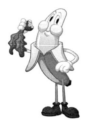

Day 9

What's in a Label?

*L*ong, long ago, people grew their own produce, made biscuits from scratch, and threw a hunk of meat on the fire. We don't have as much time to devote to our food anymore. Thank goodness for food manufacturers. They've made our lives easier. However, what exactly are we eating? Hip hip hurray for food labels. Food labels identify the food, the ingredient list, the manufacturer, nutrition information, and perhaps food safety guidelines or freshness dating.

Do you read food labels? What do you like or dislike about them?

JF: Since being a part of several diet programs, I have learned to understand food labels, serving sizes, calories, etc. It wasn't until I had fully committed to one of these programs for about one week that I realized I don't need to eat the same amount of calories as a fullback for the New York Giants in order to satiate my hunger. What I hate about food labels is that they very clearly list what I need to maintain a healthy lifestyle and I don't always appreciate the truth.

You: _____

_____

Whether you like food labels or not, it's important to *read them*. They contain valuable information that can make or break your effort to be informed about choices for healthy eating and weight loss. This chapter contains reference numbers and terms. Ignorance of the law is no excuse.

Ruth's **Rule:** *Food labels have valuable information, and you'll want to be reading them for help with healthy eating and weight loss.*

A Food Labels Primer

The purpose of the *Nutrition Facts* label is to help the public plan a healthy diet.

The Nutrition Facts label identifies:

+ the number of servings in the package
+ the serving size
+ the calories per serving
+ the amount of certain nutrients in a serving
+ and the percent daily value of a nutrient based on a 2,000-calorie diet

A label doesn't have enough room to print everything, so current labels contain the most important information. When science determined that trans fats were as bad as saturated fat, trans fats were added to the label.

If you have certain health problems, the Nutrition Facts label can be extremely beneficial. To help with weight loss, be aware of the calories.

Surveys say that when people look at a food package, they are confused. Just because there is fruit on the picture doesn't mean that the product contains fruit. A picture is worth a thousand words, but not always. Read the label.

The Food and Drug Administration (FDA) of the Department of Health and Human Services and the Food Safety and Inspection Service (FSIS) of the U.S. Department of Agriculture regulate food labels for most prepared foods under the *Nutrition Labeling and Education Act of 1990* (NLEA). Labeling for raw produce (fruits and vegetables) and fish is voluntary. Meat and poultry are regulated by the USDA, but the regulations are similar to the FDA's rules.

After 20 years, the Nutrition Facts label got a makeover. The new label reflects the latest science and makes it easier for consumers to make better choices.

Reading the Labels

Here is the original vs. the new Nutrition Facts label. Let's take a look at the new label's Servings per Container, Serving Size and Calories:

Nutrition Facts

Serving Size 2/3 cup (55g)
Servings Per Container About 8

Amount Per Serving

Calories 230	Calories from Fat 72

% Daily Value*

Total Fat 8g	12%
Saturated Fat 1g	5%
Trans Fat 0g	
Cholesterol 0mg	0%
Sodium 160mg	7%
Total Carbohydrate 37g	12%
Dietary Fiber 4g	16%
Sugars 1g	
Protein 3g	

Vitamin A	10%
Vitamin C	8%
Calcium	20%
Iron	45%

* Percent Daily Values are based on a 2,000 calorie diet. Your daily value may be higher or lower depending on your calorie needs.

		2,000	2,500
	Calories:		
Total Fat	Less than	65g	80g
Sat Fat	Less than	20g	25g
Cholesterol	Less than	300mg	300mg
Sodium	Less than	2,400mg	2,400mg
Total Carbohydrate		300g	375g
Dietary Fiber		25g	30g

Nutrition Facts

8 servings per container
Serving size 2/3 cup (55g)

Amount per serving

Calories **230**

% Daily Value*

Total Fat 8g	10%
Saturated Fat 1g	5%
Trans Fat 0g	
Cholesterol 0mg	0%
Sodium 160mg	7%
Total Carbohydrate 37g	13%
Dietary Fiber 4g	14%
Total Sugars 12g	
Includes 10g Added Sugars	20%
Protein 3g	

Vitamin D 2mcg	10%
Calcium 260mg	20%
Iron 8mg	45%
Potassium 235mg	6%

* The % Daily Value (DV) tells you how much a nutrient in a serving of food contributes to a daily diet. 2,000 calories a day is used for general nutrition advice.

Source: U.S. Food and Drug Administration.

The first bit of information on the new label is the *Servings Per Container*. It tells you how many servings are in the entire package. Some packages may only contain one serving.

By law, *Serving Size* refers to common amounts that people eat. It could be in tablespoons, cups, perhaps pieces. Keep in mind that the Serving Size doesn't mean this is how much you're supposed to eat. It is there to use as a reference. While it's valuable information, you still need to listen to your hunger cues. The information on the Nutrition

Facts label is based on a Serving Size. The Serving Size also lists the amount in grams or milliliters.

Next is the *Calories*. Some people think that the entire package contains the amount of calories listed under Calories. *No.* The calories are for *one* serving. Suppose the Serving Size is one cup, the Servings Per Container is two, and the Calories are 80 per serving. That means 160 calories for the entire container, not 80 calories. The new type size for Calories is **big** and **bold**. You can't miss it even if you tried.

Did you ever eat an entire package of something and think that the calories in one serving were the calories for the entire package? (If so, write about it below.) That's wishful thinking, or perhaps you just didn't know. From now on, remember that if there's only one serving per container, then and only then is the posted amount the calories for the entire container.

JF: The only time I really forget about the serving size is when I eat chips, crackers, or cookies. Usually the label says something like six potato chips are what you should consume per serving. I imagine the next big thing will be a television show about the super human who is able to eat only six potato chips.

You: _____

_____

Occasionally, the serving size is confusing. What if a serving is one ounce? How much is an ounce? Is it one or two handfuls? What if one serving is 12 pieces and the pieces are smashed? It's not perfect, but overall the Nutrition Label is useful. (**Hint:** Dividing the entire contents by the servings per container can be helpful when determining the referenced serving size.)

The *nutrients* that are allowed to appear on the Nutrition Facts label are listed after Calories. Nutrients must appear in a certain order. Each nutrient lists the number of grams. Under the Nutrition Facts panel, certain nutrients are mandatory. Others are voluntary.

Mandatory Nutrients	Voluntary Nutrients
Calories	Calories from saturated fat
Total fat	Polyunsaturated fat
Saturated fat	Monounsaturated fat
Trans fat	Soluble fiber
Cholesterol	Insoluble fiber
Sodium	Sugar alcohol
Total carbohydrate	Other essential vitamins and minerals
Dietary fiber	
Total Sugars	
Added Sugars	
Protein	
Vitamin D	
Calcium	
Iron	
Potassium	

Let's go over the nutrients on the new label in more detail.

Total Fat

The first nutrient on the Nutrition Facts is Total Fat. The label gives you the ability to limit unhealthy fat and choose foods with healthy fat. How much fat should you eat in a day? If you are trying to eat 1,800 calories and 70 grams of fat a day, 160 grams of fat from nachos is a bit much. Based on a fat intake of 35%, here are the numbers for fat grams per day:

Total Calories	Grams of Fat
1,200	47 or less
1,400	54 or less
1,600	62 or less
1,800	**70 or less**

Total Calories	Grams of Fat
2,000	78 or less
2,200	86 or less

The types of fats that can be included on the Nutrition Facts label are Saturated Fat, Trans Fat, Cholesterol, Polyunsaturated Fat, and Monounsaturated Fat. The Dietary Reference Intakes (DRIs) recommend total fat intake be 20-35% of your total calories. All fats contain the same amount of calories, but monounsaturated fat is the healthy fat. **Most of your fat should come from mono-unsaturated and polyunsaturated fat.** Saturated Fat and Trans Fat raise cholesterol levels. Read the label to reduce the amounts of unhealthy fat.

It's fun to calculate and compare the percent calories of fat in food, especially for foods such as milk, sour cream, cream cheese, ice cream, and hot dogs. Why eat the extra, unhealthy calories when you can choose a low-fat or fat-free version of the same food!

Here is the percentage of calories from fat in one cup of whole milk:

8 grams of Total Fat x 9 = 72; 72 (fat calories) divided by 146 Calories Per Serving x 100 = 49%

Forty-nine percent of the calories from whole milk come from fat. That's almost half fat! One cup of whole milk contains 8 grams of fat, including almost 5 grams of saturated fat. One cup of fat-free milk contains 0 grams of fat, including 0 grams of saturated fat. Do you need the extra fat?

Premium ice cream can be 55% fat compared to 13% for low-fat ice cream. One-half cup of ice cream is a one-half cup of ice cream. Instead of 140 calories from fat, you could be eating 20 calories from fat. That saves a lot of calories. It pays to read the label and choose low-fat foods.

If you eat a high-fat food, balance the rest of the meal with low-fat or fat-free foods. A meal of fried chicken, French fries, and fried zucchini is a problem. If you splurge with a really high-fat meal, balance it with low-fat or fat-free foods the rest of the week.

$\mathcal{R}$uth's Rule: *If you splurge on a high-fat food or a high-fat meal, balance it out with the rest of your foods.*

Saturated Fat

The Dietary Guidelines for Americans recommends eating less than 10 percent of calories from saturated fat. What does that mean? It depends how many calories you eat. Based on 1,800 calories, it's easy to eat more than 20 grams of saturated fat – which is 10%. If you have elevated cholesterol, go for less than 7 percent of your calories from saturated fat. Compare labels to get an idea of the amounts of saturated fat in foods. This is an important reference:

Total Calories	10% Saturated Fat Intake	7% Saturated Fat Intake
1,200	13 grams or less	9 grams or less
1,400	16 grams or less	11 grams or less
1,600	18 grams or less	12 grams or less
1,800	**20 grams or less**	**14 grams or less**
2,000	22 grams or less	16 grams or less
2,200	24 grams or less	17 grams or less

Note that 20 grams of saturated fat is less than you think. One tablespoon of butter has 100 calories and 7 grams of saturated fat. Eight ounces of prime rib could contain 33 grams of saturated fat. Saturated fat and heart attacks go hand in hand.

Trans Fat

There is no Daily Value for trans fat. Eat as little as possible. The American Heart Association recommends that you shouldn't eat more than 1% trans fat a day based on total calories. For 2,000 calories, 1% equals 2-3 grams of trans fat a day.

Cholesterol

The Dietary Guidelines 2015-2020 states that there is not a specific limit for dietary cholesterol. However, it's still important to consider and to consume as little dietary cholesterol as possible.

Sodium

According to the Dietary Guidelines for Americans 2015-2020, the recommended amount of sodium for most people ages 14 years and older should not exceed 2,300 mg day (about 1 teaspoon). Less than 2,300 mg of sodium a day is advised for people with hypertension. Reading the label for sodium is very useful because most sodium comes from canned, frozen, and processed food. In comparison, natural foods, salt added during cooking, and salt added at the table do not contribute much to the day's total amount of sodium.

Tip for Reducing Salt in Your Diet ℛ

To reduce the sodium content in canned foods by 40%, rinse the contents in a colander under running water for 60 seconds or look for foods with "reduced sodium" or "no salt added" on the label.

Total Carbohydrate

Total carbohydrates include all starches, natural and added sugars, fiber, and sugar alcohols. The Dietary Reference Intakes (DRIs) recommends that 45-65% of your calories come from carbohydrates. There are 4 calories in a gram of carbohydrate. Carbs are low in calories and are filling. They are only a problem if you eat too many. If you're diabetic, you have to watch your carbohydrates. If you have diabetes, look at the "Total Carbohydrate," not "Total Sugars" or "Added Sugars." All carbohydrates raise blood sugar.

Dietary Fiber

It's common to eat a low-fiber diet. Coffee and a donut for breakfast. A burger, fries, and a diet soda for lunch. Spaghetti and meatballs for dinner. You would be lucky to get 10 grams of fiber with this type of diet. People have a thing for not eating vegetables. They are the neglected food group. Not eating them becomes a habit. When ordering food in a restaurant, you have to make an effort to choose vegetables.

Fortunately, it's easy to add fiber to your life. Eat whole grain cereal with fruit for breakfast. A whole-wheat bread sandwich loaded with romaine lettuce, tomato, and green pepper for lunch. Baby carrots for a snack. Protein, brown rice, salad, and a vegetable for dinner. Now that's more like it.

Here are the DRIs recommendations for fiber:

Adult men 50 and younger	Adult women 50 and younger
38 grams a day	25 grams a day

Adult men over 50	Adult women over 50
30 grams a day	21 grams a day

Source: National Academy of Medicine, Food and Nutrition Board

Fiber, fiber, fiber. Fiber makes the world go round. Insoluble fiber, that is. Insoluble fiber, aka bran, goes through the intestines undigested. For insoluble fiber to "do its job," you need liquid to bulk it up for smooth sailing out to sea.

Another familiar type of fiber is soluble fiber. The label doesn't have to distinguish between the different types of fiber. It's more important to get the recommended intake, rather than focusing on the type of fiber.

Added Sugars

The 2015-2020 Dietary Guidelines for Americans advocates limiting *added sugars* to no more than 10% of your day's calories. For 1,800 calories that would be 180 calories or 45 grams of sugar. One 20-ounce bottle of soda could have 325 calories and 88 grams of sugar. Limit foods with added sugars! They contain calories and little or no nutrients.

Hint: If a serving of food contains 5 grams of added sugars, multiply 5 x 4. There are 20 calories from sugar.

Protein

There is no daily value for protein, and most people don't have a problem getting enough protein. According to the Dietary Reference Intakes, adults should get 10-35% of their calories from protein. Consuming 0.8 grams of protein per kilogram body weight is the minimum amount of protein recommended. To do the math, remember that 1 pound equals 2.2 kilograms. There are 4 calories in a gram of protein.

Be aware of the fat grams found in some protein foods. Choose lean sources of protein.

Vitamin D, Calcium, Iron and Potassium

Fiber, vitamin D, calcium, iron, and potassium are listed on the new food label because some Americans may not get enough of these nutrients. Get at least the % Daily Value for these nutrients. It may improve your health and reduce your risk of disease. Getting enough iron is important for pregnant women and people with anemia.

% Daily Value

To the right of the nutrients is the % Daily Value. The % DV is based on 100% of the daily value for each of the nutrients based on 2,000 calories. Why 2,000 calories? Well, 2,000 calories is the approximate calorie requirement for postmenopausal women. Postmenopausal women have the greatest risk for eating excess amounts of calories and fat. If you're very thin, older and not active, you will need less than 2,000 calories. If you have extra weight or are active, most likely you eat more than 2,000 calories.

Five grams of saturated fat on a food label doesn't seem like much. But the % DV for 5 grams is 23%, which is high. Therefore, 5 grams of saturated fat would be a significant amount for one serving.

In another case, 140 milligrams (mg) of sodium seems like a lot. However, 140 milligrams out of 2,300 milligrams is only 6%, which is relatively low.

Putting the % Daily Value in Perspective ∝

Here is a "Quick Guide to % DV":
• 5% or less is low   • 20% or more is high

If you forget the recommended number of milligrams that you need a day, look at the % Daily Value to see if it is a high or a low percent. The % Daily Value is an easy way for you to decide if you need more or less of a nutrient.

The Daily Reference Value (DRV) is calculated based on these numbers:

Fat	35% of calories
Saturated fat	10% of calories
Carbohydrates	55% of calories
Protein	10% (for adults and children over 4)
Fiber	14 grams/1,000 calories

Desirable upper limit for the Daily Reference Value (% DV):
♦ Eat less than 78 grams of fat.
♦ Eat less than 20 grams of saturated fat.
♦ Eat less than 300 milligrams of cholesterol.
♦ Eat less than 2,300 milligrams of sodium.
♦ Eat less than 50 grams of added sugars.

Lower limit:
♦ Eat at least 275 grams of carbohydrate.
♦ Eat at least 28 milligrams of fiber.

These recommendations came from www.fda.gov. - New changes to the Nutrition Facts Label.

Listen to the Label

If you are eating 2,000 calories a day, your goal is to stay under 100% for total fat, saturated fat, cholesterol, and sodium. You want to get at least 100% for total carbohydrate, fiber, vitamin D, calcium, iron, and potassium.

Footnote on the Label

At the bottom of the Nutrition Facts is a footnote to explain the meaning of Daily Value. The footnote reads "The % Daily Value (DV) tells you how much a nutrient in a serving of food contributes to a daily diet. 2,000 calories a day is used for general nutrition advice."

Multi-Serving Packages

The new label does the math for you. There is a dual column label on packages that contain more than one serving but *could* be consumed all at once. This is a great eye-opener for people who can't eat just one portion. In the middle column is the calories and nutrients "per serving." In the right column is the calories and nutrients "per container"/"per package". If you eat the entire contents, this is one of those times when you say to yourself, "Wow. That was a lot of calories."

Do You Have Food Allergies? ⚮

The list of ingredients is extremely helpful for people with allergies. The *2006 Food Allergen Labeling and Consumer Protection Act* requires allergen labeling for milk, eggs, fish, crustacean shellfish, tree nuts, wheat, peanuts, and soybeans.

Wording and Health Claims

One food manufacturer's idea of "light" or "healthy" may not be what another food manufacturer had in mind. In the past, a food manufacturer could claim that a deep-fried candy bar was healthy. *Not anymore.* The FDA and the Food Safety and Inspection Service (FSIS) have uniform definitions for terms so that everyone is on the same page. The terms must meet requirements. The words "free," "low," "high," "good source," "reduced," "less," "light," and "more" are regulated. Health claims can be made on the label if there's a relationship between certain nutrients and reduced risk of disease. An example of a health claim would be between sodium and hypertension.

To make the sodium and hypertension claim, a food must meet the requirements for "low sodium."

What is "Healthy"?

Even the word "healthy" means something. For an individual food to be "healthy," it has to meet certain nutrient criteria and be consistent.

Regulated terms offer uniform definitions and consistency for products with the dietary guidelines.

Free	Contains no amount or only a trivial amount of a nutrient.
Less	Contains 25% or less of a nutrient or calories than the regular product.
More	Contains at least 10% of the Daily Value more than the regular food, altered or not.
Good source	Contains 10-19% of the Daily Value for a particular nutrient in a serving.
High	Contains 20% or more of the Daily Value for a particular nutrient in a serving.

Food Labels – There for You

Food labels protect us. For healthy eating, read labels and compare nutrients. Reading the food label gives you information and helps you eat less of some foods and more of other foods. Pick out the information that's important to you.

When you're trying to lose weight, labels can help you control calories. Since the ready-to-eat foods from bakeries and delis are not required to have food labels, get an idea of the calories of similar foods with labels. Then double the amount to be safe! And don't forget to watch portion sizes. I hope that you "at least" (more than a little) have a new appreciation for food labels!

The food label is your new best friend.

$\mathcal{D}$ay 9 CHECK-IN ☑

What did you accomplish yesterday?

You: _____

_____

JF: I ate breakfast and a structured, well-balanced lunch. Not very exciting but every day can't be a box of chocolate-covered marshmallows.

What is your goal for today?

(Start reading food labels.) (Look at the number of calories in a serving.) (Limit sodium to 2,300 milligrams a day.) (Calculate the percentage calories of fat in cheese.) (Choose a "lean" protein for dinner.) (Read labels for saturated fat.) (Limit fat to 70 grams.)

JF: I will have a lean protein for dinner. I haven't been cooking a lot but when I do, I'm surprised at how little salt, butter, or oil I use. I actually know now that a plate of mostly rice is not the way to stay out of the refrigerator three hours later for snacking on processed cheese slices. (I have done that. Don't judge me.)

You: _____

_____

Day 10

Bare Bones on Calcium

I'm shrinking .... Do you ever think this about yourself? One way to prevent it is getting enough calcium.

Consuming enough calcium in your diet is essential for strong bones. Have you ever seen a piece of wood eaten by termites? It crumbles. Without calcium, your bones will deteriorate and crumble, too. Osteoporosis means porous bones (weak and crumbly). If your bones are porous and weak, falling, bending over, and even coughing could cause a bone to break.

Have you started actually shrinking? Do you know anyone who is shrinking in height? Osteoporosis can decrease a person's height as much as 2 to 8 inches!

Do you ever think about your bones?

JF: I think about my bones only when I see an old lady who is 3 feet tall, and I wonder if she ever used to be 5'4" like me.

You: _____

_____

Do you drink milk? How much? What kind of milk?

JF: Milk makes me puke. I can only drink soymilk and by drink I mean putting it on my cereal and only eating the cereal. But ice cream is totally okay. Odd, I know.

You: _____

_____

Do you eat yogurt and cheese every day?

JF: I buy every flavor of yogurt and forget that it is in the fridge. Isn't that weird? Funny how I don't forget to eat ice cream, though.

You: _____

_____

Do you take a calcium supplement? How often?

JF: I have all the vitamins I need to take but have a problem lately swallowing those gigantic horse pills!!! I mean I want to take them, but it would be easier to insert them.

You: _____

_____

You take care of your hair and wear nice clothes. To be healthy, you have to take care of your bones as well. Your body could be disintegrating on the inside, and you may not know it.

*R*uth's Rule: *Take care of your bones in order to stay healthy.*

An Essential Mineral

Calcium is a very important mineral. Ninety-nine percent of your body's calcium can be found in bones and teeth. As an adult, bones stay the same size and shape, but the calcium levels inside the bones are constantly coming and going for body functions.

People may or may not be getting enough calcium in their diet. And it's alarming to see the graphs of children and teens that show milk consumption going down and soda consumption going up. Low calcium intakes at a young age mean pain and suffering later in life.

Strong bones are packed with a lot of calcium. Boys and girls ages nine to 18 need 1,300 mg of calcium a day and at least 60 minutes of physical activity a day to build strong bones. Children's bones grow rapidly. Bones get bigger and denser until the early 20s. Bone mass starts to decline in the early 30s. It's crucial to build bones during youth. The ages of nine to 12 are a critical period for girl's bodies to get calcium deposits. If adolescents, especially girls, don't get enough calcium, their bones won't reach their peak bone mass. Girls need to build up a calcium supply so that when they get older, the loss won't be debilitating and put them at a risk for developing osteoporosis.

When you were young, did you drink milk and get enough calcium in your diet? Why or why not?

JF: I did drink a lot of milk as a child. Then this completely stopped when I was left to my own devices about my nutritional health.

You: _____

_____

Calcium is constantly needed to build and maintain bone mass. If your body doesn't have enough calcium in your blood for day-to-day body functions, it will take calcium from the bones.

How Much Do We Need?

Look at the chart below. If you or someone in your family isn't getting enough calcium every day, figure out a way to get more. One cup (8 ounces) of milk contains around 300 mg of calcium.

Daily Recommended Calcium and Vitamin D Intakes

Ages	Daily Calcium in Milligrams	Daily Vitamin D in IU
Birth to 6 months	200	400
7-12 months	260	400
1-3 years	700	600
4-8 years	1,000	600
9-18 years	1,300	600
19-50 years	1,000	600
51-70 men	1,000	600

51-70 women	1,200	600
71 and over	1,200	800
Pregnant/breastfeeding		
18 years and younger	1,300	600
19-50 years	1,000	600

Source: National Academy of Medicine, Food and Nutrition Board

Are you currently getting enough calcium in your diet on a regular basis? If not, why not? Do you even know? Keeping a food journal will help pinpoint a deficiency.

JF: I am absolutely sure that I am not getting enough calcium. Meanwhile, I am afraid to keep a food journal. I will only keep a record when I have good foods days because that would be a Post-it note, not a journal.

You: _____

_____

Did you notice that the calcium requirement increases to 1,200 mg at 50 years old for women? That daily total is the equivalent of drinking four glasses of milk a day. If you're over 50, do you drink three glasses of milk a day? How about two?

The "Silent Disease" – Osteoporosis

Attention men, women, and children. If you don't get enough calcium in your diet or you take medications affecting calcium, you may be at risk of getting osteoporosis. Eighty percent of the people with osteoporosis are women. Osteoporosis is widespread and expensive. It's called the "Silent Disease" and is a threat for more than half of people 50 years and older. You don't know that you have it until you break a bone or start shrinking. Then it's too late.

Calcium is essential during all phases of life to maintain bone mass. Osteoporosis can even occur in children ages 8-14 years. Everyone needs to be concerned. Children who are very ill at a young age can risk getting osteoporosis as they get older.

Estrogen helps deposit calcium into bones. For *women*, the lack of estrogen after menopause causes the body to lose its calcium stores. Women may lose up to 20 percent of their bone mass four to eight years after menopause. As the bones get weaker, they get brittle. The spine buckles. That's where you see people with a Dowager's Hump. The vertebrae in the spine squish together. People become shorter and get a hump. Osteoporosis is painful. Who needs it?

Women taking estrogen have strong bones. Meanwhile, the estrogen could cause other problems. However, many people would rather take a pill than drink a glass of milk or consume other sources of calcium.

Certain medical conditions and medications, smoking, and drinking alcohol are the biggest threats to *men* getting osteoporosis. By the time men are 65 years old, they lose calcium at about the same rate as women.

Sometimes older people on medications get dizzy and fall or they are frail and lose their balance. If bones are weak, any fall could cause a bone to break. A broken hip at an older age could be a deal-breaker.

If you have osteoporosis, there are drugs to make bones stronger but not without side effects. I prefer prevention. Diet is critical to prevent osteoporosis. It's never too late to start eating healthy and getting more calcium in the diet.

What about Milk?

For some reason, milk gets a bad rap. A lot of fad diets don't include milk or dairy products. There are a lot of milk misconceptions. It must be working. Fewer people are drinking milk. Milk is thoroughly tested and strictly regulated for bacteria, antibiotics, and hormones. If milk caused health problems, they would be showing up in people.

Milk is an easy way to get calcium. As a food source, milk is rich in lots of nutrients. Milk provides calcium, vitamins A and D, riboflavin, phosphorous, vitamin B-12, potassium, niacin, and protein. Milk also provides fluid.

Some people drink soda, because it is more convenient. Drinking milk could taste rather bland after a refreshing carbonated drink.

When I grew up, milk was the most common drink available. We didn't have a choice at school. I had friends who didn't drink milk. They are probably an inch or two shorter now than they were then. If people don't grow up drinking milk, it's unlikely that they would start drinking milk as an adult.

Are You Lactose Intolerant?

Some people can't tolerate milk. It's called *lactose intolerance.* You might not know that you have it. Do you get gassy a lot? The symptoms range from a little gas to diarrhea 30 minutes after drinking a glass of milk. People with lactose intolerance don't have enough of the enzyme *lactase,* which breaks down the lactose (a sugar) found in milk products. Some people can tolerate small amounts of milk at a time. Some people run to the bathroom after a latte.

If you have lactose intolerance, buy lactose-free milk. It's already been treated with lactase. Or you can take lactase pills or add lactase drops to milk or milk products. Soymilk is a good alternative. Check the calcium content. Not all soymilk is created equal for fat content and calcium.

If you're lactose intolerant, it's not an excuse to avoid dairy foods.

Even so, there are more and more foods fortified with calcium on the market.

Quick Reference for Calcium Sources

Most calcium comes from dairy foods, but there are other possibilities. Below is the calcium content for a variety of foods:

Supplements		
Calcium supplement	1	500 mg
Milk, Yogurt, and Cheese		
Low-fat chocolate milk	1 cup	322 mg
Fat-free milk	1 cup	316 mg
Low-fat buttermilk	1 cup	284 mg
Powdered milk	$\frac{1}{3}$ cup dry = 1 cup fluid	283 mg

Fat-free, fruit variety, yogurt	6 ounces	258 mg
Frozen yogurt	1 cup	206 mg
Low-fat cheese	1 ounce	118 mg
Low-fat string cheese	1 stick	222 mg
Cheddar cheese	1 ounce	201 mg
Low-fat cottage cheese	½ cup	60 mg
Ice cream	½ cup	84 mg
Soft-serve ice cream	½ cup	113 mg
Sour cream	1 tablespoon	12 mg
Cream cheese	1 tablespoon	14 mg
Soy		
Soymilk with added calcium	1 cup	301 mg
Tofu with calcium sulfate	½ cup	434 mg
Edamame	½ cup	49 mg
Fish		
Salmon, canned with bones	3 ounces	212 mg
Sardines, canned with bones	3 ounces	324 mg
Nuts and Beans		
Almonds	1 ounce (23 almonds)	76 mg
Kidney beans	½ cup	44 mg
Baked beans	½ cup	43 mg
Vegetables		
Broccoli, cooked	1 cup	62 mg
Kale, cooked	1 cup	94 mg
Mustard greens	1 cup	165 mg
Bok choy	1 cup	158 mg
Frozen spinach	½ cup	123 mg
Okra	½ cup	62 mg
Fruit		
Figs, raw	5 medium	90 mg
Oranges	1	60 mg
Fortified Foods		
Fruit juice	1 cup	349 mg

Almond Milk	1 cup	451 mg
Sugar-free, instant hot cocoa	1 packet	300 mg
Waffles	1 round, 4-inch	106 mg
Oatmeal, instant	1 packet	114 mg

Source: USDA National Database for Standard Reference, Release 28, 2016

The calcium content on products varies from brand to brand. Be sure to read the label.

Ruth's Rule: *Most calcium comes from dairy foods, like low-fat milk, cheese and yogurt, but there are also additional options.*

Considering Your Options

When you're watching your weight, choose low-fat or fat-free milk products. Fat-free, 1%, 2%, and whole milk have about the same amounts of calcium and vitamin D. Only the fat content differs. If you don't like fat-free or 1% milk, get used to it. A lot of people say, "Fat-free milk tastes like water." What's wrong with water? After a while, you'll prefer fat-free milk. Whole milk will taste like cream.

People tell me that they can't drink milk because their cholesterol is high. Fat-free milk and 1% milk have fewer calories and contain little or no saturated fat. The fat in 1%, 2% milk, and whole milk counts toward your daily extra calories.

Milk, yogurt, and cheese contain the most calcium. Cream cheese and sour cream are not good sources of calcium. Ice cream, cottage cheese, and pudding have some calcium. Fruited yogurt is healthy but contains added sugars. Plain yogurt with frozen raspberries makes a quick, delicious, refreshing, healthy, calcium-rich breakfast, lunch, or snack. Frozen berries are available year-round. Let the berries melt slightly to bring out the flavor.

Broccoli and dark green leafy vegetables contain calcium but not as much as dairy foods. For a 300 mg serving of calcium, you need to eat five cups of broccoli.

A lot of people who are trying to lose weight, especially teens and women, sacrifice the milk products in their diet as a way of cutting back calories. *Not a good idea.*

Calcium can be constipating for some people. If you get constipated from calcium, keep adding more fiber and more fluids to your diet every day.

Ways to Boost Your Calcium Intake

Here are some easy ways to increase your calcium consumption:

- Drink fat-free or 1% milk with meals. Be a trend-setter.
- Low-fat cheese and crackers
- Fat-free chocolate milk for snack
- Yogurt and fruit with granola
- String cheese for snack
- Add a lot of milk to coffee or tea.
- Make soup with milk.
- Smoothies made with milk, yogurt, or tofu
- Fat-free pudding
- Add fat-free milk to hot cereal instead of water.
- Add powdered milk to foods or beverages.
- Dip fruit in yogurt.
- Cereal with milk
- Canned salmon with the bones
- Order cappuccinos or lattes with fat-free milk.
- Have sardines for a snack. Those little bones add up.
- Fortified juice and other fortified products with calcium
- A handful of almonds for snack
- Use plain yogurt in place of sour cream (top a baked potato with plain yogurt and chives).

What calcium foods are you willing to add to your diet?

JF: I love yogurt. I will commit to eating it when I buy it. And as soon as they make calcium pills smaller than my college class ring, I promise to take those every day.

You: _____

_____

People tell me that they buy canned salmon with the bones and throw it away, because it looks gross. Drain the liquid and mash it up with a fork. The soft bones have no taste and are a good source of calcium. The bones are soft and edible because of the cooking process.

Look at the % Daily Value for calcium on the food label. If calcium is 20%, add a "0". 20% calcium equals 200 mg of calcium per serving. This _only_ works for calcium with the _old_ food label.

Some people don't like the taste of milk. Add chocolate powder or buy fat-free chocolate milk. It's delicious. Fat-free chocolate milk is a healthy way to satisfy your craving for chocolate. Sugar-free hot cocoa fortified with calcium is another satisfying way to get chocolate and calcium without the calories. Chocolate milk is a popular recovery food for athletes. It replenishes carbohydrates and adds protein.

Avoid raw milk or any unpasteurized milk products. The risk of harmful bacterial contamination is not worth it.

Supplementing Calcium

If you don't get enough calcium from food, please take a supplement. The two main types of calcium compounds are _calcium carbonate_ and _calcium citrate_. Take calcium carbonate with meals. Calcium citrate can be taken any time. If you have less stomach acid, calcium citrate is a good choice. Calcium is better absorbed if it's 500 mg or less at a time. If you're taking two a day, spread them out throughout the day. Don't take calcium and iron at the same time. Some calcium, such as oyster shell, bone meal, or dolomite without the USP symbol, may contain lead. Coral calcium may contain lead. If you're allergic to shellfish, coral calcium may be a problem. Calcium supplements could interfere with certain medications. Check with a doctor or pharmacist for interactions.

For calcium, too much of a good thing is true. **The Tolerable Upper Level (UL) of calcium from food and supplements is 2,500 mg a day for ages 19-50 and 2,000 mg a day for ages 50+ years.** Excess calcium could cause kidney stones. On the other hand, getting the right amount of calcium and adequate hydration could prevent kidney stones.

There are many questions about substances that affect calcium. The National Institutes of Health says that as long as calcium intake is adequate, excess amounts of protein, caffeine, phosphorus (found in soda), and sodium do not negatively affect calcium balance.

Vitamin D is also important for bone health. In fact, low levels of vitamin D, perhaps affecting 50% of the population, may contribute to heart disease and certain types of cancer, along with a bunch of other health problems. Your skin makes vitamin D. Fifteen minutes in the sun a day without sunscreen to some part of your body is recommended to get the sunshine vitamin. This vitamin is found in egg yolks, fortified milk, other fortified products, and fatty fish. However, it may be necessary to take a supplement for optimum levels. Be part of the in-crowd. Get your vitamin D tested.

Weight-Bearing Exercise Is Important ∞

Weight-bearing physical activity builds and maintains bones. Weight-bearing physical activity is exercise that you do on your feet. Examples include walking, dancing, taking the stairs, even push-ups. These types of activities put pressure on bones and make them stronger. Swimming builds muscles and burns calories but doesn't put pressure on bones. Tai Chi and yoga are good for improving balance, which could prevent falls.

Risk Factors for Osteoporosis

The Surgeon General is America's highest ranking public health officer. If the Surgeon General says we need to protect our bones, we should listen. The 2012 Surgeon General's Report "Bone Health and Osteoporosis" says that these factors put a person at risk for weak bones:

- ◆ Being female
- ◆ Over 65 years old

- Race – Caucasians and Asians are at higher risk.
- Smoking cigarettes (reduces bone mass)
- Drinking more than two alcohol drinks several times a week (reduces bone mass)
- Broken bone after 50 years old
- Family history of osteoporosis (could be genetics)
- Fair or poor health, including a history of anorexia nervosa
- Underweight and small frame (smaller bones)
- Never got enough calcium in diet
- Menopause before 45 years old (less estrogen)
- Low estrogen or low testosterone levels
- Not physically active
- Poor vision (risk of falling)
- Certain medical conditions (rheumatoid arthritis, renal disease, inflammatory bowel disease, hyperthyroidism, asthma, epilepsy, radiation and chemotherapy for cancer)
- Certain medications (glucocorticoids, anticonvulsants, anticlotting drugs)

Be Calcium-Savvy – For the Health of It!

Many Americans aren't consuming enough calcium or vitamin D or getting enough physical activity. Some surveys say that *over 80% of teenage girls and over 60% of teenage boys* aren't getting enough calcium. This is scary. It's very important for everyone, especially children, to get enough calcium and vitamin D. Everyone is at risk for osteoporosis. Don't be the hunched-over person being pushed around in a wheelchair.

If you have any risk factors for osteoporosis, get a *bone mineral density (BMD)* test. The sooner you know there is a problem, the more time you have to treat it.

Want More Info? ☙

For more information on osteoporosis, go to the *National Institutes of Health – Osteoporosis and Related Bone Diseases, National Resource Center* (www.niams.nih.gov/bone) and the National Osteoporosis Foundation (www.nof.org).

Drink milk. Eat yogurt and low-fat cheese. If needed, take a calcium supplement. Be good to your bones. Get enough calcium, vitamin D, and physical activity.

A food with calcium is your new best friend.

*D*ay 10 *CHECK-IN* ☑

What did you accomplish yesterday?

JF: I ate breakfast, shot a commercial, and managed to not eat everything offered on the set! I don't understand how actresses stay so thin when all the industry does is promote obesity with cookies around all day! I managed to eat just one cookie and not 12. It should have been on the news. It was such a monumental moment in our world's history!

You: _____

_____

What is your goal for today?

(Make sure the kids you know are getting three to four servings of calcium-rich foods a day.) (Buy a calcium supplement with vitamin D.) (Switch to fat-free or 1% milk.) (Buy low-fat cheese.) (Eat plain yogurt and add fresh or frozen fruit.) (Drink a glass of calcium-fortified orange juice.) (Drink a glass of milk before you go to sleep.) (Buy resistance bands or free weights and do them three times a week.) (Go outside for some vitamin D.)

JF: I will eat a whole wheat bagel for breakfast, and I am going to keep that momentum going. I might even exercise.

You: _____

_____

Day 11

Will Kill for Chocolate

*T*hings are going along fine. Then, out of nowhere, you get a craving, and you become *possessed*. Something deep within your soul takes over your mind and body until you get what you want. Nothing better get in your way or else!

A *craving* is the urgent need for a particular food. It can be difficult to focus on anything until the urge is met. You may not be hungry, but you eat anyway. Eating provides the instant gratification you're seeking.

Cravings can happen to anyone. From my experience, women tend to experience cravings on a more regular basis than men. For guys, cravings tend to be more random.

A strong craving can make you quit a diet so fast that you don't know what hit you. The degree of intensity varies from mild to strong. An occasional craving won't cause much, if any, damage. However, eating what you crave on a regular basis can cause weight to go up. It's best to understand cravings so you can do something about them. When people are motivated and in control, they don't have as many cravings and can effectively fight them off.

A Look at Your Cravings

Seeing food, talking about food, or smelling food could trigger your cravings. Does watching a commercial on television make you hungry for something? How about walking by a bakery or smelling bread or cookies being baked? Are you pregnant? Do you crave pickles and ice cream? (Actually, I have yet to meet a pregnant woman who craves pickles and ice cream.)

Do you get food cravings? Are they weak or strong? Describe how they feel to you.

JF: When my cravings get out of control, I climb into my car, pajama-clad or not, and drive to buy the item. So, bottom line, if my car gets repossessed, I will be able to control my cravings. That's probably the wrong attitude, though, huh?

You: _____

_____

What foods do you crave? Something sweet? Salty? High in fat? Crunchy? A combo of sugar and fat? Sour? Creamy?

JF: Yes. I am not trying to be funny here. My answer to all those choices is yes.

You: _____

_____

What triggers your cravings? When you have a craving, are you hungry? Do you start craving foods when you're trying not to eat them?

JF: That time of the month is my nemesis. I crave all the wrong foods when my hormones go into overdrive. I crave everything from men to shopping to food. Not necessarily in that order. Sometimes I want a man in a shoe store wrapped in bacon. I like to utilize my time wisely and multi-task.

You: _____

_____

Do the cravings come at a certain time of the day? In the morning? Afternoon? Evening? Late at night? Certain time of the month? How often?

JF: Like I said earlier, that "time of the month" is my problem. At night, I just force myself to go to sleep to combat the cravings. I have also found that keeping my kitchen and refrigerator completely barren helps, too. Not a wise tactic, but effective none the less.

You: _____

_____

People don't always connect cravings with emotions. What emotions are you feeling at that time? Are you happy or stressed? Depressed or angry? Tired or bored? Did someone say something hurtful to you?

JF: Being a performer has helped me channel a lot of my emotions into making other people happy. However, I can get very sleepy, lethargic, and anxious. I have learned that certain foods do trigger the emotions and make the feelings worse. There are times when I pray for early menopause so that the hot flashes will make me less likely to eat an entire cake.

You: _____

_____

Lastly, does eating the food satisfy you? Are you happy afterward? For how long?

JF: Eating good food prepared by others, even if it is junk nutritionally, can satisfy me. Like a decadent dessert at a nice restaurant or something a friend cooked from their heart.

You: _____

_____

If you haven't thought about cravings, keep a food craving journal. It will help you to identify what you eat in response to a craving, when, and why. Different situations may trigger different cravings.

Foods that Comfort

The foods we crave are often our *comfort foods*. Comfort foods offer emotional support for a particular situation. Food cravings that are comfort foods can make us feel happy and safe.

I asked 124 men and women in Los Angeles about their comfort foods. I've provided a sample of their answers below by their first names only. This list of participants includes people from a range of ages and different ethnic backgrounds. Many of them originated from various parts of the U.S. but others are from foreign countries.

When I asked the participants to talk about their comfort foods, their eyes immediately lit up. They smiled and started to glow. With only a few exceptions, almost everyone had an immediate answer. A lot of these people had a handful of comfort foods, and each one came up with a wonderful, detailed story. Some people had different foods for different situations.

Surprisingly, everyone was curious about the comfort foods preferred by other people. Comfort foods are only a problem when excess amounts result in excess weight. The people who mentioned these comfort foods include those who *did and those who didn't* experience weight gain from their comfort foods. Note that overlapping answers were deleted to show the variety of types of comfort foods. Chocolate was a popular choice in my survey, as it is within the general population.

Ruby	Bread
Edith	Apple pie
Eliu	Ice cream
Rona	Coffee with French vanilla cream
Dan	Cashews
Claudine	Chocolate with almonds
Lita	Potato chips
Willie	Bacon, eggs, and fried rice
Elaine	Macaroni and cheese
Vera	Korean ribs
Sonia	Almond Joy with almonds
Ruth	Carne asada
Carla	French fries
Jackie	2 McDonald's cheeseburgers with fries
Nubia	Mashed potatoes
Joy	Cake
Tonya	Fried chicken
Leela	Rice dishes
Kathy	Lasagna

Terry	Sushi
Chuck	Milk and donuts
Paul	Pizza
Yervand	Chicken kabob
Ani	Pasta
Sue	Homemade sloppy joes
Mike	Philly cheese steak
Ganna	Pastries and coffee
Aykuhe	Italian food
Galina	Sauerkraut or pickles
Diana	Cheese cake
Connie	Apples with vinegar and salt
Laurie	Mango or tamarind
Lisa	Fried potatoes with Mom's homemade salsa
Tosucha	Tortilla chips
Jinah	Shredded beef burrito
Sok	Coke
Jean	Warm, soft chocolate chip cookies and milk
Gigi	Hot tea
JJ	Clam chowder in a bread bowl
Alex	Chinese food (orange beef)
Mike	Popcorn
Rick	Low-calorie Monster energy drink

As you can see, people find comfort in a variety of different foods. Sweet. Salty. Creamy. Crunchy. Warm. Sour. High in fat. A combination of flavors and textures.

Of the 124 people, only four people didn't use food for comfort. One person chose prayer. One chose shopping. One person said that she never thought about it. And one person said that he didn't use food to feel better. This wasn't a scientific study. However, there are a lot of people who use food for comfort compared to those who don't.

*R*uth's **Rule:** *If you crave food and then can't stop eating, pinpoint the specific food that causes the problem.*

Chocolate Cravings

As mentioned, chocolate is a favorite comfort food, and many people crave it, including a good number of those I interviewed. Why? Are they addicted to chocolate? Chocolate has fat and it's creamy. Is your body telling you that you need fat? Or do you have happy memories that are linked to chocolate?

For American women, there may be some truth to the "Will Kill for Chocolate" bumper sticker. Interestingly, craving chocolate isn't universal. People from different countries crave different foods. Also, cravings can change over time.

Until researchers come up with definitive answers, know that chocolate cravings can be dealt with using similar approaches that work for other cravings. At some point, it takes discipline, craving or not. Deal with it and feel proud for not caving in. And keep reading the chapter for ideas for coping with cravings.

Cravings and the Body

A lot of research still needs to be done even in the general area of understanding food cravings overall. Are they related to brain chemistry? Well, everyone is wired differently. Some people like to sit and read. Other people like to jump out of airplanes. What drives us? Our brain chemistry differs from person to person. Could lacking or changing levels of the neurotransmitters *dopamine* and *serotonin* or of *opioids* (brain chemicals) cause food cravings? Does eating certain foods raise levels of the neurotransmitters and make us feel better? Do serotonin levels affect appetite? Maybe eating sweets or carbohydrates raises serotonin levels and makes us feel uplifted.

If brain chemicals drive some people to constantly eat, individuals still can take control of their diet. If this is you, your goal is to only eat if you are physically hungry and stop when you have had a reasonable amount. What if you always feel hungry? Eat small, frequent meals with one or two snacks. Eating only healthy food every few hours will fill you up and not out. If your brain chemistry needs a little help, antidepressants may be the answer in some cases.

Are your cravings related to changing hormones? Again, we are all different. Everyone's levels of hormones differ. Even so, perhaps changing estrogen levels *do* cause you to feel irritable or depressed, and eating a combination of sugar and fat does make you feel better. If you suspect this to be the case, the first step is realizing that something is different. If hormones cause a temporary change in your eating habits, keep it within reason and balance this with exercise.

More on Your Cravings

Do you ever crave something sweet? Then you crave something salty? Then you crave something sweet? You may end up eating *a lot* of calories. Is it hunger, a craving, or something else? It's probably *your emotions*.

Cravings may start as physical hunger and then turn into emotional hunger. Emotional eating drives us to eat more than we need. If you have a craving and you eat until you are "full" or "stuffed," ask yourself, "What's going on?" What are you feeling? Perhaps you'll find yourself thinking, "I'm not hungry. I'm lonely." What do you need? Put your thoughts into words. Will eating make you feel better? Or will you feel worse, sooner or later?

Some cravings are learned habits. We are in a certain situation with certain people that we either like or dislike. Food is introduced. The food helps us cope or offers a distraction. We remember how we felt after we ate the food. When the situation happens again, we are conditioned to remember the food and begin to crave it.

Can you think of a situation when you started craving your comfort foods? What happened? What did you eat?

JF: There are times when boredom gets me to eat the wrong foods. Situations where I feel disappointment also lure me to eat. It's as if I feel let down by an individual or situation, and I eat to feel better. Sometimes a person's best boyfriend or girlfriend is fatty foods.

You: _____

Are your cravings so strong that you feel out of control? Do you eat instead of dealing with problems in your life?

JF: If my schedule is packed, I do feel too distracted to eat too much or to eat the wrong things. Idle time is when my cravings take me to the drive-thru.

You: _____

Changing Your Behavior

If you crave a certain food at a certain time, it's probably a habit. *Good news!* Habits can be changed.

+ **First, you have to realize that you're giving in to cravings. Then, to take the fizzle out of the behavior, start making healthier substitutions (choose fewer calories and less fat).** If you crave potato chips and can't stop eating them, switch to pretzels. Eventually, the craving for chips will disappear. If you eat too many pretzels, at least pretzels have fewer calories than potato chips. Also, prepackaging the craved food or buying a smaller container might deter you from overdoing it.

+ **Do you have a strong craving for something sweet after dinner? This is a craving that can be controlled and conquered.** Let's say you eat dessert every night, and often find yourself craving something sweet during the last few bites of dinner. If you stay strong and don't give in to dessert for a few days, the craving for it will fade and go away. To ease the pain of withdrawal, limit yourself to one bite of something sweet. Or, as your new M.O., have fruit or just have one bite of dessert to satisfy that urge for something sweet. This is about creating habits that you'll want to have on an ongoing basis.

+ **Do you satisfy your craving with two pieces of chocolate or the entire package? There is a solution ...** if you like chocolate, take one small piece and make it last a long time. Look at it for a while. Smell it. Lick it. Taste it. Let it melt in your mouth. Slowly chew the rest of it. You will be surprised how long it will take to eat it and how satisfied you'll be with a small amount. *Really!*

♦ **Some people don't allow themselves to eat what they crave, become obsessed, and only think about eating. If this is you, make rules.** Give yourself a certain amount within reason. Portion out an amount and enjoy it.

♦ **Instead of giving in to cravings, challenge them. Get to know them.** Are your cravings physiological (brain chemistry or hormones)? Are they psychological (emotional, habit, environmental)? Do they make you feel better? Are they causing harm? You probably have more discipline than you think. Are you tempted to jump into traffic or dive into a geyser? *No.* It's common sense. Apply the same standards to food. If cravings cause your eating to go out of control one day, pick yourself up and start over tomorrow. It wasn't your day to lose weight.

If you didn't give in to your cravings, would you survive?

JF: Nope. I hear that a lack of candy, greasy foods, and alcohol are all the leading causes of heart disease. Wait. Maybe I have that backwards.

You: _____

Develop a Winning Strategy ❧

Analyze and identify what triggers your cravings. Is it a certain time? Can the situation or food be avoided? Keep the problem food out of sight. Make a rule to not eat it alone. When you drive by a bakery with the best pastries in the world, look the other way until you pass by it. (Out of sight. Out of mind.) Cravings are often short-term. It may not take much time before the craving passes. It may be a battle of wills. Persistence will win.

*R***uth's Rule:** *Get to know your cravings. Awareness will enable you to challenge them.*

Distractions Work Wonders!

If you have a lot of cravings, get more out of life besides food.

Find a way to distract yourself. Here are 15 ways to distract your-self from food cravings.

1. Get enough sleep. Take a quick nap. If you're sleeping, you can't eat.

2. Have a positive attitude. *You have the power to change.*

3. Go outside in the sun. Get some vitamin D. Be one with nature.

4. Relax. Do controlled breathing.

5. Be happy. Most destructive eating behavior involves negative emotions.

6. Listen to music. Let it rip. It can take you to another world.

7. Play an instrument. If you don't know how, make time for some lessons.

8. Plant a garden. Soon you'll have a lovely view from your window.

9. Buy some fresh flowers.

10. Meditate. It's relaxing.

11. Do artwork or crafts. It will keep your mind and hands busy.

12. Put on perfume or cologne. Smelling something besides food will take away the mood for food.

13. Be around positive people. It rubs off!

14. Do things that you enjoy. Get a massage.

15. Get a pet. Walk your dog. Go to a dog park.

Cravings Can Be Overcome

To a certain extent, genetics determines how we think and how our body responds. When situations in life happen, it may not be easy to deal with them. But it is possible to control your reactions to situations. Who is in charge *of you?* The weak you or the strong you?

One of you has to take control. Fill up on fruits and vegetables, instead of fast foods loaded with fat calories or high-calorie processed snack foods.

Tap Feel Good Brain Chemicals ☙

Chase away stress-causing brain chemicals (cortisol) with physical activity. Physical activity releases *endorphins*, the feel-good brain chemical. Try 30 minutes of power walking or an hour of aerobic dancing. Remember, every little bit helps. A five-minute walk in the opposite direction of the vending machine instead of an afternoon candy bar will do wonders.

If cravings are extreme, think about the consequences. Nothing in excess is healthy, whether it's food, drugs, or alcohol. Do your cravings prevent weight loss? Do you feel bad about yourself? Every time you overdo it, write down the situation, think about it, and do better next time.

Cravings can be controlled. It may seem like someone is twisting your arm, but train yourself to say no or limit the amount. If you can talk yourself into it, you can talk yourself out of it. Fewer cravings mean fewer calories. Fewer calories mean weight loss. Cravings are very individual and complicated. Give yourself permission to take action and change.

Taking control of your cravings is your new best friend.

$\mathcal{D}$ay 11 CHECK-IN ☑

What goal did you accomplish yesterday?

JF: Veggies. I ate some. Then I drank water all day when they had soda and all things sugary and luscious available at work.

You: _____

_____

What is your goal today?

(Keep a food journal targeting food cravings – what, when, and why.) (When you have a craving, try nonfood distractions [exercise, listening to music, getting more sleep, etc.].) (When you feel like eating, put a little cologne under your nose.) (Substitute a craved food with a vegetable.) (See how long you can chew one bite of chocolate.)

JF: I am going to journal all that I eat today. Also, eating throughout the day will be the way I combat my cravings.

You: _____

_____

Day 12

Lose 10 Pounds a Day!

*L*osing 10 pounds a day would be extreme, but losing 10 pounds a week would be fantastic. *Let's get real.*

Do you like to try the latest fad diets? What fad diets or weight loss supplements have you tried?

JF: Okay, we're getting real personal now. I am a reformed ephedra/ ephedrine user. I took it before the drug got banned for all the adverse health issues it caused. I was down from a size 14 to a 10 in less than two weeks and it was awesome! Now in hindsight I see that this was stupid. I could have died – but I would have been the hottest chick in the morgue.

You: _____

_____

Did you lose any weight? How much? Did you stop? Did you have side effects?

JF: I lost a lot of weight very quickly to the point where none of my clothes fit. My friends told me to stop doing what I was doing because I was losing weight too fast.

You: _____

_____

Nothing raises a registered dietitian nutritionist's blood pressure like a fad diet. On the other hand, nothing gives us a good chuckle like a natural weight-loss patch, fat-burning creams, or an ancient remedy tea for losing weight.

I will try to be nice. *Come on, people.* Do you really believe that you can lose five pounds overnight or 10 pounds in a week – safely and keep it off?

The Popularity of Fad Diets

Why do people want to lose 10 pounds in a week? I'd say that they want to lose the weight, and then go back to doing what they were doing before and be happy. Fad diets are popular because they offer a unique way to lose weight quickly. *Perfect.* Except that they seldom work. Usually people can't stick with the diets since they don't contain the foods that they like to eat. Some people may lose weight in the beginning but often gain the weight back.

Fad diets are short-term solutions. They don't teach healthy eating habits. If fad diets and weight loss pills worked, no one would have excess weight. Fad diets and diet pills can be frustrating and cost a lot of money. They may also be harmful to your health.

Weight-loss products and fad approaches to dieting have been around for a long time. New ones appear every day. *Sure, why not?* They're big business. People spend billions of dollars a year trying to lose weight. It seems that the wackier the diet, the better. Year after year, people keep trying them. When one diet doesn't work, maybe the next fad diet will be better.

Are people too trusting? Gullible? Desperate? Do they have plenty of money to spend on fad diets and magic pills that don't work? *Yes. Yes. Yes. I don't know.*

A Short History of Fad Dieting

Fad diets have been around longer than you think. Would you believe the 11th century? Legend has it that William the Conqueror tried to lose weight by going to bed and only drinking alcohol. Well, maybe if it was apple martinis.

In the early 1800s, the poet Lord Byron lost weight by pouring vinegar on his food. *Hmmm … sound familiar?* In the 1860s, a British undertaker named William Banting wrote a popular low-carbo-hydrate "diet book." *Again ... ring any bells?*

For centuries, people have tried fasting diets, liquid diets, very low-calorie diets, high-protein diets, cleansing diets, single-food diets, and food-combining diets. A lot of the current diets are fad diets from the past that have been recycled and updated. History has shown us that there have always been people looking for quick and easy ways to lose weight. There is something for everyone. Like to smoke? There's the "Cigarette Diet." Like to drink? There's the "Drinking Man's Diet." Are you a vegetarian and want to be bored to tears by your food choices? Only eat brown rice and water on the "The Zen Macrobiotic Diet."

*R*uth's Rule: *Avoid the fad diet ... even if it's been recycled and has a long history.*

Consumer Protection Is Born

Harvey Wiley, MD, is known as America's first consumer advocate. In the late 1800s and the beginning of the following century, there were many harmful products on the market. Food and drugs didn't have much government control and sometimes didn't contain what the label said they contained. Occasionally the foods contained harmful ingredients. For example, honey was diluted with cheap glucose syrup, and cough syrup for babies contained morphine. Wiley tried to introduce pure food bills but they didn't go anywhere because of strong lobbies.

In 1914, Dr. Wiley wrote an article called "Swindled Getting Slim." The article exposed misleading and fraudulent diet products. "Diet hucksters" sold products that promised quick weight loss. *Do you believe it?* At the time, there was a diet pill called "Get Slim," which contained citric acid, sugar and pink dye. There was another pill promising "permanent slenderness." *Imagine!* As long as there are people who believe in miracles, there will be people selling quick fixes.

Did you try fen-phen? Taking fenfluramine and phentermine in conjunction with one another was a popular way to lose weight in the '90s. The two prescription drugs were FDA-approved. Fen-phen worked great. People were losing weight fast and easily. Too bad some people developed heart valve disease, an unusual drug reaction. It was believed that fenfluramine or fenfluramine *in combination with* phentermine may have caused the problem. Sometimes the problems don't show up right away. It is worth taking the chance?

Even if there were a drug or supplement that actually worked for weight loss, you would still have to learn new eating habits. The drug only works while you are taking it. If you stop taking the drug and go back to your old habits, you'll gain the weight back. *Are you with me on this?*

JF: So you mean to say that after going off weight loss pills, I could gain all the weight back in less than a week? Well, sadly, I found that out the hard way.

You: _____

_____

Regulation of Supplements

There are laws for food and drugs. What about supplements? Are you among the 50% of Americans who take dietary supplements? Vitamins? Minerals? Herbs? Enzymes?

Over-the-counter diet pills? Supplements are big business. Consumers take dietary supplements for many different reasons. Lose weight. Have more energy. Detoxify the body. Sleep better. Reduce disease.

Dietary supplements are under the general umbrella of "foods," not drugs. So they are regulated differently than drugs. Supplement ingredients sold before October 15, 1994, do not need FDA review or approval before they are marketed. They are presumed safe, based on human use for all those years. For "new dietary ingredients" (an ingredient not sold before October 15, 1994), a manufacturer must notify the FDA that it is marketing a supplement with a new ingredient and must provide information on how it determined with reasonable evidence that it is expected to be safe.

Whether it's a diet pill, vitamin, mineral, herb, or something else, consumers beware! Jackie mentioned ephedra earlier in this chapter. People died taking that weight-loss herb. Diet supplements are not tested for safety by the FDA. The government steps in to ban substances after people die. Ephedra didn't turn out to be a safe weight-loss supplement.

Under an amendment to the "Federal Food, Drug and Cosmetic Act," manufacturers are now required to report all serious adverse dietary supplement events to the FDA. Hopefully, this will ensure a quicker response to get unsafe supplements off the market.

Be Savvy about Supplements ❧

Consumers need to be well informed before they purchase dietary supplements, either for weight loss or other reasons. It would be wise to know everything that you can about them. Many supplements are unnecessary, not supported by scientific research, and could have drug-like effects. Supplements do not need a doctor's prescription. However, you should consult with a healthcare professional before taking dietary supplements, especially if you're taking a prescription medicine. Also, look for "USP" on dietary supplements. It means that manufacturers voluntarily chose to have U.S. Pharmacopeia, a nonprofit, independent organization, test the dietary supplements for integrity, purity, and potency. For online resources for background on supplements, see the list of websites later in this chapter.

Health Fraud

To this day, there are many "magic" weight-loss pills being sold. Could you buy the same 1914 "Get Slim" diet pill today? You bet, and you would get the same results. Read any diet-pill advertisement. The marketing tactics are rather misleading. First of all, look at the list of ingredients. What's so special about it? A combination of common ingredients with unfamiliar ingredients does not make it special.

If you read the fine print today, you will see that the diet pills and gimmicks are in combination with a low-calorie diet and exercise. Otherwise, it would be misleading. *Hello!* If you eat less and exercise, you will lose weight *with or without* the pills.

Don't be a victim of health fraud. It could be supplements, special foods, devices, services, or programs. "Quack" companies are in business to make money and downplay regular food and peer-reviewed science. They entice you with emotional appeal. Their remedies to promote health usually don't work. Be skeptical if you see the words "fat burner," "no-risk, money-back guarantee," "secret formula," "miraculous," "patent pending," and "spot reduction."

Stay Informed - Online Resources ❧

Here are some helpful websites that contain valuable information relating to dietary supplements, health fraud, and ineffective products:

- www.ods.od.nih.gov – Contains vitamins, minerals, and botanical fact sheets.
- www.cfsan.fda.gov
- www.ftc.gov
- www.quackwatch.com – Good for health fraud.
- www.consumerlab.com
- www.usp.org
- www.supplementwatch.com
- www.nccam.nih.gov – National Center for Complementary and Alternative Medicine

My Experience with Fad Diets

When I was growing up in the 20th century, there wasn't a lot of readily available, reasonable nutrition information. I was on my own. My interest in wanting to be thin began in first grade. I was thin. But I wanted to be *thinner*. I wanted to be just like my friend, who was a stick. I would try to not eat but it didn't work. As soon as I got hungry, I had to eat.

In those days, we didn't have computers, and the television shows were limited. As a result, children spent a lot of time outside. In Wisconsin, we ran around in the summer dodging mosquitoes, swam in lakes, and rode bikes around the neighborhood. We had a lot of fresh vegetables from the garden, and my mother cooked healthy meals. In the winter, we shoveled snow. Shoveling snow is a fantastic cardio workout. During my youth, I ate healthfully and got plenty of exercise. I stayed thin (not stick thin) from a healthy lifestyle.

When I was a teen, the British model Twiggy was popular. Every teenage girl wanted to be as thin as Twiggy. A lot of the girls talked about dieting and wanting to be excessively thin. I was willing to give it a try. Succeeding was a different story. Had I known about BMI and that Twiggy's BMI was 14.5 (a BMI of less than 18.5 is considered "underweight"), I could have saved myself a lot of time and energy. Since I didn't know any better, the first diet that I tried in high school was the Apple Cider Vinegar Diet. I thought maybe this was my chance to get super thin. After the first sip of vinegar, I quit. The indigestion was too much for me. As you read earlier, the Vinegar Diet has been around for 200 years. Occasionally, clients tell me that they try to lose weight by drinking vinegar. They drink it, even though it upsets their stomach. They think that the vinegar is burning away their fat. None of them said that they lost weight.

Do people think that a diet has to cause pain and suffering to work? Do people feel like they have to punish themselves to lose weight? Apparently. I'm not surprised that people quit. Do you need pain and suffering to feel like you accomplished something?

JF: I must admit that I do believe that if one is not starving, the diet is probably not working or one is not really dieting. I realize now that consistency is the only way to train your body into understanding that things will be different and will get better as time passes.

You: _____

_____

The next diet I tried in high school came from a popular woman's magazine. I had to follow a low-calorie meal plan with recipes. We didn't have a lot of the ingredients at my house, and I didn't want to cook the elaborate lunches and dinners. By the second day, I quit because I didn't like what was on the menu.

Summers were my weakness. Every summer, I would put on 10 pounds out of boredom. I would slowly lose the 10 pounds during the school year being busy and not being able to eat whenever I wanted. In those days, we didn't have "nutrition breaks" and were only allowed to eat during lunch.

One year in college, I decided that I didn't want to gain any weight over the summer. I couldn't eat less because I got too hungry. So I kept increasing my exercise. It was a great summer. I managed to maintain my weight. I jogged one mile in the morning, swam in a fish hatchery for about 30 minutes during lunch, and then pedaled my bike five miles along country roads after dinner. That amount of exercise was needed to maintain my weight.

At the time, I didn't realize that I was eating for emotions. I would have weighed more, except in those days we didn't have such a wide variety of tasty snacks. We only had a couple of fast food restaurant choices, and people didn't eat out in restaurants as much as today. And I did manage to resist the Danish bakeries and their mouth-watering, buttery kringle pastry – except for special occasions.

Where are you coming from? Is this your highest weight? Did you have extra weight as a child? A teen?

JF: I have never been skinny but I didn't stand out as a very fat child. I had a lot of childhood girlfriends who were bigger than me. At the time, I joked around so much that I didn't focus on what I ate and didn't make an effort to not eat when I wasn't hungry.

You: _____

_____

When did your weight go up? After graduating from school? After getting married? After having kids? Job change? Menopause? Physical injury? Traumatic experience?

JF: After moving to California, I got my heaviest. I am from New York and was very mobile. I never sat still and I walked a lot. I moved to

California and now own a car; trips to the gym used to seem like trips to climb Mount Everest. My ex-husband was overweight, albeit an athlete, and we did eat together but we also worked out together. I think once I became single again, I retreated to food as a mate to console myself when lonely and bored. My relationship with food comes from my family and eating homemade, wonderful slow-cooked meals. I've eaten large portions my entire life. I've always associated mealtimes with some heavy serious foods. If you have seen it on *Animal Planet*, my mom has covered it in gravy and served it for dinner.

You: _____

_____

I wish that I had known what I know now when I was young. It would have been easier. Science is always evolving. For now, the Dietary Guidelines for Americans and MyPlate are practical and science-based sources of nutrition information. I follow them today, and they work. Looking over my own early life compared to that of today's children, I have concluded that nutrition education needs to start early in school. Lifetime habits are formed at an early age. Kids need to learn how to eat healthy right away. If kids aren't learning how to eat healthy at home, then nutrition education has to be taught in schools. It has been said that some people have eating disorders as a result of wanting to eat less and not knowing how to do it.

Lose Weight While You Sleep?

History has told us that fad diets and diet pills have been around for a long time. They may continue to be around. Unfortunately, they offer false hope. The bare truth is that if you eat too many calories from food – whether it's carbohydrate, fat, or protein – you will gain weight.

Fad diets don't work. It's impossible to safely lose a lot of weight quickly. Very low-calorie diets don't change habits and can put people at medical risk for potentially developing health complications. Weight loss should be slow and steady. You want to slowly lose fat, not quickly rob water from muscles.

Your Perfect Fad Diet ⚬

What would be your perfect fad diet? What would you call it?

JF: My perfect fad diet would be to meet for weekly weigh-ins in a funeral home, and the person who embalms and prepares the corpses for burial would be the spokesperson. The only bodies they would service would be morbidly obese people and I would have a dead fat person propped up next to the scale. The program would be called Eat 'N' Die. My slogan would be "Six-foot sub or six feet under?" Too morbid? Maybe, but I'm sure that it would be effective.

Try a "Common Sense Lifestyle Diet"

So how do you lose weight? You may not know it, but the way has *always* been around. *Common sense.* There are no pills that melt away fat or speed up metabolism. *Be practical.* Go for a healthy lifestyle, which is what this book, *The Food Is My Friend Diet,* offers. This is not a short-term diet that lasts a week, or a few months. It's a lifestyle change to adopt forever.

The Food Is My Friend Diet is a sort of "Common Sense Lifestyle Diet." It's low risk. Some discipline is required. You have to watch your portions and be aware of the calories. Follow the MyPlate eating guidelines. Rely on real food. Eat lots of fruits and vegetables, whole grains, fat-free or low-fat dairy products, lean protein, and healthy fat. Get physical activity every day. It's a matter of eating less and/or exercising more.

Is moderation and consistency too boring? Why take a chance with drugs or diet pills that could harm you? *Keep it simple.* Focus on your health. Just eat less food and get physical activity. Only eat if you're hungry. *You really can do this!*

*R*uth's Rule: *When it comes to losing weight, try a little common sense. There is no "magic" formula or approach.*

Trust the Dietitian

The Internet is flooded with "urban health myths." There is an abundance of convincing nutrition information that is inaccurate and basically crazy. Where do you go for nutrition information? A relative? A friend? The guy at the health food store? A smooth-talking "nutritionist" with an official-looking computer printout and lots of expensive supplements for you to buy?

There's a big difference between a nutritionist and a registered dietitian nutritionist. The term "nutritionist" isn't regulated. Your neighbor down the street could call himself a nutritionist. Nutritionists may or may not have formal training in nutrition. They could be self-proclaimed experts or have a mail-order credential. Nutritionists may be more interested in selling you supplements. Nutritionists might claim that they can cure a disease, use unproven tests, or promote a diet that is deficient in major nutrients.

Before you believe what you hear or read about food and nutrition information, check out the source. What are his or her credentials?

A registered dietitian nutritionist is the best person to help you learn how to eat healthy and achieve a healthy lifestyle. A dietitian lives and breathes nutrition. A registered dietitian nutritionist completes a bachelor's, master's, or doctorate degree in nutrition-related fields from an accredited university or college. Our college education is based on science and nutrition classes. RDNs complete one year of supervised training from an accredited institution and are nationally credentialed after passing a registration examination. Some states require licensing, not all. We also maintain continuing education hours throughout our careers to ensure competence. Some registered dietitians nutritionists earn specialty certifications in different areas, such as oncology, gerontological, pediatrics, renal or sports nutrition.

If you have food and nutrition questions about losing weight, gaining weight, diabetes, hypertension, heart disease, cancer, digestive problems, allergies, HIV/AIDS, gastric bypass surgery, eating disorders, sports nutrition, being a vegetarian, kidney disease, wellness, being pregnant or breastfeeding, celiac disease, food safety, or food service management, call a registered dietitian nutritionist.

A "Registered Dietitian Nutritionist" (RDN) is a nutrition expert that you can trust. For nutrition services, look for the words "dietitian" and "registered dietitian nutritionist." To find a registered dietitian nutritionist in your area, go to www.eatright.org. The Academy of Nutrition and Dietetics is the world's largest organization of food and nutrition professionals. We are qualified nutrition experts. Besides following the latest science, we offer encouragement and accountability.

By the way, if you are not totally satisfied with *The Food Is My Friend Diet,* you can have all of your weight back.

A registered dietitian nutritionist is your new best friend.

$\mathcal{D}$ay 12 CHECK-IN ☑

What did you accomplish yesterday?

JF: I sat in a coffee shop and worked for hours and did not eat. Now that is self-control. Or maybe it was the $5 coffee and the $11 muffin I was immune from.

You: _____

_____

What is your goal for today?

(Be weary of "flesh reducers.") (Get rid of your fad-diet books.) (Go to www.eatright. org for accurate food and nutrition information.) (List and evaluate your dietary supplements. Are they safe? Are they effective? Are they necessary?) (Continue eating plenty of fruits and vegetables.)

JF: My goal today is not to be tempted to call the number advertised in those commercials to inquire about lap band surgery.

You: _____

_____

Day 13

Where Are You Now? Where Do You Want to Go?

*E*very person has their own preference as to what body shape looks best to them. Some people like big bulging muscles. Some people like the bony look. Some people like a big caboose. Throughout history, bigness has meant affluence. Extra bulk was a good thing. It meant that you could afford to buy food. Today's society leans toward thinness but some people seem to be rebellious.

Back in 1959, Barbara Millicent Roberts, better known as Barbie, was a hot item for little girls. A Barbie doll was 11.5 inches tall. If dolls are 1/6 scale, Barbie would be 5' 9". Her measurements would be 36-18-33. *Not bad.* Except, if her bathroom scale was correct at 110 pounds, her Body Mass Index would be 16 (a healthy BMI is higher, from 18.5 to 24.9). She certainly was shapely, but a BMI that low is very unhealthy. Did little girls want to grow up and look like Barbie? When I was young, no one I knew talked about wanting Barbie's figure. We were more concerned about getting a date with Ken. In 1997, Barbie's waist expanded. An 18-inch waist was not realistic. Times have changed. Today, Barbie comes in all shapes and sizes.

No one is saying that you should look like a doll. What is a good body? On the thin side? A little extra padding? Statistically, excess amounts of padding are related to health problems. How much is too much? There are a variety of ways to assess your healthy body weight.

Two Basic Approaches

The first way to assess your weight is the *mirror test*. Take off all of your clothes and stand in front of a mirror. But first, take a deep breath and say, "I am proud of myself, and I feel great!" *Give yourself some words of encouragement. What do you think? Write it down.*

JF: NAKED!? Okay. WELL, MY BOOBS WERE FREE! Yup. They are huge and did not cost me a dime. You see, I have a lot of voices in my head (separate issue) but primarily the ones I hear every day tell me that I've got it going on with an occasional "You Go, Girl!" Our mirrors do show us what we can improve upon, but it's a lot easier to come from a mindset of making what is great greater, or pretty prettier. Starting from a negative is too steep a hill to climb. So many of us are so much closer to the top than we realize.

You: _____

_____

Yes, encourage yourself, but that being said … if you see ripples, rolls, or bulges, there is fat underneath the skin. This is your first indication that you're carrying extra weight.

The second way is the *pinch test*. This has been used for many years. When I was young, "pinch an inch" was a popular saying. We were always pinching ourselves. To pinch an inch, grab a chunk of your body to the right of the navel between your thumb and forefinger. Pull it away from your body slightly to make sure you haven't grabbed any muscle. If the fold is thicker than one inch, there is too much fat. Or pinch the inside of your arm. These days having only one extra inch isn't much. Nonetheless, it doesn't take much extra weight to increase your risk of disease. If you have more than one inch, you're in the right place. *Keep reading.*

Three Popular Formulas

Broca's Index is one of the earliest known formulas for calculating ideal body weight. Dr. P.P. Broca, a French surgeon, came up with this formula in 1871. It was later translated into pounds and inches.

For women, allow 100 pounds for the first 5 feet and 5 pounds for each additional inch. For men, allow 110 pounds for the first 5 feet and 5 pounds for each additional inch.

I still see this calculation being used.

In the last 60 years, there have been a number of *height/weight charts* to determine recommended body weights. The 1959 and 1983 *Metropolitan Life Insurance Company height/weight tables* were popular for many years to identify desirable body weights for longevity based on height, weight, sex, and frame size. Insured men and women (mostly middle class and white) were grouped into frame sizes. A body weight higher than the average life insurance policy holder for height, age, and sex was considered overweight. The life insurance height/weight charts were always confusing to me. Was it with or without clothes? No shoes, 1-inch heels or 2-inch heels? Was my frame small, medium, or large?

Since the 1980s, the most common way to assess body weight is the *Body Mass Index (BMI).* In 1998, the National Heart, Lung and Blood Institute (NHLBI), part of the National Institutes of Health, made BMI its standard measurement for determining healthy weights. It is now consistently used worldwide as a standard reference by government agencies and other health organizations. Body Mass Index (BMI) is a reality check. It is a measure of your weight in relation to your height to gauge body fat. It lets you know if you're "normal," "overweight," or "obese." If you keep gaining weight and you also grow in height, weight doesn't matter. Unfortunately, at some point, we stop "going up" and start "going out."

*R*uth's Rule: *The BMI can be a reality check – a reinforcement for your goal of losing weight.*

A Closer Look at the BMI

Most people seem to be familiar with BMI. Some time between 1830-1850, Adolphe Quetelet, a Belgian statistician, developed the "Quetelet Index," now known as Body Mass Index. That's right. In the mid-1800s. About the time that the first "low carbohydrate" diet became popular.

BMI is a relatively good measurement and useful for most people. Of course, there are some drawbacks. Two people with the same height and weight could look completely different depending on their bone structure, muscle mass, and body fat. BMI doesn't distinguish between fat and muscle. The statement "I'm not fat; I'm big boned" could be valid.

BMI is for adults over 20 years old. Each height has a range of numbers to take into account sex, muscle, and bone mass. It may not be reliable for older people 70 and up because of loss of muscle and bone mass. Women have a higher percentage of fat than men for the same BMI. The Body Mass Index may not be effective in people who are less than five feet tall. BMI is not effective for pregnant and breastfeeding women, body builders, or very ill people.

Children and the BMI ◌෴

Body Mass Index for children and teens 2 to 20 years old is calculated the same way as adults, except the BMI number is interpreted differently. Children grow at different rates, so the BMI is applied to the Centers for Disease Control and Prevention (CDC) 2000 growth charts according to age and sex. The BMI-for-Age Percentile compares height and weight with other boys and girls the same age. See http://www.cdc.gov/growthcharts.

Parents often think that their overweight children will naturally slim down as they get older and taller. I don't see this happen very often. Unless overweight children change their habits, the weight will usually continue to rise.

To get an accurate BMI, you need an accurate height and weight. In my many years of measuring people, not many people know their real height. Secure a measuring tape against the wall and take your height. Are you as tall as you think?

A person's weight can also be inaccurate. Some people don't have a clue to how much they weigh. Some home scales are great because you can be up to 10 pounds lighter. If it makes you happy, go for it. When you're losing weight, scales don't have to be accurate. You just need consistency. Weigh yourself on only one scale. Almost every scale will give you a slightly different weight. For BMI, the weight doesn't have to be perfect, unless you're trying to get out of the "obese" range. Then every ounce counts.

Body Mass Index Table

	NORMAL						OVERWEIGHT					OBESE									
BMI	19	20	21	22	23	24	25	26	27	28	29	30	31	32	33	34	35	36	37	38	39
Height	Weight																				
5'0"	97	102	107	112	118	123	128	133	138	143	148	153	158	163	168	174	179	184	189	194	199
5'1"	100	106	111	116	122	127	132	137	143	148	153	158	164	169	174	180	185	190	195	201	206
5'2"	104	109	115	120	126	131	136	142	147	153	158	164	169	175	180	186	191	196	202	207	213
5'3"	107	113	118	124	130	135	141	146	152	158	163	169	175	180	186	191	197	203	208	214	220
5'4"	110	116	122	128	134	140	145	151	157	163	169	174	180	186	192	197	204	209	215	221	227
5'5"	114	120	126	132	138	144	150	156	162	168	174	180	186	192	198	204	210	216	222	228	234
5'6"	118	124	130	136	142	148	155	161	167	173	179	186	192	198	204	210	216	223	229	235	241
5'7"	121	127	134	140	146	153	159	166	172	178	185	191	198	204	211	217	223	230	236	242	249
5'8"	125	131	138	144	151	158	164	171	177	184	190	197	203	210	216	223	230	236	243	249	256
5'9"	128	135	142	149	155	162	169	176	182	189	196	203	209	216	223	230	236	243	250	257	263
5'10"	132	139	146	153	160	167	174	181	188	195	202	209	216	222	229	236	243	250	257	264	271
5'11"	136	143	150	157	165	172	179	186	193	200	208	215	222	229	236	243	250	257	265	272	279
6'0"	140	147	154	162	169	177	184	191	199	206	213	221	228	235	242	250	258	265	272	279	287
6'1"	144	151	159	166	174	182	189	197	204	212	219	227	235	242	250	257	265	272	280	288	295
6'2"	148	155	163	171	179	186	194	202	210	218	225	233	241	249	256	264	272	280	287	295	303
6'3"	152	160	168	176	184	192	200	208	216	224	232	240	248	256	264	272	279	287	295	303	311
6'4"	156	164	172	180	189	197	205	213	221	230	238	246	254	263	271	279	287	295	304	312	320

Source: Adapted from Clinical Guidelines on the Identification, Evaluation, and Treatment of Overweight and Obesity in Adults: The Evidence Report

Here is the BMI calculation:

BMI = Weight in Pounds x 703 divided by Height in Inches divided by Height in Inches. (Example: 130 x 703 divided by 66 divided by 66 = 20.9 BMI)

If you don't have a calculator, take a look at the BMI chart. Find your height without shoes in the left column. Follow across the horizontal column until you find your weight without clothes. Move straight up the column to find your BMI.

Here are the different classifications of the BMI:
A BMI of less than 18.5 is "underweight."
A range of 18.5 to 24.9 is "normal" (healthy).
A BMI of 25 to 29.9 is "overweight."
Finally, 30 or more is "obese." (There are a few categories of obese, but obese is obese.)

What is your BMI? Are you "underweight," "normal," "overweight," or "obese"?

JF: I have been told by a trainer in the past that I am over 40% body fat, so essentially I am a cream-filled Twinkie with hair. I have to make a joke about this fact; otherwise, I would cry uncontrollably, so chuckle, chuckle.

You: _____

Over two-thirds of U.S. adults are "overweight" or "obese." Nearly 40% of those people are "obese." There's the potential for a lot of health problems caused by excess weight.

Obesity is a major risk factor for disease and premature death. If you're "overweight" and have health problems – such as diabetes, high blood pressure, heart disease, some types of cancer, sleep apnea, gallbladder disease, liver disease, osteoarthritis, irregular menstrual periods, or a family history of these health problems – you're wise to be working on losing weight. If you're young and in good health, but overweight or obese, I'm glad you also want to lose weight. As you get older, it will become harder to lose weight, and the health risks will become a reality.

Your goal is to slowly get back to "normal." If you were never "normal," keep losing 5-10 pounds at a time. Take a break from losing, maintain for three to six months and go for another 5-10 pounds. It may take your body a while to get used to a new weight. It also takes your mind a while to get used to eating less.

Each BMI number has a range of 4-8 pounds. BMI is a wake-up call for many of my clients. They're shocked to learn that they are "obese."

Your "WC" – Waist Circumference

Where is the "more of you to love" located? The location of body fat can be a risk factor. A good way to assess health is *waist circumference (WC)*. Waist circumference measures abdominal fat. A high waist measurement may increase your risk of heart disease and diabetes.

Are you at risk? Find the top of your hip bone. Put the tape measure around your waist, just above the top of the hip bones without clothes. Exhale naturally without sucking it in. Not too tight. Not too loose.

You are at greater risk for disease if your waist measurement is:

Men	Women
40" or more	35" or more

Source: www.nhlbi.nih.gov

What is your waist measurement?

You: _____

The BMI and waist circumference can be used together to assess health risk. According to the World Health Organization (WHO), some Asian populations may require a smaller waist circumference and lower BMI range to be in the "healthy weight" range.

The *waist-to-hip ratio* is another way to assess body composition. It may be less accurate than waist circumference.

Are You an Apple or a Pear?

If you carry extra weight in the hips and thighs, you are "pear shaped." If you carry extra weight in the stomach area, you are "apple shaped." Apples and pears are fruits. Are both healthy?

Your waist measurement is your answer. The extra "visceral" fat around your waist, making you an apple, is unhealthy. The visceral fat surrounds your organs, secretes hormones, and causes inflammation. Inflammation promotes disease. The less fat the better. It appears that apples may need to make an extra effort to lose weight and exercise for health reasons.

So ... would you say that you're an apple or a pear?

JF: I would say that I've been an accordion. When I lie down, all the fat spreads out, especially when I stretch out all the way. Sometimes you can hear noises as my joints are elongated. When I stand up, it all scrunches back into a nice rectangle-like box.

You: _____

_____

When you lose weight, you will either be a smaller apple or a smaller pear. You cannot "spot reduce" to get rid of the extra fat around your waist. It is, however, possible to firm and strengthen the muscles in the stomach area. For example, sit-ups are an important exercise to incorporate into your firming and strengthening routine. Still, as you lose weight, the "padding" covering the abdominal muscles will slowly decrease.

*R*uth's **Rule:** *Whether you're an apple shape or a pear shape, whether your weight is above the hips or below the hips, avoid excess amounts of body fat.*

Why You Should Care

Health and risk factors can be more accurately determined by body fat, not weight. If you're a professional athlete or a bodybuilder with a lot of muscle mass and a large bone structure, your BMI may put you in the "overweight" category, or even the "obese" one. Actually, you could in fact have a strong heart and be very fit in those cases. A sedentary woman may not be "overweight," but she can have a high percentage of body fat.

Certain amounts of fat are necessary in the body. There is *essential fat* and *storage fat*. Women need more essential fat than men for reproduction. Storage fat can be used as fuel, if needed. Keep the amounts of storage fat to a minimum. Fat is fluffy. Fat sits around and only burns 2-3 calories per pound a day. Muscle has a blood supply and burns as much as 5-6 calories per pound a day. Muscle is dense so it takes up less space. When you build up muscle mass, you will lose inches.

Some of the ways to measure body fat percentage include *dual energy-ray absorptiometry* (DXA), *bioelectrical impedance, hydrostatic (underwater) weighing,* and *skinfold measurements.*

A Starting Point ❦

I suggest starting with the *mirror test* and the *pinch test.* They don't require any special equipment. They can be real eye-openers and fairly accurate. For most people, Waist Circumference and Body Mass Index are simple and practical ways of assessing the body. Waist circumference is a way to measure fat. For most people, not all, BMI can help determine the risk for disease.

A Workable Plan

The Partnership for Healthy Weight Management recommends a weight loss plan with at least the minimum number of calories. To get enough nutrients, women should eat at least 1,200 calories a day. Men should eat at least 1,400 calories a day. If you follow these calorie levels, you'll probably feel a fair amount of hunger because that's not very many calories. An intake of 1,800 calories a day is more realistic and less punishing. In order to meet nutritional needs, the Dietary Guidelines for Americans states that adults should not use a calorie pattern less than 1,600 calories.

There are 3,500 calories in a pound. Eat 500 calories less a day to lose one pound a week. Five hundred calories equals approximately:

- A 6-ounce muffin
- A quarter-pound hamburger with cheese
- 1 cup premium ice cream
- 3½ cans of beer

Eat 500 calories less a day *and* exercise 500 calories a day to lose two pounds a week.

Your goal is to lose 1-2 pounds a week. *Really?* If you have been struggling to lose weight all of your life, it may not be that simple. In over 20 years of helping people lose weight, I haven't seen anyone consistently lose 1-2 pounds a week for more than a few months. Humans are not computers that can be programmed to eat 500-1,000 calories less every day. Sometimes in the beginning, there is a big weight loss – *when motivation is the highest.* Weight loss can taper off or go up a little. Sometimes the weight stabilizes for awhile. Every individual is different.

Easy Does It ℭℜ

A lot of clients have told me that when they were losing weight on their own, if they didn't lose 2 pounds a week, they thought they were doing something wrong. I suggest eating *at least 100-200 calories less a day.* You won't even know that you're losing weight, and the number on the scale will slowly go down in a few months.

Make an effort to burn an extra 100-200 calories a day in physical activity. Your excess weight may come from a lack of physical activity rather than an excessive amount of calories. Patience is a virtue. If you consistently lose ½-1 pound a week, that's fantastic.

What about Metabolism?

Maybe your metabolism is slow. A slow metabolism is a good excuse. Your metabolism varies depending on age, sex, height, size, and physical activity. Multiply your weight by 10 to determine your basal metabolism. This is a very rough estimate of the number of calories your body uses to exist. Breathing, thinking, blood flowing through the body, etc., take 60-75% of your calories. Another 10% of your calories are used for digesting and absorbing food. The rest of the calories burned depend on physical activity. These calories could vary from 200-1,000 or more, depending on the type of physical activity you do, how often, how long, and how hard.

Regardless of your metabolic rate, food is your body's fuel for all functions. Food is burned for energy, and the excess calories are stored as fat. If you have extra weight, you're eating more calories than your body needs. If you want to speed up your metabolism, move more. Physical activity burns calories and increases the size of muscle cells.

Factoring in "Muscle Mass"

People who start walking or going to the gym often blame a weight gain on increasing muscle mass. *Don't count on it.* When you feel your body, does it feel hard or more like a marshmallow? If it's more like a marshmallow, you could have more fat than muscle. In that case, an "overweight" or "obese" BMI might be valid.

Your goal is to increase your muscle mass. How's your muscle mass doing these days? Good? Fair? Or poor?

JF: I actually really enjoy lifting weights. It makes me feel strong. I could truly test my muscle mass by picking a fight with a big man in the gym but he would probably ask me out. There is a price to pay for working out in the "men's" area.

You: _____

If you're soft and fluffy, check your BMI. You may not realize the degree of your "extra." With most of the population overweight, "normal" may look rather thin to you. After determining your BMI and WC, consider lipid levels, blood pressure, blood sugar, and your family's health problems, along with your lifestyle (amount of physical activity, alcohol intake, and smoking status) to assess health risk.

What's the "Ideal" Body Weight?

I don't think that there's a perfect way of determining a person's ideal weight. There are too many factors – such as current health, genetics, smoking, total body fat, body fat distribution, muscle mass, bone structure, age, sex, and physical activity – that need to be taken into consideration for an ideal weight. However, *keeping excess fat to a minimum and increasing muscle mass would be the "ideal" situation for staying healthy.* Less fat. More muscle.

Not everyone has to look like Michelangelo's David, and Barbie has food issues. But keeping your weight within a "normal" range is recommended to maintain good health. And keep this thought in mind:

An "ideal" or perfect weight is a weight in which you are in good health.

"Ideally," choose a risk-free approach to lose your weight. Losing weight is a process. Lose the weight slowly. Eat a balanced diet. Eat fewer calories than you usually eat. Be active every day.

Lowering your BMI is your new best friend.

---

*D*ay 13 CHECK-IN ☑

What did you accomplish yesterday?

JF: The car dealership insisted on driving me home while my car was being serviced, but I insisted on walking. (What was I thinking?!)

You: _____

_____

What is your goal for today?

(Buy a tape measure.) (Measure your height.) (Measure your waist.) (Buy a scale.) (Calculate the BMI for family members.) (Set a goal to not be "obese.")

JF: I own a scale but when I'm ashamed of the day I've had, I don't like to get on it. I have to train myself to take the good with the bad and not give up when the scale is obviously conspiring against me or it **seems** as if my roommate snuck in the bathroom and recalibrated it to always be five pounds heavier than I actually am.

You: _____

_____

Day 14

Doctor's Orders

*Y*our health is the #1 reason for losing weight. Excess weight is worse than you think. The Department of Health and Human Services collects data and releases obesity statements. Just 10-20 extra pounds can increase your risk of disease and death compared to a person with a "normal" weight, especially if you're between the ages of 30-64. If you are "obese," your risk of prematurely dying increases 50-100%.

Obesity occurs in every age group, race, sex, and socioeconomic status. About 160 million Americans are overweight or obese. It's estimated that obesity kills 100,000-300,000 people a year and costs $300 billion a year. The health care costs from obesity include doctor visits, medications, hospital stays, nursing home care, and also time lost from work because of illness and disability.

Overweight adults with weight-related health problems are one thing, but what about kids? Alarming new predictions say that life expectancy will decline *for the first time ever* because of the number of overweight and obese children. It has been reported that one out of three kids born in 2000 will develop diabetes. Overweight kids will get high cholesterol and high blood pressure at a younger age. While they're growing up, these children will also endure social discrimination.

Has your doctor ever told you that you need to lose weight?

JF: Strangely enough, I have never had doctor's orders to lose weight. I have had a doctor refuse to give me a prescription for weight loss drugs, however.

You: _____

_____

How's your blood pressure? How's your cholesterol? Do you have diabetes? If you are diabetic, how often do you check your blood sugar?

JF: Diabetes and high blood pressure run in my family so I have to be careful. Especially since I would rather have a Danish instead of an apple. Or would try to intravenously have milkshakes flow through my body — if I wasn't on this new eating regimen, of course.

You: _____

_____

I'm surprised by the number of my clients in their 30s who have never had a physical exam or had their blood tested. Lack of insurance was probably a major factor. Yet the sooner you know about a problem, the sooner you can take action. People have pre-diabetes for many years without knowing it. Without warning, their vision is blurry, and they feel like they're going to pass out. Sometimes they end up in the hospital with a blood sugar of 500 mg/dl or higher (should be less than 180 mg/dl if diabetic).

Weight-Related Issues

Below is a list of known health problems related to excess weight. It was compiled by the Weight Control Information Network (WIN) – a service of the National Institute of Diabetes and Digestive and Kidney Diseases (NIDDK), National Institutes of Health (NIH).

- Diabetes
- Coronary heart disease
- High blood pressure
- Stroke
- Gallbladder disease

- Osteoarthritis
- Sleep apnea and other breathing problems
- Cancer – especially breast, colon, uterine, and kidney
- Complications in pregnancy
- Increased surgery risk
- Depression
- Early death

Do you see anything that you like?

JF: I had a single gallstone and my choices were to either change my entire diet and eat blander foods or have my gall bladder removed. I chose invasive surgery over eating right; hence the reason I am participating in this project is because I obviously have my priorities mixed up. So the answer is ... I do not like anything listed above. Now if by early death, you mean I die early in the morning when I am 102, then yes ... I like the last choice.

Don't forget about *weight discrimination*. Do you want to pay more for an airline ticket? Some overweight people don't like going out in public. They're afraid the chairs won't be big enough or a seat might break. The last injustice would be buying an extra-wide coffin.

So many problems. So little time. Here's a quick description of a few major health problems and how to avoid them.

Checked Your Blood Pressure Lately?

As people get older, hypertension (high blood pressure) is very common. High blood pressure increases the risk of coronary heart disease, stroke, congestive heart failure, and kidney disease.

High blood pressure is called the "silent killer" because it doesn't always have symptoms. Blood pressure puts force on artery walls. When you have high blood pressure, your heart works harder. Eventually, high blood pressure can enlarge the heart, form bulges (aneurysms) in blood vessels, harden the arteries faster, cause blood vessels in the kidneys to harden (causing kidney failure), and cause blood vessels in the eyes to burst, resulting in blindness.

Salt intake affects blood pressure. High salt and low potassium (found in fast food and processed food) is a bad combo for high blood pressure. Foods high in potassium are known to counteract the effects of salt in the diet. A baked potato a day keeps the doctor away. If you prefer, a cup of carrot juice a day keeps the doctor away.

Understanding Blood Pressure Readings C⅜

High blood pressure is a reading of 130/80 or higher. People with chronic kidney disease should maintain blood pressure lower than 130/80. It's essential to watch the systolic blood pressure, especially in older adults.

Blood Pressure Levels	Systolic	Diastolic
Normal	less than 120	less than 80
Elevated	120-129	less than 80
Hypertension, stage 1	130-139	80-89
Hypertension, stage 2	140 or higher	90 or higher

Source: American Heart Association, 2017

Hopefully, the *DASH diet* is catching on. DASH is "Dietary Approaches to Stop Hypertension." Studies show that the DASH diet with low amounts of sodium is just as effective as blood pressure medications. What is the DASH diet? Basically, it's rich in fruits and vegetables and low-fat dairy foods with high amounts of potassium, calcium and magnesium. If you have kidney problems, potassium may not be good for you. Check with your doctor.

High blood pressure can be prevented and controlled.

To lower blood pressure:
- Lose excess weight.
- Limit sodium.
- Eat lots of high-potassium fruits and vegetables.
- Increase physical activity.

To avoid high blood pressure:
- Limit alcohol.
- Don't smoke.
- If needed, take medications on a regular basis.

*R*uth's Rule: *Eat foods high in potassium (potatoes, carrot juice) to counteract the effects of salt in the diet. Limit high-sodium items and processed food.*

How's Your Cholesterol?

A client once told me that she could feel the cholesterol in her arteries. Most people don't know if their cholesterol is elevated, unless they have their blood tested. *LDL (low density lipoprotein)* and *HDL (high density lipoprotein)* are lipoproteins that carry cholesterol in the blood. Elevated cholesterol may be a ticket to heart disease.

You are what you eat. Look at the types of fat that you eat. Trans fats increase cholesterol. Fortunately, trans fats are being phased out. Saturated fat from butter, whole milk, cheese, and high-fat meat may increase LDL cholesterol.

Elevated LDL is a common problem. LDL (lousy) cholesterol is the bad cholesterol. LDL carries cholesterol to the arteries, where it gets stuck. Over time, the waxy, fatty cholesterol globs (plaque) start sticking to your artery walls, narrowing and hardening them. With no warning, a chunk of plaque can break off, cause blood to clot, and close off an artery. The red blood cells can't get through and voila! Heart attack or stroke. It's that simple. No blood to the heart or brain is bad for business. Keep your arteries clean.

To lower LDL cholesterol:
- Decrease saturated fat and trans fat.
- Increase monounsaturated fat and omega 3 fats.
- Exercise.
- Lose weight.
- Don't smoke.
- Increase soluble fiber.*

*Soluble fiber acts like a sponge and soaks up the LDL cholesterol. Include lots of high-soluble foods such as oatmeal, barley, and beans in your diet.

The higher the HDL cholesterol, the better. HDL (happy, healthy) cholesterol is the good type. It goes through the blood picking up cholesterol and takes it back to the liver. From the liver, the cholesterol exits the body.

To raise HDL:

+ Lose weight.
+ Don't smoke.
+ Get 30-60 minutes of physical activity most days.

Triglycerides are another form of fat. A blood test will also show if your triglycerides are elevated.

If your triglycerides are high:

+ Cut back on carbohydrates (starches), sweets, and alcohol.
+ Eat fatty fish two to three times a week to get the omega 3 fatty acids.
+ Lose weight.
+ Increase physical activity.
+ Don't smoke.

Here are the good and the bad numbers:

Cholesterol Classifications

Total Cholesterol

Less than 200 mg/dl	Desirable
200-239 mg/dl	Borderline high
240 mg/dl and above	High

LDL Cholesterol

Less than 100 mg/dl	Optimal (ideal)
100-129 mg/dl	Near optimal/above optimal
130-159 mg/dl	Borderline high
160-189 mg/dl	High
190 mg/dl and above	Very high

HDL Cholesterol

Less than 40 mg/dl*	Major heart disease risk factor
40-59 mg/dl	The higher, the better
60 mg/dl and above	Gives some protection against heart disease.

*Less than 40 mg/dl for men and less than 50 mg/dl for women puts a person at a higher risk for heart disease.

Triglycerides

Less than 150 mg/dl	Normal
150-199 mg/dl	Borderline high
200-499 mg/dl	High
500 mg/dl	Very high

Source: National Cholesterol Education Program, National Heart, Lung and Blood Institute, National Institutes of Health

Excess weight and a high saturated and trans fat diet lead to an increase in LDL cholesterol. Reduce your risk of heart disease by eating a low saturated fat, high soluble fiber diet. Keep your blood vessels open and limber. Keep the unhealthy fat low and the exercise high. Again, to lower cholesterol, lose weight, limit alcohol, and don't smoke.

Cholesterol - Know Your Family History ⌘

Heredity decides cholesterol levels for some people. Heart disease may run in your family. In that case, carefully monitor your blood cholesterol levels and blood pressure, and get regular checkups. If needed, take medications on a regular basis.

The TLC Plan

The National Cholesterol Education Program has a guide to lowering cholesterol with "TLC" – *Therapeutic Lifestyle Changes*. You can lower your LDL cholesterol with just a few dietary adjustments.

Change	How to Do It	LDL Reduction
Saturated fat	Decrease to less than 7% of calories.	8-10%
Dietary cholesterol	Decrease to less than 200 mg/day.	3-5%
Weight	Lose 10 pounds, if overweight.	5-8%
Soluble fiber	Add 5-10 daily grams.	3-5%
Plant sterols/stanols*	Add 2 daily grams.	6-15%
Cumulative Estimate:		20-30%

*Plant sterols/stanols are found in tiny amounts in vegetables, fruits, seeds, and nuts. To get 2 grams a day, it is necessary to consume enriched foods or dietary supplements.

This is an excellent example of how a few small dietary changes can make a big difference. The 20-30% reduction is similar to cholesterol-lowering drugs. If your doctor says that you need to take cholesterol-reducing medication, take the drugs in addition to making the dietary changes. As a result, the drug dosage may be lowered.

Be Informed about Diabetes

Genes, excess weight, placement of fat (abdominal), and being in certain ethnic groups (Latino, Asian, Native American, Pacific Islander, African American) put people at a higher risk of getting *type 2 diabetes*. Obesity is a leading cause of this disorder. Eighty percent of diabetics are either "overweight" or "obese." If you're carrying around extra weight, it's not a matter of *if* you'll get diabetes. It's probably a matter of *when* you'll get it.

A fasting blood sugar over 100 mg/dl and under 125 mg/dl is considered *pre-diabetes*. This is not quite diabetes but it could be in the future. *Now* is the time to take action. Lose weight. Exercise. Cut back on carbs (sugar and starches).

If a fasting blood sugar is 126 mg/dl or higher two times, you have diabetes. Once you have diabetes, it's very important to control your blood sugar.

To control blood sugar:
- Lose excess weight.
- Watch carbohydrate (starches and sugar) intake.
- Get daily physical activity.
- Take medications, if needed.
- Eat small, frequent meals and snacks with consistent amounts of carbohydrate.
- Be serious about monitoring your blood sugar.
- Keep your blood sugar values in the normal range to avoid complications.

Eating a diabetic diet is similar to eating for health and losing weight. Eat healthy foods in moderation. Carbohydrates (starches and sugar) raise blood sugar. Artificial sweeteners do not raise blood sugar. If you have diabetes, don't avoid fruit. Fruits are carbohydrates but they contain valuable nutrients. It's all about eating consistent amounts of carbohydrates. Three bananas will raise blood sugar. Eat half a banana at a time. A piece of cake will also raise blood sugar. If you want cake, skip the rice, bread, or pasta in the meal.

Most people with diabetes die from a heart attack. First of all, if you have diabetes, keep your blood pressure and cholesterol in the normal range. Actually, first of all, if you have diabetes, lose weight. As Americans gain weight, the rate of diabetes is also going up. Obesity and diabetes go hand in hand.

*R**uth's Rule:** If you have diabetes or are pre-diabetic, working on losing weight is essential.*

Break Time!

It's time for a group hug. All this information about bad health stuff is a downer. What are you feeling right now? Let it out.

JF: I am feeling aware. My ex-husband died at 41 years old of a heart attack while playing basketball. He did not eat red meat or pork, drink alcohol, or smoke, but he was very overweight. All the information above just goes to show that paying attention to everything that makes us tick is how to live a full life. Neglect in any fashion can contribute to a loss — your own life or the life of someone you care deeply for.

You: _____

_____

We're not quite done with the bad stuff, however ...

Want Cancer?

You can dramatically improve your odds of getting cancer, if you:
- Smoke.
- Don't eat healthy.
- Don't exercise.
- Carry around excess weight.

Cancer starts with a single cell going bad. It multiplies, forms a tumor, invades, and conquers. *Cancer is scary.* Heart disease is the number one killer in America, yet people are more concerned about getting cancer. People are afraid of getting cancer from pesticides and additives. But cancer is nothing new. Hippocrates wrote about cancer, and all of his produce was organic.

As with diabetes, research links excess weight to cancer. Thirty percent of certain cancers are related to excess weight, a diet high in fat, low consumption of fruits and vegetables, and little or no physical activity. That's a lot of cancer that could be prevented!

Fruits, vegetables, beans, nuts, and whole grains offer great protection against cancer because they contain antioxidants, phytonutrients, and fiber. Antioxidants keep normal cells from going bad. Most of your food should come from plant sources. Include at least 2½ cups of fruits and vegetables in your diet every day. Eat fruits and vegetables with lots of color (dark green, red, yellow, and orange), such as spinach, carrots, cantaloupes, and veggies in the cabbage family. These vegetables and fruits are good sources of vitamin C and vitamin A.

What the Ultimate Cancer Report Says

At the end of 2007, the World Cancer Research Fund International and the American Institute for Cancer Research reported their findings in "Food, Nutrition, Physical Activity and the Prevention of Cancer: A Global Perspective." It's the most comprehensive report of its kind for cancer analysis. The report took five years and involved nine independent teams of scientists from around the world, hundreds of peer reviewers, and 21 international experts, who reviewed over 7,000 studies. Its major finding: Being overweight and obese is a primary risk factor for cancer. They also determined that *cancer is preventable, even if you have a genetic predisposition.*

To reduce your risk of cancer, the expert panel made the following recommendations:

♦ **Be as lean as possible within the normal range of body weight.** Avoid weight gain and increases in waist circumference throughout adulthood.

- **Be physically active as part of everyday life.** Get at least 30 minutes of moderate physical activity a day. Aim for 60 minutes of moderate activity or 30 minutes or more of vigorous physical activity a day.
- **Limit consumption of energy-dense foods.** Energy-dense foods have an energy content of more than about 225-275 calories per 100 grams. Energy-dense foods often contain substantial amounts of fat or sugar.
- **Avoid sugary drinks.** This may help with weight loss.
- **Eat mostly foods of plant origin.** Eat a variety of at least five portions/servings of fruits and vegetables a day. Eat whole grains and legumes for fiber with every meal. Limit refined starchy foods.
- **Limit intake of red meat and avoid processed meat.** Limit red meat (beef, pork, lamb, goat) to 18 ounces (cooked) a week. Eat very little processed meat (bacon, hot dogs, ham, sausage, luncheon meat). "Processed meat" means meat that has been preserved by smoking, curing, salting, or adding chemical preservatives.
- **Limit alcoholic drinks.** Restrict alcohol to no more than two drinks a day for men and one drink a day for women. Modest amounts of alcohol may reduce the risk of heart disease.
- **Limit consumption of salt.** Avoid salty and salt-preserved foods. Limit sodium to less than 2,400 mg a day (more promotes stomach cancer).
- **Avoid moldy grains and legumes.** Steer clear of exposure to the fungi aflatoxin (promotes liver cancer).
- **Aim to meet nutritional needs through diet alone.** Dietary supplements are not recommended for cancer prevention.
- **Mothers to breastfeed; children to be breastfed.** Aim to breastfeed exclusively up to six months.
- **Don't smoke.** Also don't chew tobacco, and avoid exposure to smoke.

Advice for cancer survivors: Follow the recommendations for cancer prevention for diet, healthy weight, and physical activity, if able or unless otherwise advised.

Prevention, Prevention, Prevention

As you read this chapter, did you notice any common denominators for reducing the risk of disease?

JF: I notice the stressing of physical activity every day and not just the first Friday of the month or when it is nice outside or when you can find a workout buddy or when there is a lunar eclipse or when the Lakers win or ... I could go on. But yes, there is a common thread.

You: _____

_____

Over the years, I've observed a common thread. Eat healthy. Limit unhealthy fat. Eat lots of fruits and vegetables. Avoid excess weight. Get physical activity *every day.* Of course, both smoking and excess alcohol are a big no-no for health.

You can't control genes and aging yet. Do something about the factors that you *can* control.

And see a doctor. Your blood values could be the wake-up call that you need to start making changes. Also, don't forget to get the recommended basic screenings, such as mammograms, Pap tests, colonoscopies, and PSA blood tests. Choose to die from something else.

Most heart attacks and cancers aren't really sudden. They slowly advance over time from a poor diet and a lack of physical activity. If you can prevent, delay, or control health problems by making a few dietary and lifestyle changes and getting periodic check-ups, isn't it worth it to you?

Preventing health problems is your new best friend.

End of Week 2

Congratulations! You're halfway there. Thanks for hanging in with this program!

Time to weigh in.

Weight:_____

Two weeks isn't a lot of time to see a significant weight loss. But 1-4 pounds is possible, depending on how much you weigh. For some people, maintaining their weight for two weeks is an accomplishment. Or your focus may be to eat healthy. If you stay consistent, the weight loss will soon follow.

Keep going!

---

*D*ay 14 CHECK-IN ☑

What did you accomplish yesterday?

JF: I ate at McDonald's. But not the foods I usually eat there. I ate their grilled chicken sandwich on wheat with a side salad and low-calorie vinaigrette dressing. The person who took my money at the drive-thru looked perplexed and I hope to keep the staff at the annoyingly close neighborhood McDonald's very confused but proud of my new choices.

You: _____

_____

What is your goal for today?

(Go for a walk.) (Don't eat any processed foods for the day.) (Eat an extra vegetable.) (Eat oatmeal five times this week.) (Don't eat foods with added sugars for a day.) (Call your doctor for a blood test.) (Read food labels for sodium and saturated fat.) (Get your blood pressure checked.) (Buy a blood pressure cuff.) (Quit smoking.) (Limit alcohol to one drink a day if you're a woman and two drinks if you're a man.)

JF: I have a show tonight and I will not eat the free dinner that comes with my pay. I will eat before I leave home so as to not be hungry when I arrive. Now, as for the free alcohol? Pray for me.

You: _____

_____

Day 15

Secrets to Overcoming Weight Loss Obstacles

*J*ackie Gleason used to joke that the second day of a diet is always easier than the first. Why? Because, by then, you're no longer dieting! Ain't that the truth!

I hope you have enjoyed the last two weeks of getting healthy, and you are raring to go for another two weeks. Or have you had enough of this crazy healthy eating and exercise stuff? Are you ready to throw in the towel and try the diet craze from the early 1900s? In those days, it was supposedly easy to lose weight. They ate sanitized tapeworms. *Yummy.* Here is the claim:

"Eat! Eat! Eat! & Always Stay Thin! No diet, no baths, no exercise. FAT, the enemy that is shortening your life, BANISHED!"

Of course, back then and today, many people learn the hard way that fad diets aren't all they're cracked up to be (for more on this, see Day 12). And even when dieting the smart way (as with *The Food Is My Friend Diet*), we discover that the process of dieting can have obstacles. First of all, you might not lose weight very quickly. Second, if you don't lose weight fast enough, you might quit. Third, once you lose the weight, you might not be able to maintain the weight loss. *It happens.*

Be a Maintainer, Not a Re-Gainer

Whenever you read weight loss statistics, it says that most people gain back all of the weight within five years. That's discouraging! You suffer. You lose weight. Then the weight slowly begins to creep back on after several months or several years. Why bother? Have you lost weight and gained it back? How did you feel?

JF: It *is* discouraging to lose weight, then gain it back, and it makes me feel sad. Kind of like if I eat a French fry, my pants will explode (which happened, by the way). Gaining back weight needs to not feel like a complete failure but a chance to start over. Like when I get my eyebrows waxed and the eyebrow lady waxes off too much and leaves me with a look of permanent surprise. I never get angry at her. I know that if I relax and just carry on, the hair will grow back and I can start again. That is how I should feel about my weight. It's not the end of the world if I gain back some of it. I can always start over.

You: _____

_____

One of the definite disadvantages of losing weight is that you could gain it back. Maintaining weight loss can be challenging! Hopefully, there has not been enough time for you to lose and regain any weight in the last two weeks. But my advice is that after you're done being a "loser," you should become a "maintainer" – not a "re-gainer."

"Energy In" vs. "Energy Out" ᙇ

When the "energy in" *equals* the "energy out," you are maintaining your weight. Maintaining weight is different than losing weight. When you are maintaining weight, you can eat more calories than you did while you were losing. However, not too many more!

Secret #1 is:
Find the balance between equal amounts of "energy in" and "energy out" versus too much "energy in."

If you tend to regain weight, be prepared this time. You can't say, "I don't care. I'm going to eat and drink whatever I want." You work very hard at losing weight. Don't gain it back! Stick with this book and you'll learn how to eat healthy, take off those unwanted pounds, and then stay at your desired weight.

The Power of Patience (Really, It Helps!)

You're learning everything you need to know to safely lose weight. It's important to not quit and give up. Do the best you can. Keep a positive attitude. Set a goal. Take one small step at a time to change your habits. Be successful. Take another step. *Slowly build successes.* You will lose the weight.

It's important to know that when you eat fewer calories, sometimes it takes a while for the weight (fat) to exit the body. Too many people don't have enough patience. It's possible to gain three pounds in a week. It may not be possible to lose three pounds of fat in a week. Your body may go into starvation mode and try to hang on to the weight just in case you don't get any food for a while. Your body is just trying to look out for you.

I've noticed that it often takes two to three days of eating less before the weight loss shows up on the scale. By that time, a lot of people quit. On the other hand, when people eat a lot and think that they got away with it, after a few days, the scale will indicate that they've added on some extra weight.

More Secrets You Should Know

For some people, it's easy to lose weight. They are very disciplined and enjoy following a diet plan. However, when this type of dieter quits their diet, the lost weight finds them again. They can't maintain their desired weight. Basically, *if you go back to eating the same amount of food as before or get less physical activity, you'll gain the weight back.*

The truth hurts! Well, here's more … know that if you gain weight, you are most likely simply eating too many calories. People get used to eating a certain amount of calories for their weight. When you lose weight, you have to adjust to eating fewer calories for your new lower weight.

If you think you're exercising a lot and start to regain weight, you need to eat less or exercise even more to lose weight. Besides being active throughout my day, I walk three miles daily to maintain my weight. That's *just to maintain.* For some people, walking three miles a day may seem like a lot. But that's what I've discovered I need to do to match my "energy in" and "energy out" quotient.

Once people hit thirty, they peak and may head down the road toward aging. At forty, people may need to eat less and exercise more to stay the same weight. At fifty, people may need to continue making adjustments and eat less. Be aware that maintaining your weight can be a constant struggle, especially as you get older.

To Recap ◌

Secret #2: When you lose weight, you have to adjust to eating fewer calories for your new lower weight.

Secret #3: If you think that you're exercising a lot and start to regain weight, you need to eat less or exercise even more to lose weight.

Secret #4: As you age, you may need to continue making adjustments and eat less.

In the past, why did you gain weight back when you wanted to be maintaining?

JF: I would gain weight back when I didn't eat enough during the day and by day's end I was hungry enough to eat my houseplants. The concept of grazing throughout the day works for me, and it's the best way for me to keep control of my cravings, emotions, and calories.

You: _____

_____

*R*uth's Rule: *To maintain weight loss, you need to know the insider secrets ... then apply them.*

The Real Reasons People Become Re-Gainers

Weight can be very sneaky. *Every bite counts.* If you're a nibbler, nibbles all day long add up. A bite of cake every time you go into the kitchen adds up. A piece of candy every few hours can add up. Extra spoonfuls of sugar and creamers to coffee drinks add up. Usually, you don't even notice that you're eating so much. However, a food journal will keep you aware of the extra bites. You'll see that avoiding or indulging in little 25-50 calorie bites can make or break weight-loss efforts.

Is it too hard to maintain your new low weight? Are you always hungry? Maybe your *satiety hormones* aren't working as well as they should. Does it take a long time to feel "just right"? Do you end up eating until you feel "full" or "stuffed"? When you eat a reasonable amount of food and want to keep eating, try slices of cucumber. They're mostly water, and the slices will be crunchy and filling. You won't end up eating too many calories and ultimately gain weight.

Do you feel in control for a while, but emotional eating takes over? The longer you've been comforting yourself with food, the harder it will be to change your behavior and lose weight. Your mind and body may want to gravitate to the way things were. Keep working on expressing your emotions. What are you feeling? What do you need? Write in your journal when you need to get the emotions out and there's no one available to chat with you.

Special occasions can slow down the process of losing weight. How about relatives visiting from out of town? Birthday parties for family and friends? Holiday goodies? It's enough to make you forget your focus.

After you lose weight, does your body feel strange? Were you used to your old weight? Maybe the soft padding on your body made you feel comfortable. Is it scary to feel bones that you never felt before? Maybe you're getting more attention, and you don't know how to handle it. Think about being able to comfortably fit into and button your designer jeans. Relax and enjoy. *It's the new you.*

In the last two weeks, have there been obstacles that prevented you from losing weight? Do you see any events that could interfere with eating less in the near future?

JF: This may seem odd but I've found that dating makes it hard for me to lose weight or maintain. Men can seem to eat anything they want. So when they take me out and order everything on page 3 of the menu, they expect me to join in and eat, drink, and be merry. Social eating is my biggest issue. So my plan to succeed is either to become a day trader and never leave the house again or to learn some habits that I can take with me when I am out and about.

You: _____

_____

If there have been obstacles, move on. Make a game plan for future events. (For lots of ideas, see Day 22.) Focus on the present. Forget the past. Who needs regrets?

Go at Your Own Pace

There's no set pattern for losing weight. Most people make a lot of changes and lose a lot of weight in the beginning. Some people are slow and steady. They make small changes and gradually lose a pound here and a pound there. Some people have trouble losing weight. They might lose a little and gain a little.

Some people keep trying to lose those last five pounds. Consistently losing ½-2 pounds a week may not be a realistic goal. Losing one pound a month may be slow but it's better than gaining. It may be a challenge to lose ½ pound a month. If you're persistent, you will keep losing. The key is to not give up.

Discouraged and Don't Care?

Maybe you've decided that you don't like to eat healthy. Would you rather eat greasy burgers and fries and cake instead of fruits and vegetables? Are you compelled to eat a donut on National Donut Day? Is eating a piece of cheesecake more important to you than feeling and looking better and being healthier? Or are the sacrifices that you're making worth the rewards of maintaining the weight?

In the last two weeks, is your enthusiasm starting to wear off? Did you stop being motivated? Have you ever quit a diet because you didn't care anymore?

JF: Wow, what a mind reader you are! I am working hard to stay motivated. I've had some life-altering occurrences in the last few weeks that in the past would have triggered some eating binges. But I now look at change as a way to improve and that includes treating food as my friend and not as my crutch or enemy. I have quit many diets in the past because they seemed restrictive or just too expensive. This diet is a lifestyle with guidelines, not just a public weigh-in.

You: _____

_____

How do you care when you don't care? Do you have any reasons for not caring?

JF: My reasons for not caring have always centered around overconfidence. Just because I can look adorable in a size 14 doesn't mean I should stagnate in my efforts to look better and be healthier.

You: _____

_____

If you don't care, it will be difficult to lose the weight. Have a heart-to-heart talk with yourself. Are you capable of maintaining the changes (by eating less, eating healthy, exercising more)? Will the benefits from changing habits and losing weight outweigh the present situation?

Depressed? Self-Destructive? How to Cope ∞

If you're depressed, can you lose weight? I think that it's possible. Gaining additional weight could make you *more* depressed. If you're feeling depressed, seek help from mental health professionals. In the meantime, continue to set eating and exercise goals. Tell yourself: "I'm depressed and want to eat. But that's okay. I want to lose weight. It's important to me to not regain the weight."

Or maybe you have a self-destructive personality? Just when you lose the weight, you sabotage your efforts and gain the weight back. Get to know yourself. Acknowledging your actions is a step in the right direction. Talk yourself into wanting to eat less.

Since every person is unique, everyone's approach to losing weight is slightly different. Whatever the approach (different degrees of eating less and exercising more), your reasons for losing and maintaining are crucial. Are you at risk for disease? You should be in it for the long haul. It's not healthy to be a yo-yo dieter.

Maybe it's more fun to eat and drink whatever you want. You're very busy with work, and you don't have time for exercise. Well, you're not alone. I've heard it a thousand times. You have a goal to lose weight and keep it off. *Find reasons to care* and make that your priority.

More Reasons People Ditch Diets

Do you eat because you feel sorry for yourself? Maybe you have problems with your job or your relationships. Do you have a child addicted to drugs or in jail? Don't eat out of self-pity. Eating won't change the situation.

Are you losing your focus? Take a look at the people around you. Notice the size of their portions. Count the number of margaritas that they drink. What types of foods are they eating? Analyze their situations. How can you learn from what they're doing, whether it's positive or negative? Do you think you can do better?

Back to Basics ∞

Always remember this rule ... *if you're not hungry, don't eat!!* Eat until you feel "just right." If you're not hungry, no food goes into your mouth. If you only eat when you're hungry and you're not losing weight, what you think is "just right" is too much.

Strategies for Success

When you're losing weight, what you're thinking can be just as important as what you're doing. Below are some strategies that will support your progress.

* ◆ **The rate and amount of weight that you lose is not as important as maintaining a healthy lifestyle.** Keep eating more fruits

and vegetables. Eat less high-fat and added-sugar foods. Get physical activity *every day.*

♦ **If you have a choice between "fat-free" and "sugar-free," choose fat-free.** Fat has more calories than sugar, so you'll be getting fewer calories with fat-free. Of course, a fat-free *and* sugar-free food is even better. Check the label for total calories.

♦ **Don't compare yourself to *anyone else* or how fast you think you should lose weight.** The time it takes to lose weight and the amount of weight lost is very individual.

♦ **Get in the mindset that *less food is better.*** You're not depriving yourself. You are eating smaller amounts of healthy food. If you want to indulge, enjoy something besides food. Or select a food you like that is healthy and low in calories – like blueberries.

♦ **If you're still trying to lose weight but can't, know that it's okay. Maintain for a while.** Maintain your new weight for a few months and get used to eating less at your new weight.

Losing Weight in the Real World

Here's another secret you should know: *the slower you lose the weight, the better.* You will be less likely to regain it. If your progress is slow, it will be more of a lifestyle change – not a desperate attempt to lose weight quickly. It would be easier to maintain weight if:

♦ You stayed at home by yourself all day and all night and didn't have any tempting food.

♦ Your personal chef only gave you small portions of healthy food.

♦ Your friends, family, or work didn't coax or hassle you.

♦ You had your own fully equipped gym and big yard filled with fun stuff to do.

♦ You didn't have a care in the world.

Unfortunately, the real world doesn't always cooperate. If you start gaining weight, is anything different? Analyze the situation. Find a solution.

- Did you start eating too much at social occasions?
- Did you stop your exercise plan?
- Did you start skipping meals?
- Did you start eating unhealthy snacks?
- Did you start drinking too much alcohol?
- Did you go out and eat too much for breakfast, lunch, or dinner?
- Did you stop planning meals?
- Did your portions become too big?
- Did you eat until you were "full" or "stuffed"?
- Did you eat too many "high-fat" foods or "high-calorie" desserts?
- Did you start eating for emotional reasons?
- Did you stop being motivated?

Know Your Red Flags / Green Flags

If you find yourself gaining weight, get out the Red Flags and wave them vigorously. And to stay on track, remind yourself regularly of helpful strategies (the Green Flags).

Red Flag / Green Flag Combos

Red Flag: You go to a party and stuff yourself like there's no tomorrow.

Green Flag: Fight back by allowing yourself to be a little hungry the next day. It's all about balance. Get back to less "energy in" and more "energy out."

Red Flag: You think you're eating way more chocolate than you should today.

Green Flag: This isn't your day to eat healthy. Don't worry about getting enough fruits or milk for the day. If you try to get all of the day's nutrients, you will gain weight.

Red Flag: You relax with family and friends on weekends and eat whatever you want.

Green Flag: Maybe you need to cut back on how you're indulging over the weekend. Weight gain on weekends could cancel out the weight lost during the week.

Red Flag: You eat less on the weekends, when you're relaxed and don't feel hungry, then "stress eat" during the work week.

Green Flag: Be aware of what's happening.

Red Flag: You find yourself gaining 2-3 pounds.

Green Flag: Don't wait until tomorrow. Start cutting back *right away!* Think about what caused the weight gain. Keep trying to eat a little bit less every day and get a little more physical activity every day.

More Green Flags

- **Unless you're on Death Row, save some food for tomorrow.** There's plenty of food and drinks. Try not to overeat.
- **It may be helpful to weigh yourself more often or notice how your clothes fit.** Stay within 2-3 pounds of your goal weight. Decide on an upper limit, and don't go any higher.

Remember, you can enjoy whatever you're eating and drinking – just not in excess amounts. This is a healthy lifestyle.

Reward & Encourage Your Successes

Try giving yourself short-term rewards for small weight losses. These rewards should be things that make you feel good. Pick something small and fun. The possibilities include:

- A movie
- A haircut
- A book
- A magazine
- A manicure
- A tube of lipstick
- A trip to the mall
- A visit to the driving range
- Some new free weights

Do you have a small reward that will motivate you to lose a couple of pounds?

JF: Okay, don't judge me, but I want to pierce my belly button. I also want a tattoo on my ankle. I want all the "hot girl" accessories.

You: _____

_____

What Are You Doing Right?

It's amazing to see the changes that my clients make in a short amount of time. Two weeks isn't much time, but what changes have you made in your routine? What are your successes, even if you haven't come as far as you'd like? How do you feel about these new changes?

JF: I'm proud of the fact that I have gotten to know water so well. I also listen to my body when I'm not getting what I need. I actually have a feeling come over me when I haven't had vegetables in a long time, or I haven't been eating right. Then I listen to my body and correct or add what's missing from my day.

You: _____

_____

Maybe the last two weeks have been super easy for you. Are you staying on track? Are you still highly motivated? What has helped you do so well?

JF: I am motivated. I am working on the *highly* motivated part. To get there, I have to have good old-fashioned discipline and that is just annoying.

You: _____

_____

Maintaining your weight may be difficult. However, it's very important for a healthy lifestyle and essential to end a life of yo-yo dieting. *Relax. Take it slow.* You're getting to know yourself and learning how to lose weight successfully.

Putting It All Together

You're special. *You can do it!* Your goal is to reach your targeted weight and stay there.

To that end, fill out the "Putting It All Together" items below after reviewing the sample version. It's everything that you'll need to stay focused, on one page.

Your maintained weight loss is your new best friend.

WEEKLY REMINDER

Your Reasons for Losing Weight

You should be reminding yourself every day why you want to lose weight. This is your once-a-week reminder.

Why do you want to lose weight? Are your reasons different now that you're halfway through this book?

JF: I want to be healthy inside and out. I want to live a long life and, most importantly, I want to get my belly button pierced (and feel good about others seeing it!).

You: _____

_____

Putting It All Together

Why do you want to lose weight?

I have prediabetes.

I feel depressed and sluggish from the extra weight.

When I walk, my thighs rub together.

What mental and physical triggers make you eat?

When I am lonely and bored, I crave sweets.

To keep up with my high-stress job, I drink a lot of coffee. The caffeine makes me eat fast.

GOALS:

What are problems that need to be changed? What are you going to do?

I eat for my emotions. I will only eat if I am hungry. I will drink 4 ounces of water before meals.

I eat fast. I will chew each bite 10 times. I will eat my meals on a salad plate.

I eat too many sweets. I will limit sweets to 100 calories a day. Or I will replace sweets with fruits.

My arms jiggle. I will do weights for my arms three times a week. MWF.
I will also do 40 sit-ups a day.

If you had a magic wand to make your life perfect ...

What do you want?

I want a job with more money. I want a job with health insurance.

What do you need?

I need more friends.

What is your motivation for losing weight?

What is a short-term reward?

I want more energy.

I am going to Florida for a wedding.

When I lose 10 lbs., I am going to do online dating.

Putting It All Together

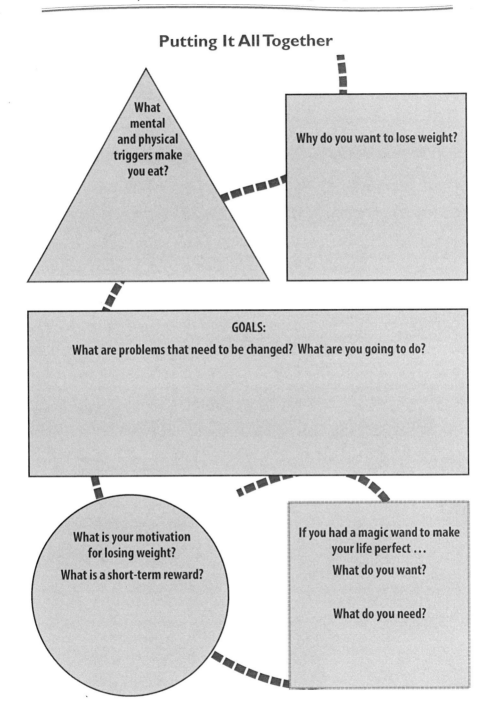

*D*ay 15 CHECK-IN ☑

What did you accomplish yesterday?

JF: I talked to someone when I had a huge craving. Talking to another person dealing with similar challenges made me realize that if I make a call instead of making a sandwich, I might not want that sandwich anymore. I've learned that it's very effective to talk it out.

You: _____

_____

What is your goal for today?

(Pick a strategy from the chapter to use today for staying on track.) (Give yourself encouragement five times a day.) (Start every day with a deep, cleansing breath. Look forward to something.) (Watch out for the nibbles.) (Cut up slices of cucumber.) (Look into buying tapeworms – just kidding!)

JF: My goal is to research those tapeworms online because if it was a bad idea but worked, I guarantee that it still exists somewhere. I will be googling antiquated and deadly ways to lose weight as soon as I am done writing today – just to feel good about what I am doing (and to have material for my stand-up routine).

You: _____

_____

Day 16

What's For Dinner?

"I'm hungry. What's for dinner?"
"I don't know. What do you want?"
"I don't know."

*S*ound familiar? *Decisions, decisions.* Three meals a day. Breakfast, lunch, and dinner, over and over, day after day. It can get old. Maybe you get tired of making and eating the same thing. Maybe you don't want to bother making your own food, so you go out.

Whatever your situation, to lose weight, it's better to keep a relatively consistent routine of portion sizes and number of calories for each meal. To meet that goal, it's a little easier to have fewer food options. You know that you're getting the same number of calories for breakfast with one cup of oatmeal. All bets are off if you eat eggs one day, French toast the next day, something else the following day, etc.

Actually, eating the same food day after day isn't entirely necessary. Variety is possible if you follow a *meal pattern.* For example, eat two grains, one protein, and one fruit for breakfast. That could be a bowl of whole grain cereal, some walnuts, and a small banana. Or it could be two pieces of whole wheat toast, an egg, and some strawberries.

Following the *MyPlate meal patterns* help you stay within a certain number of calories without actually having to *count* calories. It provides "built-in" moderation. Following a pattern also provides balance to ensure that you're getting enough essential nutrients for good health.

A lot of people eat whatever looks good to them. They often don't think about their weight, the calories, or their health. Have you been known to eat this way?

JF: I am guilty of not caring about what I eat when I'm very hungry. It's kind of like I am possessed by aliens and these aliens don't seem to know what calorie-counting is.

You: _____

_____

Let's compromise between what you usually eat and what will help you lose weight and be healthy. I'm confident that you'll be able to eat foods that you enjoy and still lose weight. Some modifications may be necessary. To lose weight and be healthy, you should eat foods that are lower in calories and rich in nutrients. You also have to eat some foods in smaller quantities.

Learn to Think Ahead

Clients tell me all the time that they don't know what they should eat, whether it's breakfast, lunch, or dinner. You've already learned what foods to eat and how much to eat to be healthy. Putting it all together takes some planning and also persistence. You can plan ahead and make a sandwich for lunch. However, if everyone's going out for Mexican food, will the sandwich sit in the refrigerator? Your answer probably depends on the situation.

When it comes to your meals, here's the million-dollar question: Are you willing to make occasional sacrifices? Warm, greasy, salty, crunchy tortilla chips and salsa can be very persuasive. They can also pack on the pounds.

JF: Sacrifice seems like the hardest thing in the world to make when a bad habit has become such a part of my life. I think asking to not take a shower for a month, shave my head, or roll around in a pool of live snakes would be easier, but I may just be being dramatic. Eat more salads? Yes, I can do that.

You: _____

_____

Do you cook? Food made at home is usually lower in calories compared to the food in restaurants. Therefore, it would be helpful to know your way around the kitchen. It doesn't take that much culinary skill to make basic meals. Meals can be low-calorie, healthy, and still be delicious. Sometimes this will require making a few modifications or substitutions to a recipe or your usual way of preparing a meal. As an added bonus, it's less expensive to make your own meals.

Basic Meal Patterns

It seems that everyone who sees me for weight loss wants a food plan. What if I love asparagus, and they hate it? The food plan goes out the window. Instead, I give clients a meal *pattern*. They fill in the blanks with their preferences.

Here is a sample 1,800-calorie meal pattern with equivalents and a sample meal plan:

1,800-Calorie Meal Pattern #1

Breakfast
2 grains
1 cup dairy
½ cup fruit
1 ounce protein

Snack
1 cup dairy

Lunch
2 grains
2 ounces protein
2½ teaspoons oil
½ cup vegetables
1 cup fruit

Snack
1 grain
1 cup dairy

Dinner
2 ounces protein
1 grain

Sample meal plan with 1,800 calories

Breakfast
1 cup cooked oatmeal; sprinkle with cinnamon
1 cup fat-free milk for oatmeal
½ cup frozen blueberries
½ ounce almonds (12 almonds)

Snack
1½ ounces string cheese

Lunch
2 slices rye bread
2 slices (2 ounces) ham
1 tablespoon mayonnaise
½ cup baby carrots
1 small (2½-inch-diameter) apple

Snack
3 cups air-popped popcorn
1 cup low-fat yogurt

Dinner
2 ounces broiled chicken with garlic and lemon
½ cup brown rice

1 cup vegetables	2 cups salad with raw leafy greens
2½ teaspoons oil	2 tablespoons salad dressing
1 cup vegetables	1 cup fresh or frozen broccoli
+ 170 extra calories	3 small cookies

Here is another 1,800-calorie meal pattern with three meals and no snacks.

1,800 Calorie Meal Pattern #2

Breakfast
2 grains
½ cup fruit
1 cup dairy
1 ounce protein

Lunch
2 grains
2 ounces protein
2½ teaspoons oil
¾ cup vegetables
1 cup fruit
1 cup dairy

Dinner
2 grains
2 ounces protein
1 cup dairy
¼ cup vegetables
1¼ teaspoons oil
½ cup vegetables
1 cup vegetables
1¼ teaspoons oil

+ 170 extra calories

Sample meal plan with 1,800 calories

Breakfast
2 slices whole-grain wheat toast
½ banana
1 cup low-fat yogurt
1 tablespoon peanut butter

Lunch
1 cup whole-grain pasta
2 ounces water-packed tuna
1 tablespoon mayonnaise
¾ cup sliced cucumbers
1 orange
1 cup low-fat soy milk

Dinner
1 hamburger bun (2 halves)
2 ounces lean hamburger
1½ ounces low-fat cheddar cheese
1 slice each of tomato and onion
1 tablespoon Thousand Island dressing
½ cup baked beans
1 (8-9 inch) ear of corn
½ tablespoon soft margarine

1 can beer

How did I make these plans? I wrote down the foods that I like and made them fit into the meal pattern. I also included the foods from the *MyPlate's guidelines for eating healthy.* Do you remember that on Day 3, we reviewed the MyPlate recommendations? Below is a recap for your convenience. Feel free to revisit Day 3 if you want more of a refresher.

Review of the MyPlate Guidelines

1,800 Calories a Day = 6 grains, 2.5 cups vegetables, 1.5 cups fruits, 3 cups dairy, 5 ounces protein foods, 5 teaspoons oils, 170 Extra Calories.

- **1 grain** = 1 slice bread, 1 cup dry cereal, or ½ cup cooked rice, pasta, or cooked cereal
- **1 cup vegetables** = 1 cup cooked or raw vegetables or juice, 2 cups raw leafy greens
- **1 cup fruit** = 1 cup fruit or 100% juice, ½ cup dried fruit
- **1 cup dairy** = 1½ ounces cheese, 1 cup milk or yogurt, 2 ounces processed cheese
- **1 ounce protein foods** = 1 ounce lean meat, poultry, or fish, 1 egg, 1 tablespoon peanut butter, ½ ounce nuts or seeds, ¼ cup beans, ¼ cup tofu, or 2 Tbsp hummus
- **Oils** = 1 Tbsp oil = 3 tsp; 1 Tbsp soft margarine = 2½ tsp; 1 Tbsp mayonnaise = 2½ tsp; 1 Tbsp mayonnaise-type salad dressing = 1 tsp; 2 Tbsp Italian dressing = 2 tsp; 2 Tbsp Thousand Island dressing = 2½ tsp. (Confused about oil? Remember that for 1,800 calories, you are aiming for 5 teaspoons of oils daily, using the MyPlate equivalents.)

These meal plans are close estimates to 1,800 calories. The calories may be a little higher or lower depending on the products, measuring techniques, and the size of the fruit. The food plans give you an idea of the types and amounts of foods to eat. Both sample meal plans contain a fair amount of food because low-calorie, high-fiber foods have a lot of bulk. They have plenty of calcium, protein, and fiber. They are also low in fat. These food plans contain balance, variety, and moderation. They have all of the nutrients that you need to be healthy. As a bonus, they also include around 170 calories to enjoy, as you wish.

Eighteen hundred calories is a good food pattern for most people trying to lose weight. You may choose a food pattern with fewer or more calories, depending on how much you weigh and your activity level. If you stop losing weight at a certain pattern, choose one of the MyPlate meal patterns with fewer calories. Keep using the pattern as a guide at home, at work, when eating out, and while traveling, to the best of your ability. You don't have to be perfect.

*R*uth's Rule: *A meal pattern is a great way to plan what you're going to eat, while creating nutritious meals you'll like within targeted calorie goals.*

It's Your Turn

It's time to make your own meal plan. Use Meal Pattern #1 as a sample. Start by filling in the blanks with the foods that you like to eat. For example, "I have to eat pancakes for breakfast." Make it fit within the pattern. Have two small pancakes, instead of a stack of five big pancakes. Maple syrup counts as some of your extra calories. Fill in all of the blanks. See where you can make low-calorie substitutions. Perhaps you could choose sugar-free syrup instead of maple syrup to save your extra calories.

Feel free to experiment with the meal pattern. If you want to eat small, frequent amounts throughout the day, take out the food groups from the meals and make them snacks. Maybe one day you want more protein for dinner. Then take out a carbohydrate so that the total calories remain relatively constant.

Dealing with Combination Foods ౿౩

Meal Plans #1 and #2 contain individual foods. Many foods are *combination foods*. Combination foods contain more than one food group. For example, a beef stew with beef and vegetables. Sushi has fish and rice. Pizza has crust, tomato sauce, vegetables, and cheese. When you look at a combination food, break it down into components. How many grains, protein foods, vegetables, and oils in a taco? It could contain 2 grains (2 tortillas), 2 protein foods (2 ounces of chicken), 1 vegetable (onions and salsa), and 6 oils (fried tortilla).

1,800-calorie meal pattern	Your meal plan
Breakfast	**Breakfast**
2 grains	_____
1 cup dairy	_____
½ cup fruit	_____
1 ounce protein	_____
Snack	**Snack**
1 cup dairy	_____
Lunch	**Lunch**
2 grains	_____
2 ounces protein	_____
2½ teaspoons oil	_____
½ cup vegetables	_____
1 cup fruit	_____
Snack	**Snack**
1 grain	_____
1 cup dairy	_____
Dinner	**Dinner**
2 ounces protein	_____
1 grain	_____
1 cup vegetables	_____
2 ½ teaspoons oil	_____
1 cup vegetables	_____
+ 170 extra calories	_____

Easy Meal Improvements

Sometimes people don't know if their meals are healthy. Let's say that this is a typical lunch:

Lunch at Home

♦ Bologna sandwich on two pieces of white bread with mayonnaise
♦ Bag of chips
♦ Apple juice
♦ Candy bar

There are many possibilities for improving this lunch. Basically, this meal is high in fat and sugar, low in fiber, and lacking nutrients. To lower the calories and fat and to make it nutrient-rich, here are a few suggestions:

Improvements

- 1 or 2 slices of whole-wheat bread, depending on your grain status for the day
- A low-fat bologna or a slice of leftover chicken breast from last night's dinner
- Mustard or fat-free mayonnaise instead of regular mayonnaise
- Add romaine lettuce, spinach leaves, a tomato slice, and a few dried cranberries to the sandwich
- Orange juice fortified with calcium, or fat-free chocolate milk
- Apple

Here's a typical lunch from a restaurant:

Lunch at Restaurant

- 6 ounces hamburger on a white bun
- Slice of cheddar cheese, a piece of lettuce
- A big glob of Thousand Island dressing on the burger
- Fries covering half of the plate
- 16 ounces soda or lemonade

How do you make it a healthier restaurant meal?

Improvements

- Only eat 2-4 ounces of the hamburger.
- If it's a giant bun, tear off some of the bun.
- If possible, choose a whole-grain bun.
- Skip the cheese.
- Scrape off some of the dressing from the burger.
- Think about sharing the hamburger with someone.
- Order a salad with dressing on the side instead of fries.
- Drink water, iced tea, diet soda, or fat-free milk.

Bing. Bang. Boom. You have cut 500 calories, maybe more!

Do you see what you have to do to lower the calories and increase the nutrients?

JF: Yes, I do see it. When I follow a meal plan, I am full for a longer period of time. And the most miraculous thing of all is that light mayonnaise tastes exactly the same as regular mayo! I might alert the news of this finding.

You: _____

_____

Getting Up to Speed

Modifying your meals is all about making healthier choices. Instead of 6-8 ounces of fatty corned beef, pastrami, or salami, choose 2-3 ounces of lean roast beef or turkey and more veggies. Instead of pepperoni or sausage pizza, choose vegetable or chicken pizza. It contains more nutrients and less unhealthy fat. Don't forget to watch portion sizes.

I strongly recommend taking the time to make a meal plan, which can include eating out. Just fill in the blanks. It eliminates the question, "What's for dinner?" and does away with high calorie, unhealthy choices.

If you like variety, make a meal plan for three or four weeks. If you like to keep it simple, make a plan for one week to get you started and keep repeating it. Stick with the same two or three breakfasts and lunches to make it easier in the beginning.

This takes some thinking and may feel like a chore. But you know what they say, _learn by doing_. "Give a man a fish; you have fed him for today. Teach a man to fish, and you have fed him for a life-time." (Author unknown) "Teach a man to cook fish and to make a meal plan with fish two times a week, and you have improved his health." (Author – me)

Once you get the hang of it, planning meals is easy. The goal is not to be dependent on someone else's meal plan. Your plan will have your personal food preferences. It will include all of the necessary food groups, including important nutrients. _Be creative. Make it your own._

I like to follow a meal pattern because I don't have to count calories. The closest I come to counting calories is the 170 calories for a treat every day. If I go over the 170, I will eat one less grain. One hundred seventy calories is a lot easier to count than 1,200 or 1,800 calories for an entire day. After a while, you can calculate the amounts in your head: 6 grains, 5 ounces protein foods, 2½ cups vegetables, 1½ cups fruits, 3 cups dairy, and 5 teaspoons oil, depending on your meal pattern.

Another Approach - The "New American Plate"

Meal patterns should contain approximately 45-65% carbohydrates, 10-35% lean protein, and 20-35% fat. *Percentages* are another way to think about what to eat. However, percentages are hard for me to visualize. I have never taken the time to calculate the percentages of nutrients. I do, however, try to estimate them.

An easy way to estimate the percentages is to follow the American Institute for Cancer Research's *"New American Plate."* Here's how it breaks down:

- Seventy percent of your plate is plant-based. (Plant foods reduce your risk of disease.)
- Vegetables, fruits, whole grains, and beans cover two-thirds of the plate.
- Meat, poultry, fish, or low-fat milk products are the remaining 30% of the plate.
- The protein section is about the size of a deck of cards.
- Rice or pasta looks like half of a baseball for each grain.

The New American Plate is an easy, practical way to visualize healthy eating and is very similar to MyPlate.

Are you eating healthier? Was your last meal 70% plant-based? Do you need to make improvements? Was there too much protein? Not enough? Too many grains? Not enough? No vegetables? A lot of fried foods? Too many sweets? Too much alcohol? Was it just right?

JF: Many of these questions sound like if I answered yes, it would have been a deliciously deadly meal. However, I am learning to eat healthier day by day. And when emotional eating is an issue, do I remember that a glass of wine is healthier than a bottle? Of course … fingers crossed behind back.

You: _____

Healthy eating may seem rather bland compared to what you are used to eating. However, it's probably more natural and less processed. Eating healthy and cooking healthy can be easy and tasty.

Substitutions for Healthier Recipes

Are you ready to step into the kitchen and modify some recipes? A few simple changes can make almost any recipe healthy. *Healthy cooking limits the amount of unhealthy fat, sugar, and salt and uses healthy fats.* If you have a recipe that contains two cups of cheese, eight ounces of cream cheese, and one cup of sour cream, it may sound like creamy, cheesy goodness. But, as far as the saturated fat and calories go, it's not so good.

How can you cut out some of the calories? Instead of two cups of Monterey Jack cheese, choose one cup of low-fat mozzarella cheese. Instead of full-fat cream cheese and sour cream, choose fat-free or low-fat versions. There will be a significant decrease in saturated fat and calories with these types of modifications. There will be little difference in taste and texture.

Making substitutions to recipes can increase the nutrients and also decrease the calories. Take out the bacon and add peppers. Throw in extra vegetables any time for more nutrients. A package of thawed, drained spinach added to a jar of spaghetti sauce will add oodles of nutrients.

Let's take a look at a yummy recipe for spinach and artichoke dip. It's warm, bacony goodness. It's also a heart attack on a cracker.

Spinach and Artichoke Dip

1 (10 ounce) package frozen chopped spinach, thawed and drained
1 (6½ ounce jar) marinated artichoke hearts, drained and chopped
2 tablespoons butter
½ cup red onion
1 tablespoon minced garlic
1 teaspoon salt

½ teaspoon freshly ground black pepper
1 cup heavy cream
1 cup shredded Monterey Jack cheese
3 strips of cooked bacon
½ cup Parmesan cheese

Preheat the oven to 350 degrees. Melt the butter in a sauté pan. Sauté the onion. Add the garlic, salt, and pepper. Add the spinach, artichoke hearts, Monterey Jack cheese, and bacon. Stir in the cream. Pour mixture in baking dish. Top with Parmesan cheese. Bake for 20 minutes or until bubbly. Served with slices of baguette bread.

This recipe is delicious but has too many calories from unhealthy fats. To make the dip healthier, cut out and/or reduce the fat, choose a healthier fat, and add more fiber in the form of vegetables. Below is a healthy version of the recipe with a few ingredient changes.

Low-Fat Spinach and Artichoke Dip
1 (10 ounce) package frozen chopped spinach, thawed and drained
1 (9 ounce) package frozen artichoke hearts, thawed and chopped
3 tablespoons olive oil
½ cup chopped red onion
½ cup chopped red bell pepper
½ cup shredded carrot
1 tablespoon minced garlic
1 teaspoon freshly ground black pepper
½ teaspoon thyme
1 cup skim ricotta cheese
1 cup shredded part-skim mozzarella cheese

Preheat the oven to 350 degrees. Heat the oil in a sauté pan over medium heat. Sauté onion, red pepper, and carrot until vegetables are soft. Add garlic, pepper, and thyme. Mix in spinach, artichoke hearts, ricotta cheese, and mozzarella cheese. Pour mixture into a baking dish. Bake for 20 minutes. Serve with pieces of whole-grain crackers or raw vegetables.

The modified recipe is bursting with flavor and health. It's low fat and loaded with fiber and calcium, yet colorful, comforting, and tasty. *Win-win.*

Do you see what I'm saying? The dip is healthier with only a few changes. Instead of butter, heavy cream, and Monterey Jack cheese, use olive oil, skim ricotta cheese, and mozzarella cheese. Use frozen artichoke hearts to cut out some of the oil calories from the marinated artichokes. Don't bother adding the salt. There's plenty of sodium in the cheese. The bacon and Parmesan cheese can be eliminated. There are enough flavors from the vegetables. The healthier version is different, but it still tastes great.

Try It, They'll Like It

Some people seem stuck on tradition. I had a client who made a decadent, very high-fat stuffing for Thanksgiving. Her relatives demanded that she make it every year. She knew it wasn't healthy and wanted to change. One year, she took out the high-fat foods and added vegetables and other healthy ingredients. She couldn't believe it. No one noticed. Moral of the story: *Change is good.* You may like it more, or you might not even notice.

Here are some ingredient substitutions that you can make to lower calories and increase health.

Healthy Ingredient Substitutions

I cup butter or margarine in baking	½ cup applesauce or ½ cup pureed prunes and ½ cup oil
I egg	2 egg whites or ¼ cup egg substitute
3 eggs	2 eggs
I cup sugar	¾ cup sugar
Butter or stick margarine	Equal amounts of soft margarine
Solid fat in baking	Use olive or canola oil (for ⅓ cup solid fat use ¼ cup oil).
All-purpose flour	Whole-wheat flour or blend oatmeal to make oat flour. Use in place of half of the all-purpose flour.
Pastry dough	Graham cracker crust
Frosting	Sprinkle with powdered sugar
Mayonnaise	Fat-free or low-fat mayonnaise
Sour cream	Fat-free sour cream or plain yogurt
Cream cheese	Low-fat or fat-free cream cheese

Ground beef	Extra-lean ground beef or ground turkey
Bacon	Turkey bacon
Ricotta cheese	Part-skim ricotta cheese
1 cup shredded cheddar cheese	1 cup reduced-fat cheddar cheese
1/2 cup beans in soup	1 cup beans (to increase vegetables)
1 cup green beans in casseroles	2 cups green beans (doubling the amount)

Look for these terms on the labels: "Free," "low," "light," "reduced," "lean" and "extra lean."

Every little bit less helps.

Healthy Food Substitutions

White rice	Brown rice, wild rice, barley, or whole grain pasta
Sour cream or butter on baked potatoes	Plain Greek yogurt, salsa, or Italian dressing (2 tablespoons of butter on a baked potato adds 200 calories and 23 grams of fat.)
Regular ice cream	Low-fat ice cream
Salad dressing	Low-fat or fat-free dressing or balsamic vinegar or lemon juice with pepper or salsa
Pasta with vegetables	Make it vegetables with pasta (1/2 the amount of pasta and double the amount of vegetables).

Experiment the next time you whip up something in the kitchen ...

- **ELIMINATE** high-fat ingredients (bacon, cheese, sour cream). Eliminate the salt.
- **SUBSTITUTE** healthy fat (olive oil, canola oil, or sunflower oil, instead of butter, margarine, or lard). Choose a low-fat, fat-free or low-sodium version (fat-free sour cream or fat-free cream cheese). Use applesauce instead of the fat in baking. Switch to a whole grain (barley, whole-grain pasta). Choose ground turkey or a leaner hamburger. Use part whole-wheat flour instead of all white flour.

◆ **MODIFY** the recipe to add more nutrients. Add oatmeal, more vegetables, beans, powdered milk, dried fruit, and whole grains. Use half the amount of certain ingredients (cheese, oil, meat, pasta).

Now you know how to make a recipe lower in calories and healthier. Can you think of ways to modify a favorite recipe and make substitutions?

JF: I sure can! Whole wheat pasta for this Italian food lover. Plus, I can mix vegetables into just about everything I cook or eat.

You: _____

---

*R*uth's Rule: *Don't be afraid to modify recipes for healthier, more nutritious food that tastes great without extra calories and fat.*

Play with a "5-Ingredient" Cookbook ⁓

Some people don't cook. However, there are millions of cookbooks. Try a "5-ingredient" cookbook. These cookbooks are helpful if you don't cook and don't have a lot of ingredients. Even with only five ingredients, it may be necessary to make a couple of modifications and substitutions to increase the nutrients and decrease the calories and fat.

For your cooking convenience, buy prepared foods, such as pre-cut or shredded vegetables, pre-washed spinach, shredded low-fat cheese, precooked chicken, or jars of minced garlic, chopped frozen onions, frozen fish, and frozen vegetables. To get the most out of cooking, double the recipe, divide up the leftovers into serving-sized portions, and freeze them. You'll have a healthy meal ready to go any time.

Now You're Ready

The next time someone asks you, "What's for dinner?" you will be ready. Following MyPlate meal patterns makes eating easy. Fill in the blanks with foods that you enjoy.

Watch out for the extra carbohydrates, fat, alcohol, and sweets. When you're losing weight, aim for around 170 calories a day of the "extras." If you can live without the "extras" or can't control the amount consumed, don't eat them. The less you eat of them, the more weight you will lose.

Your goal is to instantly analyze a recipe or a meal and decide what it needs or doesn't need so that nutrients increase and calories decrease. You're in the driver's seat. Enjoy healthy, nutritious, and balanced meals.

A meal pattern is your new best friend.

ⅅay 16 CHECK-IN ☑

What did you accomplish yesterday?

JF: My gym membership expired. You know the gym I never went to? So I joined a lower priced gym that I can walk to from home. My primary issue was the commute to the gym and now I have no excuse!

You: _____

_____

What is your goal for today?

(Plan your meals for a week.) (Choose a recipe to modify – eliminate ingredients and/or make substitutions.) (Follow a meal pattern for breakfast.) (Make a low-fat, high-fiber lunch.) (Eat a two-thirds plant-based dinner.)

JF: I will write out my meal plan and shopping list so that I can purchase the foods I need to have a productive, healthy week.

Meanwhile, I need to stop eating emotionally!! I need to find an activity that takes me away from putting a spoon in the ice cream and lifting the spoon to my mouth. Maybe the new gym will help.

You: _____

_____

Day 17

Just Call … I'll Be There

*H*ave you ever thought, "I shouldn't be eating this" – while nibbling a treat? In hindsight, truth be told, that's the most likely reason you're not losing weight. We don't want to admit the extra calories we're wolfing down. I had a client tell me that she only ate one meal a day (protein and vegetables for dinner) and couldn't lose weight. Later she said she was in denial. She didn't want to admit that the pint of ice cream she was eating after dinner prevented her from losing weight.

Believe it or not, some people don't have a clue that the bags of dried pork rinds and the 6 to 10 beers they indulge in over the weekends are the reasons they're stuck at a certain weight.

Life is a struggle. Losing weight is a struggle. It's hard to cope by yourself. If you don't have to do it alone, why should you? When attempting to lose weight, it can be beneficial to have a support person – even a support team. If you need support to achieve your goals, *ask for it.*

*R*uth's **Rule:** *Having support to meet weight - loss challenges can help you be successful.*

What Challenges You?

Since everyone's situation is different, everyone has different obstacles and challenges. The first step is to identify the problem areas in your social environment.

For some people, *family* is the biggest challenge.

- Does your family go out for dinner *a lot* ... because no one makes dinner?
- If you eat dinner at home, are the meals high in fat, low in nutrients, and missing vegetables?
- Is your home full of high-calorie snack foods?
- Is someone in your household pressuring you to eat more than you want?
- Does everyone sit around all night, watch television, and munch on snack food?
- Is there someone who likes to go out for dessert?
- Are the family dynamics dysfunctional? Do you use food to cope?
- Is food the focus at home?
- Are family gatherings and holiday celebrations loaded with lots of unhealthy food?
- Do your relatives drop by with pastries and other goodies?

Why don't relatives ever pressure you to eat vegetables? When do you hear, "Come on. Have some more broccoli." It's always, "Have another chocolate chip cookie."

Does your family sabotage your efforts to eat less or eat healthy?

JF: Funny you should ask ... I am just returning from a family vacation and let's just say that if it is fried, had parents, tastes sweet, or would stick to a wall if you threw it against one, my family served that to me. In other words, my family's cooking is AWESOME! It's just not conducive to wanting single-digit sizes in your closet.

You: _____

_____

For other people, *work* is the biggest challenge.

- Lots of businesses want employees to hang around work. Does your employer provide free soda and unhealthy snacks?
- Some workplaces don't have refrigerators or microwaves for employees to use. Is going out for lunch the only option?

- Do co-workers have bowls of candy on their desks?
- Are there vending machines with no healthy choices?
- Does the cafeteria have too many high-fat, high-sodium foods?
- Are there always cookies and donuts at staff meetings?
- Do you feel pressure at work and eat to relieve stress?
- Is there no time to take a break, causing you to overeat at meals?
- Do co-workers want you to go out for lunch?
- Are business meals at restaurants a regular part of your job?

Does your work sabotage your efforts to eat less or eat healthy?

JF: Well, since I work for myself, the answer to that is yes!! I sabotage myself when I don't cook or shop, and I eat foods served by people wearing little hats. Fast food is a big problem. This is the reason I spend most of my time now washing dishes because cooking has become a regular part of my life.

You: _____

For some people, *friends* are the biggest challenge.

- When you go out with friends, do they push you to drink more alcohol than you want?
- Do your friends only socialize around food?
- Do you feel obligated to eat too much with your friends so you'll be "big" like them?
- When you go to the movies, do your friends like to "pig out" on snacks?
- If you don't follow your friends' behavior, do you worry about what they'll think?

How do friends sabotage your efforts to eat less or eat healthy?

JF: The excuse-making Jackie would say that all my friends are evil. However, the truth is that I do it to myself. My real friends offer encouragement when I attempt to eat properly.

You: _____

What about *you?* Maybe you're also your worst enemy. Are *you* your biggest challenge?

+ Do you put yourself down?
+ Are you too hard on yourself and set unrealistic goals?
+ Are you too easy on yourself and don't set limits, especially after a stressful day?
+ Do you not care?
+ Are you self-destructive?
+ Do you use food to comfort yourself?
+ Do you always have an excuse?

What have you done to sabotage your efforts to eat less or eat healthy that you're willing to admit?

JF: I will admit that I drink wine and then ignore the fact that alcohol makes one defenseless against junk food. I will admit that when I'm dating, I make excuses for my eating by saying I ate what he ate. I will admit that I have too many things to admit and will just move on now because I'm making myself upset.

You: _____

_____

Is everyone and everything a challenge? It is, to some people. Maybe this is the time to get rid of toxic relationships. You could say, "If you're not going to be supportive while I'm trying to lose weight, then bye-bye." *Ouch!* That's a little cold and, quite frankly, not very realistic. You have to live with your family and go to work. It's better to be diplomatic and ask for their support. You have the power to make things happen.

Solutions for Home

OK, first of all, you don't have to be a victim of the status quo at home. Make some changes! Here are possible solutions:

+ If you're the grocery shopper, delegate the grocery shopping to someone else who won't buy the goodies that tempt you to go off your program.

- Only keep healthy foods around.
- Keep all of the temptations in one place. If necessary, have them locked up or hidden.
- Only have goodies around that you don't like. (However, in a pinch, you'd be surprised what you'll eat. I've known clients to take a bite of a candy bar, throw the candy away, and then get it out of the garbage and eat it.)
- Make a family policy to not use food as a reward or a bribe. An "A" on a report card shouldn't be an excuse to get a donut or ice cream. Instead, go to the zoo, go bowling, play miniature golf, or give them a big smile and a hug.
- Limit the number of meals at restaurants. Go out one time a week.
- Have a family member tell you, "Food won't solve your problems. Is there anything that I can do?"
- Instead of watching television every night, take a class with a family member.
- Have a "no dessert" policy at home, except for special occasions.
- Have a family member dish up your plate.
- Have a family member take a more aggressive role. If you're seen eating chips, it may be someone's job to take them away.
- On the other hand, maybe when someone tells you what to do, it makes you eat more. In that case, tell the person to not say anything.

Pick a problem. Decide what would help you.

For example, you might say, "Kim, I'm trying to lose weight. There are always potato chips in the house. When you go shopping, would you please not buy chips? They're too tempting for me. Once I start eating them, I can't stop. If you have to buy chips, would you put them away somewhere that I can't find them?" This is a real-life situation. This is a reasonable request.

Who do you want to support you at home? What do you want them to do?

JF: I live on my own so let's just say I want to support myself every day and not give up when I give in. GO, TEAM JACKIE! NOW PUT THE DONUTS DOWN! See? I feel good already.

You: _____

_____

Solutions for Work

Since people spend a lot of time at work, it would be good to have a healthy environment there. The workplace has the potential to *promote health*, instead of causing problems. Until your company is in compliance, take action into your own hands.

Here are some solutions for work:

◆ If the break room has too many temptations, volunteer to do the shopping. Only buy healthy snacks. You'll do everyone a favor.

◆ Form a health committee. There's strength in numbers. You're not the only person who wants to cut back and eat healthier.

◆ Promote the stairwells at work for climbing. Put up pictures of scenic views. Start a "Take the Stairs" club. If the stairs are normally locked for safety reasons, open them up during the lunch hour.

◆ Walk during lunch with co-workers.

◆ Form a group of employees for 5K or 10K charity walk/runs.

◆ Create a company team for baseball, softball, or volleyball.

Has this ever happened to you? The woman in the next cubicle loves to make people happy. She keeps a big bowl of candy on her desk. People drop by her desk a couple times a day, *including you*. It takes a strong person to resist mouth-watering sweets day after day, especially when your project is past its deadline. At that point in time, your willpower is not at its peak. Try talking to your co-worker.

You could say, "Alice, I'm trying to lose weight. I know some of the other people on the floor are also trying to lose weight. We're too tempted by your candy. Would you mind not bringing it to work or keep it out of sight?" It's not unreasonable to ask people to cooperate. No one really needs candy every day. If it's there, people are going to eat it.

Who do you want to support you at work? What do you want them to do?

JF: I work for myself and I want to be the support I need. Being around a lot of people is actually a shield for me and a way for me to avoid dealing with myself. I flourish socially when around as few as two people, and by flourishing, I mean I eat whatever is around as a way to socialize. I need to be the support I want.

You: _____

Solutions for Friends

The area of your friendships is another place where you can be a positive influence.

Here are some solutions for friends:

- Instead of going out with a friend for dessert, go for a walk together. If physical activity isn't practical, choose to eat fewer calories. Share a pastry. Order a beverage without calories. The point is being with the person, not an excuse to blow your caloric intake for the day.
- Find a weight-loss buddy who also wants to lose weight. *Support each other.*
- If you have food cravings or feel like bingeing, arrange to call someone.
- Bring healthy foods to holiday potlucks thrown by friends.
- If going to a restaurant is your excuse to eat too many carbs, ask your support buddy to remind you to watch the bread and butter or chips and salsa. Or have your support buddy remind you to order salad instead of French fries.
- When you play cards with friends once a month, limit the treats to one sweet per person. It doesn't have to be a feast. Who wants sticky, smudged cards?
- When you go to the movies, decide ahead of time to only watch the movie – not eat snacks.
- Decide with your support friend whether Happy Hour is worth the free high-fat appetizers. Have a friend remind you to only order one drink.
- When you go out, ask your support friend to share a meal.

- Talk to friends about accepting "No, thank you" as your final answer.
- Take a friend to a farmers market or enroll in a stress reduction class together.
- Some people don't and won't exercise alone. Find an exercise buddy. Will they go to the gym with you? Be a dance partner? Take a walk or jog with you? Rollerblade on the path along the beach? Shoot hoops at the park? Go to the batting cage? Play golf? Take your dogs for a hike?

Has this ever happened to you? Your best friend likes to go to restaurants and bars. Sometimes you aren't hungry and don't feel like drinking. You end up having a big meal and three or four beers. You are not losing weight, and you're getting discouraged.

You could say, "Steve, you're my best friend. I like getting together with you but I'm trying to lose weight. My blood pressure is up, and the doctor says that I have to lower my cholesterol. Instead of going out for dinner a few times a week, let's go to the driving range and hit a bucket of golf balls. I would also like to go to the batting cage." Getting the physical activity would be good for both of you. Being with friends shouldn't only be about eating and drinking. You can still talk, get exercise, and have fun, too.

Do you have a friend who could give you support? What do you want them to do?

JF: I look to men I am intimate with to support me. When cooking, loving, laughing, and spending time with a man I care about, I usually let all guards down and eat because I am content and happy. That's when I seem to crave the extra ranch dressing.

You: _____

_____

Motivating Yourself

You're with yourself all day long. Who better to get on your side?

How can you help yourself?

- If you love food, accept that you eat more than you need. Maybe a light will go on, and you won't feel like you have to eat so much.
- Try to recreate how it felt the last time you lost 20 pounds. When willpower is in control, it's a great feeling.
- Are you in a bad mood? Angry? Frustrated? Bitter? Tell yourself that food won't change anything. It hasn't resolved problems before, and it won't this time.
- When you're by yourself and want to eat, find a distraction. Do something to stop thinking about food. Take a bubble bath. Call a friend who makes you laugh.
- Do you eat in secret? Eating in a restaurant can offer support with accountability.
- Do you feel deprived? Allow yourself a 100-calorie prepackaged treat (cookies, mini-muffins) every day.
- Think about something to take away your appetite. Have you ever seen survival shows where the person is forced to gouge out a dead animal's eyeball for food? Remembering something totally gross can take away any trace of appetite immediately.
- Get professional help. You don't have to feel isolated.
- Talk yourself out of eating by telling yourself, "This doesn't taste that great" (even though it's your favorite). Taste can be psychological. Retrain your palate to not like sweetened, salty, or greasy food.
- If you won't exercise by yourself, join a running club or a hiking club. Go to the driving range. Buy a gym membership – and use it. Join the YMCA or YWCA.
- Do you always have excuses for "going off your diet"? Someone is mad at you? Pressure from work? Too many bills? Health scare? Stop making excuses to eat every time something happens. There will always be something to keep you from being consistent. *No more excuses.* Stop feeling sorry for yourself.
- Does your life need structure or consistency? Make rules. Allow yourself three meals a day.

- Some people find it helpful to join a support group to vent. Other people find it annoying to listen to other people whine. Decide for yourself what works for you.
- When you feel like eating and you're not hungry, persuade yourself to first gulp down a beverage with no calories.
- Feeling stressed? Take five minutes to relax, breathe, and remind yourself why you want to lose weight.
- Be the president of your own fan club. Not many people eat perfectly. The last thing you need is to criticize yourself. Give yourself a break. Work on being positive. You have the ability to change, regardless of everything else going on in your life.

Has this ever happened to you? You tell yourself, "I know that I'm trying to eat healthier and lose weight. And I'm doing great at home and work. But when I go to parties and conventions, I can't resist eating too much free food and drinking too much free wine. I would like to make a rule. I can sample a small portion of the food and have a no-calorie drink. I can even make a game out of eating a limited number of calories. But I won't pig out any more at these events."

What can you do to help you? How can you support yourself?

JF: I can talk it out when I feel like turning to food for companionship. And I can learn to get up, get out, and meditate or exercise when I feel like I am living outside of myself and think junk food will make me feel better.

You: _____

_____

Keep in mind that sometimes you can't do it all yourself. Nice people love helping others. Look for someone who can offer understanding and encouragement. The more help you get, the easier it will be for you to lose weight. Tell a friend or co-worker to help you stay on track when you're tempted by free offerings at parties and conventions.

S.O.S. – Seek Out Support

In times of trouble, it's especially easy to fall back on your old habits. The recurring theme is *ask for help*. What obstacles in your life are preventing you from achieving a healthy weight? Who are the problem people? What are the problem situations? Figure out who could be on your side. Think about what you want them to do, along with when, where, and how they can support you.

- Do you want someone to keep you motivated?
- Do you want to ask someone to not sabotage your efforts?
- Do you want someone to eat healthy and exercise with you?
- Do you want someone to say "no" for you?
- Do you want someone to stay out of it?
- Do you want someone to hold you accountable to your goals?
- Do you want someone to be a cheerleader and give you encouragement?
- Do you want someone to listen to you so you can vent?
- Do you want someone to ask you how you feel?
- Do you want someone to ask you if you need anything?

If you communicate, cooperation is possible. No one can read your mind. Use your words, and people will understand where you are coming from and flock to your aid. If someone turns out to be a hindrance, don't get stuck. Find someone else to help you. A person willing to support you is like a person throwing you a life preserver. Put it on. Their support and encouragement can help you. It could save your life.

A supportive person is your new best friend.

$\mathcal{D}$ay 17 CHECK-IN ☑

What did you accomplish yesterday?

JF: After breakfast, I got right to work, instead of focusing on what to eat every minute of the day. Staying busy is how I keep my head out of the refrigerator.

You: _____

_____

What is your goal for today?

(Ask a family member to stop buying unhealthy snacks or to hide them in your home.) (Tell a friend who is sabotaging your efforts that you can't go to lunch with them every day.) (Have a friend remind you that you're trying to eat less.) (Find an exercise buddy.) (Ask a co-worker to walk with you at lunch or play tennis with you on weekends.) (Tell a relative to not offer you food.) (Carry fruit with you to avoid buying candy in the afternoon.) (Tell yourself that you're doing a great job.)

JF: Eat the food I cooked rather than get into my car and drive to eat food that will only make me feel guilty afterwards.

You: _____

_____

Day 18

Fruits and Veggies ... The Art of Eating Enough

"Eat your fruits and vegetables." Did your mother tell you this?

Survey after survey shows that adults and children aren't eating enough fruits and vegetables. In fact, some surveys show that 87% of Americans aren't getting the recommended amounts. The Dietary Guidelines for Americans recommends eating 2½-6½ cups of fruits and vegetables a day in accordance with 1,200-3,200 calorie levels. People seem to know the importance of eating fruits and vegetables. Yet when it comes down to it, they aren't eating as much as their bodies need.

It would be a good idea for someone to tell more mothers to eat their fruits and vegetables. If mother isn't buying, serving, and eating lots of produce, it's unlikely that she is encouraging her family to do so. Consequently, fruits and vegetables may not be part of a child's lifestyle now and later in life.

When you were young, did fruits and vegetables show up as a regular part of your meals? Did you eat them?

JF: Nope. Fruits and veggies were never put in front of me as a requirement. My parents never made me eat them. They left a lot of my food choices up to me and I chose cheese.

You: _____

_____

What is your current status of fruit and vegetable consumption?

JF: I have vegetables a few times a week, usually when they are accompanied by other foods like steak and something in gravy. Forgive me, Father for I continue to sin because I don't like vegetables. However, I do know how to make them tasty so this is an area I need to work on.

You: _____

_____

Fruits and Veggies Are Nutritious

Fruits and vegetables are loaded with vitamins, minerals, fiber, phytonutrients, and fluid. These nutrients are essential for your health. The nutrients in fruits and vegetables can reduce your risk of high blood pressure, stroke, elevated cholesterol, heart disease, type 2 diabetes, some types of cancer, diverticulosis, neural tube birth defects, kidney stones, bone loss, and cataracts. Eating fruits and vegetables can even help you lose weight since they fill you up with fewer calories.

Fruits and vegetables are good sources of vitamin C, vitamin A (carotenoids), folate, potassium, and fiber. By the way, "folate" is found naturally in food. "Folic acid" is the synthetic form of folate found in supplements.

Vitamin C helps heal wounds, keeps teeth and gums healthy, and increases the absorption of iron. Sources of vitamin C include citrus fruit and juices, such as oranges and grapefruits, along with leafy greens, broccoli, red and green peppers, kiwi, pineapples, mangoes, melons, berries, tomatoes, cabbage, Brussels sprouts, and potatoes.

Vitamin A protects against infection and is good for eyes and skin. Sources of vitamin A include orange fruits and vegetables, such as cantaloupes, yams, carrots, pumpkin and squash, along with dark leafy greens, tomatoes, and red peppers.

Folate helps form red blood cells and protects women from having a baby with a brain or spinal cord defect. Sources of folate include cooked dry beans and peas, oranges, spinach, and fortified grain products.

Potassium helps maintain normal blood pressure. Sources of potassium include potatoes, spinach, squash, bananas, oranges, cantaloupe, cooked dry beans, tomatoes, peaches, prunes, apricots, kiwi, mangoes, papayas, and avocado.

Fiber isn't only "nature's broom." Besides being filling, high-fiber foods lower cholesterol and decrease the risk of coronary heart disease. Sources of fiber include all types of beans and most fruits and vegetables. Don't peel apples, pears, or potatoes. Important fiber and nutrients are in the skin.

For Variety, Occasionally Juice Your Vegetables ○る

Juicing is an option for fruits and vegetables. Green apples and celery is a refreshing juice with a gorgeous color. If the juicer only squeezes out the juice, you'll miss out on nutrients and fiber from the pulp.

What fruit or vegetable best describes your personality? Why?

JF: Wow. This is an interesting question. I think broccoli best describes me because it's only during the last couple of years that people have been adding broccoli to everything and seeing how it can be added to most meals. Like broccoli, I adapt easily to different environments. I am also delicious when covered with melted cheese.

Turn to Real Food

It doesn't seem logical that people could be both overweight and malnourished. However, if a person eats mostly high-calorie fried foods and processed foods with little or no nutrients, their body could easily have excess weight and be lacking necessary nutrients. Since getting your blood tested for vitamin and mineral deficiencies is not routinely done, there may be some nutrient deficiencies that have gone undetected. If you think that you can pop a pill to be healthy, think again.

Taking a vitamin is not the same as eating fruits and vegetables. A multivitamin/mineral supplement contains only certain vitamins and minerals. If a person relied on taking supplements in place of food, it would be too hard to know what and how much of every vitamin and mineral is needed to get the proper amounts found in food. High doses of some supplements may increase the risk of certain cancers. For example, studies have found that high amounts of vitamin A and beta carotene supplements may increase the risk of lung cancer in current and past cigarette smokers.

Real food – starting with fruits and vegetables – is your best line of defense for healthy weight and a reduced risk of disease. Fruits and vegetables are low in calories, especially veggies.

For a variety of nutrients, get a variety of fruits and vegetables with a variety of colors and flavors. Name a color and pick a fruit or vegetable to eat.

- **Red:** Cherries, tomatoes, strawberries, raspberries, cranberries, apples, pomegranates, radishes, red cabbage, red peppers, rhubarb
- **Orange:** Oranges, carrots, apricots, pumpkins, peaches, cantaloupe, sweet potatoes, yams, tangerines, papayas, persimmons, nectarines, mangoes, kumquats
- **Green:** Broccoli, green beans, avocado, kiwi, figs, peas, asparagus, spinach, bok choy, cabbage, collard greens, kale, honeydews, mustard greens, peppers, Brussels sprouts, okra, romaine lettuce, limes, cucumbers, zucchini, lima beans, parsley, capers, bitter melons, artichokes, chives, chayote, celery, endive, sugar snap peas, edamame, watercress, split peas, lima beans
- **Purple:** Eggplant, grapes, plums, beets, boysenberries, kidney beans
- **White:** Onions, parsnips, pears, garlic, jicama, turnips, cauliflower, potatoes, tofu, bean sprouts, cherimoya, ginger, kohlrabi, shallots, great Northern beans, lychees
- **Blue:** Blueberries
- **Pink:** Watermelon, pink grapefruit, guava
- **Yellow:** Bananas, corn, durian, grapefruit, squash, lemons, pineapple, gooseberries, star fruit, rutabagas
- **Brown:** Mushrooms, dates, prunes, raisins, beans, lentils

The list goes on … there are hundreds of fruits and vegetables.

*R*uth's **Rule:** *Eating fruits and vegetables from a wide rainbow of colors enables you to ingest a broad range of nutrients.*

Freshness, Quality, and Nutritional Value

Do you only eat "fresh" fruits and vegetables? When fruits and vegetables are fresh, they contain the most nutrients. The fresher, the better. However, fresh may not be "fresh." Heat and air can reduce nutrients. If vegetables sit around for a long time, some of the nutrients may decline. Some of the nutrients in fresh produce are lost during shipping. Avoid limp and bendable vegetables that have been sitting on the counter all day. When you get home from grocery shopping, cut off the tops of carrots and radishes. They will retain more nutrients and last longer. Most vegetables should be refrigerated. Ripen fruits at room temperature. Then refrigerate them.

Cooking Methods Affect Nutrient Content ∞

How do you cook your veggies? Boiling them in a lot of water for a long time until they are mushy leaches out the B and C vitamins. Put a steaming rack in your pot, boil the water first, and then add the vegetables for cooking. Keep a lid on the pan to cook the vegetables faster. Quickly steaming or microwaving vegetables will retain more nutrients. Cook vegetables in big pieces and don't peel them, for more nutritious food. Stir-frying carrots in a little oil makes the fat-soluble vitamins more available. Cooking tomatoes breaks down the cell walls and makes the lycopene more available.

If your produce usually stays in the refrigerator for some time, choose more frozen and canned fruits and vegetables to avoid waste. Processing plants are near the fields. The produce is picked at peak freshness and frozen or canned in a short amount time, so the nutrients are retained. The nutrients in fresh, frozen, and canned fruits and vegetables are relatively similar. In fact, certain frozen and canned vegetables have more nutrients than fresh vegetables. For example, processed tomato products have more lycopene than fresh tomatoes. The vitamin C in frozen food is comparable to the vitamin C in fresh produce.

Look at the "for best quality use by" date on the can. Canned food has a shelf life of at least two years. Canned food should remain safe, if maintained at moderate temperatures of 75 degrees or below. If you have an emergency food bin, rotate the food every year or two, so that if you need it, you'll feel comfortable eating it. According to the Canned Food Alliance, rust and dents in cans are okay, as long as the can is not leaking. If the can is leaking or bulging, *do not* eat the food or you could die from botulism bacteria.

Do you make soup? If you can boil water, you can make soup. It doesn't have to be a large amount to feed an army. Make two to three servings at a time. Boil water. Add vegetables and seasonings. Done. The nutrients lost in the water will be retained in the soup. Make a meal by adding chicken and/or beans.

Don't Like Fruits and Veggies?

Are French fries with ketchup your two favorite vegetables?

JF: Okay, this question is like asking me if I tend to breathe all day. French fries, I think, are the answer to most of life's problems. If I walked in on my husband cheating and he had a plate of fries by the bed, I would grab a handful of the fries before I set the bed on fire.

You: _____

_____

Like Jackie at the beginning of the chapter, clients frequently tell me that they don't like fruits or vegetables. Every fruit and vegetable has a different flavor. *Keep trying them. Be creative.*

Fresh, frozen, canned, or dried are all options, and even juice. I had a client who disliked vegetables. He was willing to swig down a can of vegetable juice every day. That's a fast way of getting vegetables. Eventually, this client found more and more vegetables that he would eat.

If you're not a fan of fruits and vegetables, start making small changes to your usual eating habits. Gradually lean toward a plant-based diet. Try going "vegetarian" once in a while. Here's a note of caution. As you begin to eat more fruits and vegetables, eat less of other foods or you will gain weight. Your goal is to eat fewer calories, lose weight, and be healthy.

Adjust your choices in fruits and vegetables to personal preferences. Like juicy? Choose peaches, oranges, watermelon. Like crunchy? Choose broccoli, apples, carrots. Like smooth and creamy? Choose squash, bananas, beans. There's something for everyone.

Here are more ideas:

+ Chop up carrots and put them in spaghetti sauce.
+ Salsa is a great way to get more vegetables. Instead of chips and salsa, team salsa up with raw vegetables such as celery, jicama, cucumbers, and carrots.
+ Not a fan of salsa? Get used to eating raw vegetables by dipping them in a little hummus, bean dip, guacamole, or low-fat dressing.
+ How about baked sweet potato "fries" (slice like French fries and bake)?
+ How about minestrone or tomato soup for lunch?
+ Try pureeing broccoli and carrots and add them to mashed potatoes.

If all you eat is hot dogs, pizza, and pancakes, you're asking for trouble. I once had a client who only ate these foods. There's no getting around it. You need fruits and vegetables to be healthy.

Getting Kids to Eat More Veggies

Do your kids refuse to eat vegetables? Keep introducing small amounts of different vegetables prepared in a variety of ways. Encourage one bite or a spoonful at a time. Don't force your kids to eat *every* vegetable. Each individual has personal tastes and preferences. With all of the choices, no one has to love every vegetable. The pressure could backfire.

Give your kids choices. Ask them if they want carrots or corn. Eat the vegetables yourself. Others will follow. They are watching you. Try combining the vegetables they avoid with ones they like so they have a familiar flavor. Let your kids select the vegetable for dinner and let them prepare it. Avoid using dessert as a reward for eating vegetables. This could lead to the over-consumption of calories. They may end up being too full for dessert but will eat it anyway.

Avoid Being "Sneaky" ❦

If your kids don't like vegetables, should you be sneaky and disguise them? I say no. Children learn trust from their parents. Hiding vegetables in foods and not telling them could cause deeper issues later in life. Camouflaging carrots by blending them in soup, and then telling them you made healthy soup with carrots is a different story. Be honest with them. After they like the carrot soup, introduce carrots in another way.

Everyone likes an English muffin pizza with a happy face made out of vegetables. Keep introducing vegetables associated with positive experiences to your children. Sometimes kids have issues with textures. Some kids don't like creamy textures. Or maybe their loose teeth don't allow them to eat hard, crunchy fruits and vegetables. Find out what they're willing to eat and encourage them to try. Some kids prefer raw vegetables versus cooked vegetables and vice versa.

I would suggest that everyone only eat breaded, fried zucchini dipped in Ranch dressing on special occasions – *if ever*. It's mostly fat calories. Frying at high temperatures kills nutrients.

Instead of deep-fried, serve vegetables raw, steamed, grilled, baked, sautéed, boiled, blanched, roasted, stir-fried, stewed, or microwaved. Vegetables can be tossed, dipped, shredded, pureed, juiced, chopped, or stuffed. Plain or spicy. Mix it up. There are plenty of choices. Add garlic to potatoes for some zing and more nutrients. Thank goodness for microwaves. It only takes a few minutes to microwave fresh or frozen vegetables.

Brussels Sprouts, Anyone?

I hate to ask, but ... when was the last time you ate Brussels sprouts?

JF: Brussels sprouts? I have eaten a few bean sprouts sprinkled around in shrimp fried rice. But never any sprouts flown in from Brussels.

You: _____

_____

For some reason, Brussels sprouts get a bad rap. Brussels sprouts are a delicious cruciferous vegetable. Cruciferous vegetables are in the cabbage family and include other vegetables, such as broccoli, kale, bok choy, cauliflower, Brussels sprouts, and, of course, cabbage. These vegetables get their name from their four-petaled flowers, which look like a cross. Cruciferous vegetables may offer protection against cardiovascular disease and be linked to lower cancer risks, specifically colorectal cancer. Have you ever known anyone with colorectal cancer? I hope that you'll look at Brussels sprouts in a new light. Roast or stir-fry them in a little olive oil, garlic, and salt. You will change your mind. When was the last time you had a parsnip? Keep broadening your horizons.

Fruits and Vegetables Can Be Convenient

As you've been reading, it's common for people to not eat sufficient fruits and vegetables. Sometimes they don't eat vegetables because they don't have time to prepare them. Below are ways to make eating produce more convenient:

- **Start microwaving frozen or raw vegetables or heat up a can of vegetables.** Potatoes, sweet potatoes, and yams only take a few minutes to cook in the microwave.
- If you don't want to take the time to wash an apple, **buy packaged apple slices.**
- **Short on time for making a salad? Make enough for two days. Or buy pre-washed salad greens.** Mix pre-shredded red cabbage, baby carrots, and cherry tomatoes into the pre-washed

salad greens for a quick and colorful salad. Add a little dressing before eating.

- **Keep a supply of frozen fruits and vegetables in the freezer and canned fruit and vegetables in the pantry.** Frozen and canned vegetables don't have to be washed or chopped. Choose canned fruit with "no added sugar" and packed in water or juice. Fruit is naturally sweet.
- **Don't forget about beans.** All canned beans count as a vegetable – garbanzo beans, kidney beans, etc. Add them to soup or salads.

Do you not make the effort to eat veggies? Before you know it, the day is over, and you didn't eat any vegetables. Weeks go by fast, too. Vegetables may be forgotten. For your health, you need to make the effort to include fruits and vegetables in your meals. Make consuming fruits and vegetables a priority.

Think Produce Is Expensive? ☞

Do you skip eating fruits and vegetables because of the expense? A USDA report showed that fruits and vegetables per serving are less expensive than candy bars and other snack foods. Fruit can usually be bought in bulk for less money. Sometimes certain markets have less expensive produce than big chain supermarkets. It pays to look around. Also, watch the store circulars for special pricing on featured items at the chains.

Influenced by Advertising?

Some people don't eat fruits and vegetables because they would rather eat other foods. *Chips? Cookies?* Billions of dollars are spent every year on food advertising. Did you know that the majority of advertising money is spent on foods that you don't need, compared to a teeny, tiny amount of money spent on promoting fruits, vegetables, whole grains, and beans? Will eating processed food, candy, or soda improve your health? *I don't think so.*

Are you influenced by ads? Do you need fancy marketing to tell you to eat fruits and vegetables?

JF: Fancy marketing entices me to try new things, but it's not influential enough to convince me that a bowl of steamed veggies is better than a bowl of strawberry ice cream.

You: _____

As Fresh as Your Own Backyard

Have you had the opportunity to taste the difference between a store-bought tomato and a fresh tomato recently picked off the vine? An orange just picked from a tree is incredibly sweet. Nothing beats the flavor of recently picked fruits and vegetables.

If you have a yard, plant some crops. Gardening is a rewarding way to get physical activity. It's a win-win. And there's nothing healthier than growing and eating freshly picked vegetables. While I was growing up, half of our backyard was a garden. At the time, it seemed more like a mosquito patch. My mother would pick green beans from the garden and cook them for dinner within minutes.

Wondering how to get involved?

- **Start small.** Ask friends and relatives about the plants they've had success with in the past. Find a sunny spot.
- **If you don't have a yard or small patch of dirt, try container gardening.** A cherry tomato plant in a pot works well.
- **Growing an herb garden on the windowsill is a step in the right direction.** Fresh herbs are loaded with important nutrients. Add the fresh herbs to salads. Try basil, oregano, dill. *Yum.*
- **How about hydroponics?** You can grow vegetables indoors in water. The food has the same nutrients as food grown in dirt. *No fuss. No muss.* Sounds intriguing, doesn't it?
- **Is there a community garden near you? If not, start one.** A community garden is a good way to socialize and learn gardening tips from fellow gardeners.

Growing your own fruits, vegetables, and herbs brings a whole new appreciation to the meaning of fresh and flavorful. Plus, it's very educational for children to see how vegetables are grown. It's amazing to see a zucchini grow six inches overnight. It makes you feel proud to eat fruits or vegetables that you cultivated yourself. Gardening also keeps you busy. There's always time for television some other day.

Tough Schedule? Rely on Your Local Farmers ☙

Another way to get closer to fruits and vegetables is to visit a *farmers market*. Going to a farmers market is a fun family activity. It's inspiring to know that you bought produce directly from the farmer. I remember going to farmers markets with my mother during the summers in Wisconsin. There were farmers from small farms in the area, and they sold their crops out of the backs of their rickety old pickup trucks. The vegetables were still covered in dirt, and they were really cheap. Sometimes all we had for dinner was super sweet corn on the cob and raspberries fresh from the farm.

Will you commit to growing your own fruits, vegetables, or herbs? What are you willing to do?

JF: I've always wanted to grow a huge vegetable and herb garden. I now live at a place where I have a huge yard to do so. So yes, this is a commitment I am happy to say I am excited about. Now just point me to the big, hunky, shirtless man who is going to cut down the grass in my yard so that I can start this project.

You: _____

_____

Lots of Choices

If you like to cook, you can create zillions of great-looking and delicious-tasting dishes using fruits and vegetables. How about roasted beets and blood oranges with fennel or chicken salad with peach and mint salsa? If you have the time and interest, the sky's the limit for beautiful food.

These easy, helpful hints will help you expand your usual intake of produce:

- Keep a bowl of fruit in the kitchen or on your desk at work.
- Store a container of cut-up vegetables in the refrigerator.
- Top pancakes and waffles with fresh or defrosted fruit instead of syrup and butter.
- Stir-fry vegetables in a little olive oil. Then add a little teriyaki sauce.
- Order orange juice at fast-food restaurants and bring along an apple instead of ordering fries.
- Load sandwiches with dark green lettuce, spinach, tomatoes, zucchini slices, onion, avocado, or shredded carrots.
- Freeze grapes or berries and eat as snacks.
- Make your own pizza with whole-grain crust and add whatever vegetables you want.
- Add shredded carrots, cabbage, or peppers to tacos.
- Add fresh or canned vegetables to prepared soup.
- Top chicken with fruit salsa instead of a cheese sauce.
- Make fruit smoothies – mix milk or juice with plain yogurt, fruit (fresh or frozen), and ice.
- Grill vegetables (tomatoes, onions, corn, eggplant, green and red peppers, mushrooms or yellow squash). Baste with olive oil and season with herbs and spices. Try grilled pineapple or other fruit.
- Cut up an apple and dip in peanut butter for breakfast, lunch, or a snack.
- Substitute cooked spaghetti squash for pasta and serve with marinara sauce.
- Nibble on blueberries instead of chocolate.
- Turn baked potatoes into a main dish. Top potatoes with chopped vegetables and low-fat cheese or salsa.
- Add fruits to vegetables (pineapple chunks to coleslaw or mandarin oranges to salads).
- Eat fresh fruit cobbler for dessert instead of cake.
- Eat two different vegetables at dinner, or a vegetable *and* salad.
- Add raisins or chopped apricots to couscous, bulgur, or barley.

- Add chopped broccoli, shredded carrots, and zucchini to meat loaf or lasagna.
- When you go out to eat, ask what fruits and vegetables are available instead of French fries.
- Be the one to bring fruits and veggies for appetizers and desserts to work, family gatherings, or parties.

Here's a winning approach: Pick a vegetable and plan your meal around it, instead of planning your meal around the protein. Do you like pinto beans? Is it cold outside? Make vegetarian chili. Chop a small onion and sauté it in a little olive oil. Add a can of stewed tomatoes, some chili powder, two cans of pinto beans, and a can of corn. *Voila.* Lunch or dinner. Or try two different kinds of beans – like black beans and kidney beans. You can also add other spices like oregano and cumin. If you want meat, the chili could be made with just one can of beans and lean ground turkey or beef.

What are you going to do to eat more fruits or vegetables during meals and for snacks?

JF: I will buy some. And by buy some, I don't just mean a head of lettuce, but also other vegetables of different colors and types. I promise to eat them before they turn into little green, moldy science projects.

You: _____

_____

*R*uth's Rule: *With a dash of creativity, there are countless ways you could be eating more fruits and vegetables.*

What You Should Know about Food Safety

Foodborne illness or "food poisoning" can happen to anyone. Although the U.S. food supply is safe, any food has the potential for contamination. What does food safety have to do with losing weight? Being sick is not a recommended way to eat fewer calories.

There are two types of bacteria, *spoilage bacteria* and *pathogenic bacteria.* Many of us have found spoilage bacteria on food lost in the refrigerator. It looks freaky. There's no way we are going to eat it. Then there's pathogenic bacteria. You can't see, smell, or taste this type of bacteria.

Since you'll be eating more fruits and vegetables, it's important to practice safe food handling to avoid eating harmful bacteria. *Salmonella* and *E. coli* are the most common bacteria that contaminate raw fruits and vegetables. Produce can get contaminated from chickens or animals in the field. The symptoms can start from 8 to 72 hours for salmonella to 1 to 8 days for E. coli 0157:H7 after ingesting the bacteria. Salmonella can cause typical flu symptoms of nausea, diarrhea, chills, fever, headache, even death. E. coli 0157:H7 can cause bloody diarrhea, cramps, vomiting, kidney failure, even death.

It's important to take food safety seriously. The FDA and USDA offer precautions to reduce the risk of getting sick.

Here are some tips to remember.

- When you're in the grocery store, don't buy bruised or damaged fruits and vegetables. Bacteria can get into the cracks.
- Don't let raw juices from meat, chicken, and fish cross-contaminate the produce in your grocery cart.
- Before and after handling food, wash your hands with warm water and soap for 20 seconds.
- Keep counters clean.
- Keep fruits and vegetables separate from raw meat, chicken, and fish in the refrigerator.
- Don't cut up raw chicken or meat and then cut up vegetables using the same cutting board and knife. Use separate cutting boards. Wash cutting boards in hot, soapy water or put plastic cutting boards in the dishwasher.
- Thoroughly rinse, not soak, fruits and vegetables under cold running water to remove any dirt or bacteria before eating them.
- Use a produce brush to scrub produce such as potatoes and cucumbers.
- Don't forget to wash off melons, pineapples, and avocados before cutting. Otherwise bacteria on the rind could enter the fruit from the knife. Produce washes are not necessary or recommended.

- Cut off the outer leaves from lettuce and cabbage to remove dirt and potential pesticides.
- Make sure that your refrigerator is 40 degrees or cooler. Cold temperatures slow down the growth of bacteria. To ensure the proper temperature, place a thermometer in the middle of the refrigerator on the back wall. The freezer temperature should be 0 degrees or cooler.
- The FDA doesn't recommend eating raw sprouts, such as bean, alfalfa, clover, or radish. The sprouts may contain salmonella that cannot be washed off.

Watch Out for Mold ∞

Should you eat moldy fruits and vegetables? Molds are fungi. Most fungi have a root, a stalk, and spores on top of the stalk. The roots may grow deep into the food. If you find mold on firm fruit and vegetables with low moisture content, such as cabbage, cut off an inch around and below the mold. Don't get the mold on the knife, or it could contaminate the rest of the fruit or vegetable. If there is mold on soft fruits and vegetables, such as peaches, throw them away. The mold may also be growing below the surface. If you find a moldy fruit or vegetable in the refrigerator, clean the area and any nearby produce thoroughly.

Bacteria. Mold. Scary stuff. Fear should not be a deterrent for eating fruits and vegetables. Take precautions. No one wants to get sick from eating healthy foods. It's not worth taking a chance. Occasionally, there are problems that are out of our control.

If you're new to the food safety scene or want reliable resources to protect yourself, www.foodsafety.gov is a great website for current food contamination problems and general information on food safety. It is the "gateway to government food safety information." From there, you will find www.fsis.usda.gov. CFSAN is the FDA's Center for Food Safety and Applied Nutrition, and FSIS is the USDA's Food Safety and Inspection Service. FSIS inspects and protects the U.S.

food supply. They also provide information to consumers about safe food handling so that you can reduce your risk of foodborne illness.

The Question of Pesticides

Afraid of pesticides? The Environmental Protection Agency (EPA) approves, regulates, and sets tolerances for crop chemicals. The Food and Drug Administration (FDA) tests most foods for pesticide residues. The USDA tests for pesticide residues in meat, poultry, and eggs. If the stringent health, safety, and environmental standards are met, there should only be minimal, acceptable amounts of pesticide residues on the surface, if any.

The benefits of eating fruits and vegetables outweigh the potential risks. Aside from environmental issues, there are more health problems from excess body fat than pesticide-related problems. Low-fat, high-fiber diets (with lots of fruits and vegetables) may reduce the risk of cancer.

Do you only eat organic food? Thirty years ago, people used to go through the dumpsters of grocery stores, dig out the old produce, and sell it as organic. Today, the term "organic" is regulated and in compliance with the Organic Foods Production Act and the National Organic Program. Organic produce should have less or no pesticide residues but definitely could contain bacteria. Most foodborne illnesses are caused from bacteria.

All produce should be thoroughly rinsed off with water before eating.

Getting Your Share

How much fruits and vegetables should you aim for during meals and snacks? Let's take a look:

Breakfast:	½ cup berries on cereal
Snack:	one large (2¾" diameter) peach
Lunch:	1 cup salad greens with ½ cup cherry tomatoes and sliced cucumbers
Snack:	½ cup baby carrots (about 6) with hummus
Dinner:	½ cup broccoli, 1 small ear (about 6") of corn

This is not extreme eating. This is 1½ cups of fruits and 2½ cups vegetables. This meets the requirement for 1,800 calories a day. Yet even with this reasonable amount, almost 90% of Americans aren't getting the minimum.

Don't forget to include *MyPlate's vegetable subgroups*. Based on 1,800 calories, the **weekly vegetable intake** includes:

- 1½ cups of dark green vegetables (broccoli)
- 5½ cups of red/orange vegetables (carrots)
- 1½ cups of cooked dry beans and peas (pinto beans)
- 5 cups of starchy vegetables (potatoes)
- 4 cups of the rest of the vegetables

These amounts add up to a total of 17½ cups of vegetables (2½ cups of vegetables a day equals 17½ cups a week). If it seems like a lot right now, gradually increase the amounts you eat.

Let's Hear It for Pumpkin ◖♀

When was the last time you ate pumpkin? Pumpkin is a nutritional powerhouse. Pumpkin isn't only for pie. What would you like to make with canned pumpkin? Bread? Muffins? Soup? Pancakes? Pudding? A spread? How about pumpkin mashed potatoes? Or a pumpkin pie without the crust? Adding pumpkin to your meals is a great way to eat orange vegetables.

Have Produce on Your Side

I hope you have found solutions to obstacles that may have prevented you from eating enough fruits and vegetables. Every time you eat, look at your plate. Half of your plate should be filled with fruits and vegetables. Think vitamins, minerals, and fiber in glorious, living color. Remember the Golden Rule: "Eat when you're hungry. Don't eat if you're not hungry." Even if you're eating the healthiest food in the world, don't feel obligated to finish it just because it's good for you.

Eating the recommended amounts of fruits and vegetables is filling and low in calories. If you are serious about losing weight and being healthy, eat fruits and vegetables. It's not that difficult. Hang in there for the long-term health benefits.

Now you can tell mother a thing or two.

Fruits and vegetables are your new best friends.

---

*D*ay 18 CHECK-IN ☑

What did you accomplish yesterday?

JF: I ate a lot of fish and vegetables and no junk food.

You: _____

_____

What is your goal for today?

(If you don't eat fruits and vegetables, start by eating one fruit and one vegetable today.) (If you think you don't like fruits and/or vegetables, look through this chapter for an item you might enjoy today.) (If you're not eating enough fruits and vegetables, start eating two fruits and two vegetables today.) (Bring a fruit to work.) (Eat a vegetable for snack.) (Make a recipe with canned pumpkin.) (Try roasted Brussels sprouts.) (Make a salad with two or more vegetables.) (Pick a color for the day. Eat an "orange" fruit or vegetable for breakfast, lunch and dinner.) (Buy some dirt, a pot, and some seeds. Plant some vegetables.) (Go to a farmers market.)

JF: To continue to cook. I have been cooking a lot and eating my own creations and loving it actually.

You: _____

_____

Day 19

Paper or Plastic? A Supermarket Tour

*S*ince the food we eat doesn't magically appear on our plates, we have to go out and buy it. People either love or hate shopping for groceries. These days, there is a variety of places to shop for food. To name a few: chain grocery stores, upscale gourmet stores, convenience stores, farmers markets, ethnic markets, liquor stores, warehouse stores, health food stores, discount stores, mom-and-pop markets, and now even online delivery.

Shoppers like convenience. Grocery stores have pharmacies, movie rentals, banks, coffee bars, even chain restaurants under one roof. If grocery shopping is pleasurable for you, you will spend more time in the store, and that means you'll spend more money. That's okay, unless you're spending a lot of money on high-calorie food items.

Where do you usually shop? Do you love to spend time in the grocery store? Do you go up and down every aisle looking for deals and reading labels? Do you like to try new products?

JF: I actually dread going to the supermarket because the entire trip sometimes feels like a fight between me and coffee cake. I usually shop at a neighborhood grocery store and occasionally I bump into someone watching me talk myself out of buying donuts.

You: _____

_____

A trip to the grocery store can be a disaster for someone trying to lose weight. Are you disciplined in the grocery store?

JF: I am most disciplined when I shop with a set budget to spend. If I'm having a particularly lucrative month and go to the market without a budget, I explore the world of Hot Pockets and soda. That's likely to be diet soda, but it's still not the kind of food one should eat to maintain a healthy lifestyle.

You: _____

_____

To eat healthy and lose weight, it's important to buy foods that are *high* in nutrients, *low* in calories, *high* in fiber and *low* in fat. It's the highs and lows of grocery shopping.

Hang on to your hats. We're going on a supermarket tour. You can add the fine art of grocery shopping to your list of accomplishments. The purpose of the supermarket tour is to help you choose healthy food so that you can make healthy meals. And, of course, eating healthy meals will help you lose or maintain weight and reduce your risk of disease.

*R*uth's **Rule:** *Shop for foods that are* **high** *in nutrients,* **low** *in calories,* **high** *in fiber and* **low** *in fat.*

Shopping Fundamentals

I strongly recommend planning your meals and making a *grocery list* before you go shopping. Your grocery list is an important tool to use for successful grocery shopping. Here's another pearl of wisdom. Don't go shopping hungry. I guarantee that you'll end up with a cart full of sugary and salty goodies if you do.

Grocery stores are in business to sell food. Today's stores stock more items than the general store from the pioneer days. You may see more than butter, bacon, and pickles to lure you. Manufacturers pay extra money to place their items at the ends of the aisles. The unhealthiest foods for you are usually at eye level. The average person who is trying to lose weight can easily succumb to the dangers of buying unhealthy, high-calorie foods conveniently placed throughout the store.

Don't worry about it. Every time you go shopping, buy more and more healthy foods. Healthy foods are low in saturated fat, trans fat, sodium, and sugar. Before you know it, healthy food will taste delicious to you. Gradually cut out the less healthy foods. Rome wasn't built in a day.

Are there problem areas for you in the grocery store? Salty snacks? Frozen desserts? Candy? Bakery? Alcohol?

JF: The alcohol section of the grocery store is indeed very tempting. With that said, my main nemesis is sweets, anything with sugar in excess. When I cut back on sugary foods, I usually drop weight very quickly. In other words, when I eat all the foods that are good for me, the fat on my body leaves in anger because it feels neglected.

You: _____

Learn from Other Shoppers ❧

Are you a thrill-seeker? Check out what other people are putting into their carts. It gives you an idea of what other folks are eating. Do they load up their carts with fruits, vegetables, and other healthy foods? Do they have an abundance of foods with sugar, fat, or salt? Look, but be nice. I've seen people glare disapprovingly at other shoppers.

Your Tour Begins

It's time for some fun. Grab a cart. Our goal is to buy high-fiber and low-fat foods. We will be buying lots of fruits and vegetables, whole grains, lean proteins, healthy fats, and low-fat or fat-free dairy products. Don't forget: you're allowed a small amount of "extra calories" a day. So there's some room for a treat or two. You've already learned how to read a label. All the pieces of the puzzle are coming together. The fewer calories you buy, the fewer calories you will eat.

Bakery

Eyes forward. Keep walking until you get to the produce department. Avoid looking at the tasty-looking bakery items on either side of you. *Out of sight. Out of mind.* A lot of times bakery goods look better than they taste. Is it worth a second on the lips and forever on the hips? Talk yourself out of it. *Nope. Not today. Too many calories.*

Produce Section

Relax and enjoy. You're in the produce department. It's cool and refreshing. Take a look around. There's a rainbow of colors. Red. Orange. Green. Yellow. Even purple. That's a good thing. Where there's color, there's a lot of vitamins, important minerals, fiber, and phytonutrients. Fill your cart. All of these foods are relatively high in nutrients and low in calories. Fruits and vegetables are not considered a source of fat. Strawberries contain a little bit of fat in the seeds. Don't worry about the 200 seeds in the average strawberry. It's the good kind of fat.

Fruit makes a great dessert. It is low in calories compared to processed desserts. When was the last time you had a kiwi? *Try one.* Wash it ... cut it in half, scoop, and eat. Or eat it skin and all. Kiwis are loaded with nutrients and fiber. Are you getting enough vitamin A? Worry no more. There are plenty of foods with vitamin A in the produce section. Are you brave enough to try kale? No time like the present.

> ## Quick Unscramble Quiz ଔ
>
> *Name a healthy dark green, leafy vegetable. Unscramble to find the answer. NPASICH*
>
> _____
>
> _____
>
> _____
>
> _____
>
> (For the answer, go to the Frozen Food section that follows.)

There are people who don't like fruit, and there are others who don't like vegetables. If my clients don't like vegetables, I ask them to name the vegetables that they eat. They usually have five or six choices. Potatoes and corn are vegetables. Start with the vegetables that you like. Combine them with new ones. Then eat the new ones by themselves. It's never too late to eat veggies. Eating vegetables should be a habit. Start with small bites. What vegetable doesn't taste good stir-fried in a little olive oil and garlic or teriyaki sauce? Some people like to pour BBQ sauce on vegetables.

Clients also tell me that they buy fruits and vegetables but they end up rotting in the refrigerator. *Easy to do.* I've seen it happen. As soon as you get home, cut vegetables up and bag them in small serving sizes. *Problem solved.* When you open the refrigerator, you'll have snacks ready to go for a few days. Make sure they are at eye level, or they could get lost. Eat fruit for snacks. Pile slices of vegetables on sandwiches.

Many fruits and vegetables are high in vitamins A and C, potassium, and fiber. Eating fruits and vegetables may reduce the risk for heart disease and certain cancers. Make sure your cart has plenty of fruits and vegetables for. breakfast, lunch, dinner, and snacks.

What is your favorite cruciferous vegetable? (Broccoli, cauliflower, kohlrabi, Brussels sprouts, cabbage, bok choy, kale, wasabi, watercress, turnips, rutabaga?)

JF: Cruciferous?????? And I never knew what bok choy was. Kohlrabi? Are we still doing the word scramble? Because the only word that I really know here is broccoli.

You: _____

_____

You can't go wrong in the produce section. Of course, you don't want to buy more fruits and vegetables than you can eat in a week.

Give New Veggies and Fruits a Tryout ℃

The next time you go to the grocery store, pick out a new fruit or vegetable to try. Experiment with produce you've never eaten. Spend some time in the produce section and get to know it. For additional ideas for eating more produce, see Day 18.

Next to the fruits and vegetables is the refrigerated juice section. There are many choices and flavors of juice. Drinking juice can add a variety of nutrients to your day, such as vitamin C, calcium, folate, and potassium. Choose 100% juice. Eight ounces of juice equals 1 cup of fruit. Four to eight ounces of juice adds nutrients without too many calories. Drinking 22 ounces of juice is another story — too many calories.

Dairy Case

The dairy section is important. Many people, including children, aren't getting enough calcium in their diets. Linger in this section. Are you getting your share of calcium? What are you willing to start eating? Whole and 2% fat dairy foods contain more fat and therefore more calories. One percent fat and fat-free dairy foods have the same amount of calcium but contain less or no fat.

Milk, yogurt, and cheese are excellent sources of calcium and protein. Yogurt makes a great afternoon snack. Plain yogurt with slices of fruit is refreshing and delicious. Look at the different types of milk and yogurt. Have you ever tried low-fat buttermilk? It tastes great and is low in calories.

Sometimes cheese is near the dairy case. What are your choices? Cottage cheese is a good source of protein and calcium. Ricotta cheese makes a great spread for rye bread. There are many other types to try.

Regular cheese is made from whole milk so it contains more saturated fat. Read the labels and look for cheese that is *reduced fat, low fat, part skim,* or *fat-free*. Who needs the extra fat calories? Be aware of the sodium in cheese. Low-fat foods, including low-fat and fat-free dairy foods, are an important part of healthy eating. When you have a choice, buy the lowest fat version.

You might find the tofu nearby. Tofu is a complete plant protein. A stir-fry made with tofu and veggies is a quick, healthy, and tasty breakfast, lunch, or dinner. Tofu is very versatile and can be used in smoothies, main dishes, even desserts.

Don't Forget to Read Labels ଓ

Keep reading labels for important information. Low-fat means no more than 3 grams of fat per 100 calories. If a food is high in fat, avoid it. Or balance the day with less or no fat. If you're eating 2,000 calories a day, a Daily Value of 5% or less is low in fat.

Frozen Foods

What dark green, leafy vegetable is healthy? The answer to the unscramble quiz is SPINACH. In addition to the Produce Department, this nutritious veggie can also be found in Frozen Foods. Frozen spinach is very convenient. It can be added to spaghetti sauce or other dishes. It is a super healthy enhancement.

Frozen foods are handy, especially for people who don't have a lot of time to cook. They are content to stay in your freezer until you're ready for them. Frozen fruits and vegetables retain their nutrients.

Frozen desserts taste good but may contain lots of calories. When emotions give you a call, you might grab a spoon and head for the freezer. Fortunately, there are many low-calorie frozen snacks available. The 100-calorie ice cream treats taste great. Frozen juice bars are an energizing, low-calorie snack or dessert. As long as you limit snacks to one a day, it's not a problem.

Have you ever started eating frozen chocolate cake (without bothering to defrost it) and kept eating until it was gone? First you cut a piece and eat it. Then you shave off some frosting from the next piece. The piece is started so you might as well finish it. Before you know it, there's nothing left.

JF: Why frozen when I can bake a delicious cake from scratch? And yes.

You: _____

Frozen meals are quick and convenient. They may also contain a lot of fat, sodium, and sugar. *Read the labels.* At least the portion sizes are controlled.

265

Grocery Shelves

Red alert! Proceed with caution. **Candy, cookies, and snacks** are around the next corner. These are empty *calories.* If you're losing weight on 1,800 calories, the extra calorie amount is only 170 calories a day. There are no nutrients in this aisle. In this section, our eyes are often bigger than our stomachs. If you desire something sweet, graham crackers and gingersnaps are tasty (but not too sweet), and they contain fewer calories than a lot of the packaged cookies.

When you're watching your weight, it's better to avoid sweets for a while. Look straight ahead and quickly walk down the aisle. *Stay strong.* If it's too much of a temptation, don't even walk here. Too many of these foods can add excess weight. *Move on.*

You can breathe a sigh of relief. Across the aisle are the **rice cakes and crackers.** Some crackers contain more fat than others. Rice cakes are crunchy, low-calorie snacks. Look for the words "whole grain" and check the grams of fiber on cracker packages.

Further down the aisle is the **coffee and tea.** The processed coffee and tea beverages in cans and bottles can contain a lot of other things, including sugar calories. Making your own iced tea from tea bags is easy and natural. Herbal tea over ice is a delicious way to hydrate.

Next is the **oil and bread** aisle. Buy heart-healthy oils and save some room in the cart for heart-healthy nuts. Choose monounsaturated fats like olive and canola oil. Most of your fats should be monounsaturated. Try walnut oil to add flavor to a salad. Healthy oils still have calories, but they're better for your health. Use oil in small amounts. Here's your chance to buy low-fat or fat-free versions of mayonnaise. Tangy mustard would be another option with very few calories.

Want to drop 10 pounds in a year without even trying? Instead of using a tablespoon of butter or oil for cooking or flavoring, season with an herb, a spice, or vinegar. An extra tablespoon of butter or oil every day can put on an extra 10-12 pounds a year.

Bread and other grains are important for energy, vitamins, minerals, and fiber. Look for bread, rolls, buns, English muffins, even bagels and pita bread that say "whole grain" or "whole wheat" on the package. Look at the total number of grams of carbohydrate. Brown bread still raises blood sugar. Choose bread that contains 3 grams or more of fiber per slice. Most grain foods are low in fat. Want something sweet? Instead of a sweet roll for breakfast, whole grain toast with a fruit spread is sweet and satisfying.

The aisle with **herbs and spices** is interesting. Most people stick to a few favorite spices. Trying new herbs and spices can offer a variety of flavors without the sodium. It's fun to experiment. Find a recipe with a new, ethnic flavor and expand your horizons.

Now we are in the **nut, dried fruit, canned fruit, and juice** aisle. This is a healthy aisle. Nuts are a good source of protein and healthy fat. A handful of nuts makes a great snack. If you have high blood pressure, buy unsalted nuts.

Dried or canned fruit is a good choice for fruit. Dried fruit and canned fruit don't spoil and can be transported easily. Both are available year-round. Watch the sugar content in canned fruit. Fruit packed in natural juice has fewer calories than fruit with heavy syrup. Buy 100% juice in bottles or cans, not "fruit drink" or "fruit punch." Fruit nectars have higher amounts of sugar than fruit juice. Fruit drinks and punch contain diluted amounts of juice with added sugar. By the way, frozen juice concentrate is 100% juice with the water taken out. No sugar is added.

Next is the **salad dressing, canned goods, and pasta** aisle. Choose a salad dressing with a healthy oil like olive oil. Make the most of the healthy fats but watch the portion size. Drizzle or dip. Don't pour. For variety, choose a reduced-calorie dressing. Salad sprays are a fun way to use less salad dressing.

Canned meats can be convenient. Salmon and tuna are a great way to get protein and omega 3 fatty acids. Buy tuna packed in water, not oil. Try salmon and tuna in the pouches. Tuna in a pouch doesn't seem as fishy as tuna in a can, and can openers are not necessary. Rinse tuna to reduce the sodium. Eat foods with omega 3s two times a week to protect your heart, eyes, and brain. If cooking fresh fish isn't your thing, here's a chance to get fish and omega 3s.

Need a quick meal? Canned soup is a great way to go. It's easy and convenient. If your fresh vegetables stay in the refrigerator until they're unrecognizable, choose canned vegetables. Keep a supply of canned tomatoes and other canned vegetables, such as mushrooms, in your pantry to throw together a last-minute meal.

Check the date on canned foods and store them in a clean, cool, dry place. Canned food should be consumed within two years of processing. After two years, there may be color and texture changes.

Buy lots of beans. All types of beans. They are an excellent source of inexpensive protein, complex carbohydrate, and soluble fiber, but deliver no fat. If your vegetable consumption is low, include beans more often.

Try This Fridge Routine Before Shopping ❧

Here's a tip. Before you go to the grocery store (or every week), go through the food in the refrigerator. Throw away leftovers that are more than a few days old and produce that is past its prime. This will save you some surprises a few weeks down the road. Who needs mold spores turning into a science fiction character in the produce crisper! Have you ever found something in your refrigerator that was so mushy and fuzzy that you couldn't identify it? Where's *CSI* when you need it?

If you're running low in stock, pick up some whole wheat pasta and brown rice. Grains are low in calories. However, it would be prudent to measure your portion sizes. One half cup isn't much. Watch the fat/oil that you add to the grains. It can add *a lot* of calories. This is an opportunity to try a new whole grain and increase your fiber. Tip: Store brown rice in the refrigerator. Brown rice is a whole grain and can go rancid.

Next is the **cereal** aisle. Look for "whole grain" cereals. If you buy a pre-sweetened, whole-grain cereal at eye level on the shelf, try mixing it with another whole grain cereal without sugar. Putting a small amount of sweetened, whole grain cereal in a bag makes a sweet, healthy snack. It's sweet, crunchy, a whole grain, and not as many calories as a brownie.

Feeling a little sluggish? There are a lot of good-tasting bran cereals on the grocery shelves. They do their job with gusto. Don't forget to put oatmeal in your cart. Old-fashioned oatmeal doesn't contain artificial colors or flavors. There's nothing healthier than a bowl of high-soluble fiber oatmeal with fruit and nuts for breakfast. *Life is good.*

A whole grain, high-fiber granola bar is a healthier choice than a candy bar from a vending machine. Granola seems healthy. Read the label. Granola can contain saturated fat from coconut oil. Eat small amounts of granola or mix it with another cereal. Avoid foods like donuts, croissants, and sweet rolls (processed, high fat, and high sugar). *Too many calories!*

Meat Department

Along the back of the store is the fresh meat department. There are many different choices, including beef, pork, lamb, chicken, turkey, and fish. There are processed meats, such as bacon and sausage. A lot of meat counters have precooked protein for convenience. Consider the price and sodium content. The meat department contains important protein but there is the potential for saturated fat in its offerings. Watch the white stuff (visible fat).

Choose *lean* and *extra lean* sources of protein. Limit choices of processed meats and always choose lower-fat versions of hot dogs, bacon, or sausage. Full-fat bacon and sausage contain *a lot* of saturated fat. Canadian bacon has a lot less fat than bacon but still contains a lot of sodium.

Look for cuts of meat with the words *tenderloin, sirloin, round,* or *flank steak.* Buy 95% lean ground beef. When you cook meat, trim off the visible fat and remove the skin from poultry. Ground turkey used to be ground up with the skin. Read the label for the fat content. A high-fat meat would be a prime grade, a rib cut, bacon, and fatty corned beef. Fresh and frozen fish is a good low-fat source of protein. Breaded and fried seafood contain a lot of fat calories. How do you flavor your fish? Cocktail sauce is fat-free versus tartar sauce, which contains fat. Canned and smoked fish can be high in sodium.

Toiletries and Supplements Aisle

On the same aisle with your shampoo and toothpaste, you'll find vitamins and other supplements. No special supplements or products are necessary for a healthy diet. If you buy a multi-vitamin/mineral supplement, choose one without iron – unless you're anemic. Be educated about any supplements that you're taking. Don't take a supplement because your cousin or a guy at the gym is taking it. Do the research and decide if it's right for you. You might save yourself some money and avoid side effects.

Adult Beverages

Limit your selections in the alcohol section. For health reasons, drink alcohol in moderation. When you're losing weight and eating healthy, the calories from alcohol should be considered. Mixed drinks have more calories than beer or wine.

What Did You Learn?

How are you doing so far? What new things did you learn?

JF: I am maturing in my eating. It's still hard to change a lot of bad habits. However, I've learned that I can be just as full, eat healthy foods all day, and not feel deprived. And if I stay in my house and never go out again, I can have complete self-control.

You: _____

_____

Grocery Check-Out Stand

It's time to unload the cart and pay for the groceries. If you're hungry and have to wait in line, a candy bar is going to sound outstanding. Resist the temptation. Buy sugarless gum or sugarless mints instead.

That concludes our supermarket tour. We've covered all the major food groups. Our cart is filled with plenty of fruits and vegetables, whole grains, lean sources of protein, low-fat and fat-free dairy products, and healthy fats. There is a variety of colors, flavors, and nutrients. Not many of the foods contain fat, sodium, and sugar.

Congratulations! Well done.

Healthy Shopping on a Budget ରେ

If you're on a tight budget, it's possible to eat healthy with careful planning. A combination of beans and rice is an inexpensive protein. Cut up fruit for dessert, instead of buying expensive cakes and pastries. Rather than eating high-processed snacks, make your own popcorn. A bag of unpopped popcorn goes a long way. Popcorn is a whole grain and is low in calories. All of these examples are low in calories, nutritious, and can be less expensive than processed foods.

Now You're Ready

Your food choices impact your health. The next time you go grocery shopping, march proudly into the store. You have the power to reduce your risk of heart disease, diabetes, and cancer. Follow MyPlate guidelines and buy a variety of foods to get all of the necessary nutrients. Fill your grocery cart with health and vitality. Healthy eating tastes great.

If in doubt, read the food label. Think moderation, low fat, and high fiber. With your newly acquired supermarket tour knowledge, you can start changing your shopping habits. What you buy is what you eat.

A grocery list is your new best friend.

$\mathcal{D}$ay 19 CHECK-IN ☑

What did you accomplish yesterday?

JF: I had oatmeal and fruit for breakfast and didn't feel deprived. I felt full for hours until it was time for lunch. This oatmeal thing is brilliant and I wonder if the rest of the world has caught on.

You: _____

_____

What is your goal for today?

(Go grocery shopping with health in mind.) (Stick to a grocery list.) (Look for sales.) (No nibbling while shopping; chew gum instead.) (Check out other people's grocery carts – for good ideas and things to avoid.) (Try low-fat cheese.) (Only buy high-fiber, low-fat foods.) (Try a new fruit or vegetable.) (Try a new whole grain.)

JF: To make my list, use coupons, and continue to shop like a responsible adult woman and not like a hungry, pimple-faced teenager.

You: _____

_____

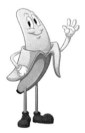

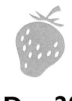

Day 20

All About Protein

*T*he three major macronutrients that provide calories are protein, fat, and carbohydrate. Today's topic is protein, and tomorrow's will be fat. On Day 26, we'll look at carbohydrate. Meanwhile, *pump it up.* Meat, poultry, fish, dry beans and peas, eggs, nuts, and seeds are all sources of protein.

Protein Basics

Protein is essential for growth, for building and repairing muscle mass, and for protecting the immune system. There is protein in *every* cell in the body. Protein is made up of 20 amino acids. During digestion and absorption, dietary proteins are broken down into the amino acids. The amino acids become the building blocks for all of the body's components. Amino acids include *nonessential amino acids* and nine *essential amino acids*. The human body can make the nonessential amino acids. The essential amino acids must come from food.

Beef, turkey, chicken, fish, pork, lamb, eggs, milk, yogurt, cheese, goat, ostrich, etc. are considered complete proteins or "animal proteins," and they contain all of the essential amino acids. Basically, anything that can walk or swim and its byproducts are complete proteins.

If you aren't eating complete proteins, you have to mix and match incomplete proteins to make a complete protein. Incomplete proteins or "plant proteins" are lacking or low in one or more of the essential amino acids. Plant protein includes grains, beans, nuts, seeds, and vegetables.

In the old days, vegetarians were advised to combine the incomplete proteins at one meal, such as beans and rice, beans and corn tortillas, rice and black-eyed peas, pita bread with hummus, or rice and lentils. These days, it's okay to eat a variety of incomplete proteins throughout the day. Your body will put them together, as needed.

Soy – A Complete Protein ℞

Grains, such as rice, are low in the amino acid lysine. Beans are low in the sulfur amino acids cysteine and methionine. Soybeans contain higher levels of cysteine and methionine. Therefore, soy protein is a plant that is considered a "complete" protein.

How's your protein intake? Do you like to sink your teeth into a juicy steak or bite off a creamy piece of tofu?

JF: I can't believe the words tofu and steak are in the same sentence! I think a piece of steak is better tasting than tofu. However, I hear that tofu is delicious when it's seasoned properly or when you're tied to a chair, have a gun pointed at your head, and you're forced to eat it.

You: _____

How Much Do You Need?

The National Academy of Medicine's Food and Nutrition Board analyzes data taken from the latest research to determine appropriate amounts of nutrients for human beings. These amounts are based on age, sex, physical activity, and nutritional needs to prevent the risk of chronic disease. The RDA for women is 46 grams of protein a day. For men, the RDA is 56 grams of protein a day. The Board's RDAs meet the needs of 97-98% of people. The Recommended Dietary Allowance for adult men and women is based on 0.8 grams of protein per kilogram of body weight. The protein RDA for pregnancy and breast feeding is based on 1.1 grams per kilogram.

Let's review an example of how this plays out. A person weighing 150 pounds is 68 kilograms (150 divided by 2.2 = 68 kilograms). We then multiply 68 x .8 and get 54.4 grams. So this person would need 54.4 grams of protein a day to meet a sufficient nutrient intake level.

Here's another approach to your protein needs. The National Academy of Medicine's adult Acceptable Macronutrient Distribution Range (AMDR) for protein is 10-35% of the total calories. The AMDR is also associated with reducing the risk of chronic disease, while providing sufficient intakes of essential nutrients.

Based on an intake of 1,800 calories a day, 10% protein would be 180 calories of protein or 45 grams. In contrast, 35% protein would be 630 calories of protein or 158 grams. A range of 45-158 grams of protein is quite large. Actually, 15% is a common recommendation for protein. Based on 1,800 calories, 15% protein would be 270 calories or 68 grams of protein a day.

Most foods contain some protein. Here are some examples:

- 3 ounces chicken, 26 grams of protein
- 3 ounces lean ground beef, 22 grams of protein
- 1 cup pinto beans, 12 grams of protein
- 1 cup milk, 8 grams of protein
- 1 large egg, 6 grams of protein
- 1 slice of bread, 3 grams of protein
- 1 cup cereal, 2-8 grams of protein, depending on the cereal
- 1 large banana, 1.5 grams of protein

Here's a third option. Following MyPlate guidelines makes it easy to get enough protein. For the 1,800-calorie meal pattern, *MyPlate recommends 5 ounces of protein from meat, poultry, fish, eggs, beans, nuts, and seeds a day.* Five ounces of protein isn't much compared to what most people are used to eating. Five ounces of chicken breast is 43 grams of protein. Keep in mind that the 5-ounce recommendation of protein is from the protein foods group. You'll get more protein from other food groups, such as milk, bread, fruit, etc.

*R*uth's Rule: *I've found three ways to be helpful in targeting protein consumption: the RDA of 0.8 grams of protein per kilogram of body weight, a goal of 15% of calories, and the MyPlate recommendation of 5 ounces a day for an 1,800-calorie diet.*

The Relationship between Muscle and Protein ෬

Big muscles come from strength training and extra calories, which includes a little more protein. In this pursuit, carbohydrates are the main fuel. If you want to increase muscle mass, you only need an extra 2-4 ounces of protein a day. Eating protein doesn't build muscles. Exercise builds muscles.

It's interesting to know that muscle is composed of 75% water, 20% protein, and the remaining 5% is fat, carbohydrate, and minerals. When people go on high-protein/low-carbohydrate diets, the rapid weight loss is primarily water from muscles.

When you eat beef or other red meats, you are eating muscle.

Lowdown on Lean Beef

Let's talk about beef, which contains a lot of important nutrients. Beef is an excellent source of protein, vitamin B12, zinc, selenium, and phosphorus. Beef is a good source of niacin (B3), vitamin B6, iron, and riboflavin (B2).

There are 29 cuts of beef that meet the government guidelines for "lean." For a 3-ounce serving, "lean" is less than 10 grams of total fat, 4.5 grams or less of saturated fat, and less than 95 milligrams of cholesterol. *On average, the 29 cuts of lean beef have amounts of saturated fat similar to a skinless chicken breast!*

Lean beef is low in saturated fat. Some cuts of lean beef contain less saturated fat than skinless dark meat chicken. If you're watching your cholesterol, feel confident about eating beef that contains the words *"round"* (eye round, top round or London broil, bottom round, round tip, or sandwich steak) and *"loin"* (sirloin or tri-tip steak, tenderloin or filet mignon, top loin or New York strip steak), as well as *flank steak* – also called London broil, chuck shoulder, arm roasts, and at least *90% lean ground beef.* Ninety-five percent extra lean ground beef would be leaner. Note that 95% lean ground beef has almost half the amount of fat calories as 80% lean ground beef.

Reducing Fat in Meat Choices

Red meat and poultry may present a problem if they contain high amounts of saturated fat. Saturated fat adds needless calories and clogs arteries. Limit your intake of higher fat protein sources, such as 75-80% ground beef, regular sausage, duck, hot dogs, bologna, and salami.

The difference between USDA Prime, Choice and Select grades is the marbling. Marbling is the white fat in the muscle tissue. *Select has the least amount of fat.* Look at the differences in the percentage of fat in these grades of *beef*:

♦ USDA Prime   above 8%
♦ USDA Choice   4-8%
♦ USDA Select   3-4%

In case you didn't notice, you can save a lot of saturated fat by choosing Select grades. By the way, Kobe beef is 20-25% fat.

The leanest cuts of *pork* are *pork loin, tenderloin, center loin,* and *ham.* Pork tenderloin has the same amount of total fat as a skinless chicken breast and only a little bit more saturated fat. Pork is an excellent source of protein, thiamin (B1), vitamin B6, phosphorus, and niacin (B3). Pork is a good source of riboflavin (B2), potassium, and zinc. Pork tenderloin is considered an extra lean source of protein. Choose lean cuts of *lamb – leg, arm,* and *loin.*

To limit saturated fat, choose lean and low-fat sources of meat and poultry. Broil, grill, or bake instead of frying to reduce calories. Brown hamburger and drain off the fat before adding other ingredients. Don't forget about lean cuts of buffalo, ostrich, and emu. They are low in fat.

Eggs Are Back!

Eggs are our buddies, again. Eggs are an inexpensive, high quality protein. One egg equals 1 ounce from the protein foods group. They contain almost every nutrient, except vitamin C. That's amazing. One yolk contains 184 milligrams of cholesterol, but they are low in saturated fat.

Avoid eating raw eggs. One in 10,000 eggs may have salmonella. There could be raw eggs in protein drinks, homemade mayonnaise, homemade ice cream, homemade eggnog, Hollandaise sauce, or Caesar salad. Eggs should be cooked until firm to avoid salmonella problems. FYI: Hard-boiled eggs should not sit out for more than two hours to avoid potential salmonella contamination.

Some enhanced eggs may contain 150 milligrams of the omega 3 fatty acid DHA because the chickens are fed algae. Some egg yolks contain more vitamin E, lutein, and zeaxanthin than regular eggs. Lutein and zeaxanthin are carotenoids, a type of antioxidant, found in the retina and lens of the eye. Ongoing research is looking at the relationship between lutein/zeaxanthin and the eye diseases macular degeneration and cataracts. Egg yolks are also an excellent source of choline, which is important for the heart, nerves, and the brain. Many Americans are lacking choline in their diets.

Other Choices: Try Fish

There's more to fish than tuna. Tuna and shrimp are the most commonly consumed fish. Shrimp has more cholesterol than most fish, but *shrimp* is lower in saturated fat than meat or poultry. Salmon is gaining popularity.

Did you know that there are different types of *salmon*? There are five types of Pacific Salmon. There's *Sockeye* (the most intense red color; it's good for lox and sashimi), *King* or *Chinook* (the biggest), *Coho* or *Silvers* (commonly used in foodservice), *Chum* (the meatiest and firmest in texture), and *Pink* or *Humpback*. Pink salmon is the smallest and most abundant of the Alaskan salmon. Pink Salmon is the lightest in color of all the salmon and is frequently chosen for canned salmon. Red Sockeye is another salmon commonly canned.

Speaking of fish. A lot of people don't eat fish because it tastes fishy. A fish is a fish. Expand your fish intake by trying different types of fish in restaurants. If you like a certain type of fish, find a recipe and make it at home. *Red snapper* is an example of a delicious, mild-flavored fish. *Alaskan Pollock* is used to make surimi – fake crabmeat. Slowly get used to eating more types of fish. By the way, fresh fish should not smell or taste fishy.

Afraid of the PCBs in *farmed salmon?* Farmed salmon may or may not contain polychlorinated biphenyls (PCBs). More than half of salmon fillets are from farmed fish. However, the risk of PCBs in farmed fish may be low. Farmed salmon has more fat than wild salmon. To decrease potential PCBs, trim off the fat and don't eat the skin. Broiling, grilling, and baking allow the fat to be cooked off. Wild (Alaskan) salmon is also an option.

A Concern: Mercury in Fish

Afraid of mercury? And who isn't. Almost all fish and shellfish have trace amounts of mercury. The mercury isn't the same type of mercury in thermometers or the type of mercury used to fill teeth. The mercury in fish is *methylmercury.* Mercury from industrial pollution falls from the air into streams and oceans and turns into methylmercury in the water. For most people, fish consumption doesn't pose a health risk. However, this type of mercury can harm an unborn baby or the nervous system of young children.

The Department of Health and Human Services (HHS) and the Environmental Protection Agency (EPA) list the mercury levels in commercial fish and shellfish. *King mackerel, shark, swordfish, and tilefish (from the Gulf of Mexico) have the highest amounts of methylmercury.*

39 mcg (micrograms) of mercury a week is the total allowable amount for a pregnant or breastfeeding woman who weighs 124 pounds. Tilapia is low in mercury, but it also has less omega 3 fatty acids. Tuna steak is albacore tuna. Albacore or white tuna has more mercury than light or chunk tuna. Fish sticks and fish sandwiches from fast food restaurants are made from low mercury fish.

	Mcg of Mercury per 4 ounces	EPA + DHA mg (omega 3 fatty acids) 4 ounces cooked
King Mackerel	110	450
Shark	151	1,250
Swordfish	147	1,000
Tilefish (Gulf of Mexico)	219	1,000
Salmon: Atlantic, Chinook, Coho	2	1,200-2,400
Salmon: Pink and Sockeye	2	700-900
Rainbow trout	11	1,000-1,100
Tuna: White, canned (albacore)	40	1,000
Tuna: Light, canned (chunk)	13	150-300
Shrimp	0	100
Sardines: Atlantic and Pacific	2	1,100-1,600
Tilapia	2	150

Source: Appendix 11. Dietary Guidelines for Americans, 2010

Fish Advisory for Women of Childbearing Age ❧

The U.S. Food and Drug Administration and the Environmental Protection Agency issued a consumer advisory for selecting and eating fish or shellfish for breast feeding mothers and women who are or might become pregnant.

Do not eat shark, swordfish, king mackerel, marlin, orange roughy, bigeye tuna or tilefish (from the Gulf of Mexico). Eat 8 to 12 ounces a week of a variety of low mercury fish, such as shrimp, canned light tuna, salmon, pollock, and catfish. Up to 4 ounces of albacore (white) tuna or fish with higher mercury levels may be eaten in a week.

If you fish, check the local health department for advisories about the mercury levels of fish caught in local lakes, rivers, and coastal areas. If there is no advice, you can eat up to 4 ounces of local fish per week but no other fish during that week.

This advisory is for women at risk and young children. Portion sizes for children differ. The general population may also follow these guidelines. The benefits of eating fish outweigh the risks.

The meat and potatoes days are over. Think outside the barn. Fish is high-quality protein and is low in saturated fat. Eat fatty fish rich in the polyunsaturated omega 3 fatty acids EPA and DHA. EPA and DHA may be linked to a reduction in heart disease. You'll learn more about omega 3s in a minute.

What fish would you like to try? Anchovies, sardines, or trout? How about herring? Instead of a hamburger, how about a salmon burger? It is delicious.

JF: I do agree that salmon is delicious. I also agree that fish is a wonderful alternative to red meat. I think my problem is paying for dinner. If the meal is on me, then I will order a sensible salmon dinner. If someone else is paying, I tend to want to order the biggest steak that the restaurant can slaughter and fit on a plate.

You: _____

The Wonderful World of Beans

Going vegetarian is a good way to get protein without the unhealthy fat. Do you ever "spill the beans"?

Beans contain protein and complex carbohydrates. They are high in fiber and low in fat. Beans are an excellent source of folate and a good source of potassium, iron, magnesium, manganese, and copper. This economical source of protein contains calcium, antioxidants, and phytonutrients. Beans come in many colors, shapes, and flavors. MyPlate recommends eating one and one half cups of beans a week.

Small red beans, red kidney beans, pinto beans, and black beans are four different beans on a list of "Top 20 Power Foods" containing powerful antioxidants. Eat more beans and less protein with saturated fat to decrease your risk of heart disease and certain cancers. In America, pinto beans take first place as the most-consumed bean. Navy beans take second place.

What are your favorite beans?

JF: I am shocked that I have an answer to this. My favorite beans are black beans.

You: _____

_____

Beans are either fresh or dried. Fresh beans are usually sold in their pods, such as green beans. So what are "dry" beans or "dried" beans?

Beans, peas, and lentils are from the legume family. Legumes produce seeds, which are the beans (or pulses) in a pod. "Dry" or "dried" beans are harvested when the seed pod is *dry* and the seeds (beans) are hard. Examples of dried beans are pinto beans, great Northern or navy beans, kidney or red beans, black beans, lentils, garbanzo beans, split peas, black-eyed peas, and cannellini beans. "Dried beans" are the hard beans in a package that you soak in water and cook. Beans in a can, such as garbanzos (chickpeas), are also "dried" beans.

Bean Facts ❧

- Beans may reduce your risk of heart disease and certain cancers.
- Beans are high in soluble fiber, which lowers cholesterol.
- One cup of beans contains 13 grams of fiber.
- The fiber in beans can help stabilize blood sugar levels.
- Beans are the only food in MyPlate listed as both a protein and a vegetable.
- Beans count as a vegetable but not at the same time as protein.
- One-half cup of cooked beans equals ½ cup of vegetables.
- One-quarter cup of cooked beans equals 1 ounce from the protein foods group.
- Soaking beans increases the size three times.
- One cup of dried beans equals 3 cups cooked beans.
- One-half cup of beans contains 6-7 grams of protein.
- Lentils and split peas do not have to be soaked before cooking.

If flatulence isn't your thing, soaking and cooking beans removes about 50% of the gas-producing carbohydrates. Here's the quick-soak method. Add three cups of water for every cup of beans that you're cooking. Boil for 2-3 minutes. Turn off stove, cover, and let stand for 1-2 hours. Change the water. Boil and simmer beans until tender, about 45-60 minutes.

Soybeans, the complete protein mentioned earlier, are very versatile. They can be made into milk, oil, flour, and many different soy products. Choose tofu products containing calcium. Two ounces of tofu (1/4 cup) or 1 ounce of cooked tempeh is considered a 1-ounce equivalent from the protein foods group. Whole natural soy foods may have more health benefits than foods made from processed isolated soy protein.

Ways to Eat More Beans ∞

- Add beans to salads, as a source of protein.
- Make bean or lentil soup for a main course.
- Serve bean dip instead of a sour cream dip. Serve with whole grain crackers.
- Add beans to pasta to increase the protein.
- Add beans to quesadillas.
- Make baked beans as a side dish for more fiber.
- Mix beans with chopped vegetables and add salad dressing for a quick salad.
- Add beans to baked potatoes.
- How about a hummus sandwich (made from garbanzo beans) with grated carrots and chopped tomatoes in pita bread? Two tablespoons hummus equals 1 ounce from the protein foods group.
- How about beans instead of fries?

Beanery Cooking

When I was young, by myself, and hungry, I would heat up a can of pork and beans and make a bean sandwich. It wasn't my first choice.

At the time I felt like the orphan kid Oliver. Now I see the health value of what I was eating. Bean sandwich, anyone?

There are hundreds of recipes using beans for appetizers, soups, main dishes, and desserts. Pureed beans can be used to make brownies, even mock pecan pie. Any bean is healthy. Soybeans, kidney beans, black beans, garbanzo beans, red beans, pinto beans, cannellini beans, cranberry beans, fava beans, and navy beans are just a few types. Chili with beans is warm and comforting, as are split pea soup and lentil soup. One cup of split pea soup, lentil soup, or bean soup is considered a 2-ounce equivalent of protein from the protein foods group.

Here's a healthy, tasty snack. Drain and rinse a small, 8-ounce can of garbanzo beans. Heat up a fry pan and add a couple tablespoons of olive oil. Stir-fry about 5 minutes until lightly browned. Sprinkle with garlic and onion powder, curry, or another favorite spice.

Nutty Protein

What is your favorite nut? Almonds, Brazil nuts, cashews, hazelnuts (filberts), macadamias, pecans, pine nuts, pistachios, walnuts, or peanuts?

JF: I am addicted to pistachios. If I ever find a 40-pound bag, I will buy it and eat all those pistachios in one sitting. Probably not a good idea, though, huh?

You: _____

_____

I wouldn't be able to decide. I like *all* of them. There are two groups of nuts. Tree nuts and peanuts. Technically, peanuts are a type of legume from the pea family but we will consider them nuts.

A lot of people are afraid to eat nuts. They think that nuts will make them gain weight. *Nuts are good for you.* Most nuts come from trees, so we know they don't contain cholesterol (which comes from animal sources). When you're trying to lose weight or maintain weight, include nuts – just watch your portion size. Nuts are a major source of my protein for breakfast, lunch, and snacks.

One half ounce of nuts is equal to 1 ounce from the protein foods group. One ounce of nuts equals ¼ cup or a small handful. If you look at a handful of macadamia nuts or walnuts, the sizes aren't consistent. For one ounce of nuts, use a ¼ cup measuring cup instead of counting the individual nuts. One tablespoon of peanut butter is equal to 1 ounce from the protein foods group.

Nuts are a source of protein, fiber, vitamins such as folate, thiamin, niacin, vitamin E and vitamin B6, and the minerals magnesium, copper, zinc, iron, selenium, phosphorus, calcium, and potassium. Nuts contain many phytonutrients; examples include flavonoids, isoflavones, ellagic acid, and phenolic compounds.

There is an FDA "qualified" health claim for nuts and heart disease. "Scientific evidence suggests but does not prove that eating 1.5 ounces per day of most nuts as part of a diet low in saturated fat and cholesterol may reduce the risk of heart disease." The nuts included in the claim are almonds, hazelnuts, peanuts, pecans, pistachios, and walnuts. One and a half ounces of nuts equals 1/3 cup.

The National Heart, Lung and Blood Institute recommends 4-5 servings a week from nuts, seeds, and dried beans, as part of the DASH (Dietary Approaches to Stop Hypertension) diet. Potassium, calcium, and magnesium are important minerals for controlling blood pressure.

You would think that a nut is a nut. But check out the differences, especially in number of nuts, protein grams, and fat grams:

	1 ounce	Calories	grams Protein	grams Total Fat	grams Carbohydrates
Almonds	23	164	6	14	6
Brazil nuts	6	187	4	19	3
Cashews	18	157	5	12	9
Hazelnuts	21	178	4	17	5
Macadamias	10-12	204	2	21	4
Peanuts	32 pieces	161	7	14	5
Pecans	19 halves	196	3	20	4
Pine nuts	167	191	4	19	4
Pistachios	49	159	6	13	8
Walnuts	14 halves	185	4	18	4

Source: USDA National Nutrient Database for Standard Reference, Release 28, 2016

Nuts have varying amounts of protein, fat, carbohydrates, and nutrients. Nuts seem high in fat but it is mostly monounsaturated fat, except for Brazil nuts, peanuts, pine nuts, and walnuts. Brazil nuts and peanuts are about half monounsaturated fat and half polyunsaturated fat. Pine nuts and walnuts have more polyunsaturated fat. Monounsaturated and polyunsaturated fats are the healthy fats.

Nuts and Their Nutrients

Every type of nut has different health benefits. Eat a variety of different ones. Are they high in calories? Consider what you're getting for your calories. Protein and healthy fat. Is that better than a big slab of prime rib? *Yes.* Let's look at the nutrients in nuts. (Note: A rating of 10-19% DV [Daily Value] is "good." Twenty percent or more DV is a "rich in," "high," or "excellent" source.)

+ **Almonds** are related to the peach and the plum family. They are a rich (excellent) source of alpha-tocopherol *vitamin E.* One ounce of almonds provides 7.4 milligrams or about 50% of the Daily Value for vitamin E. Besides vitamin E, almonds are an excellent source of riboflavin (B2), copper, magnesium, and manganese. Almonds are a good source of fiber and phosphorus. Almonds contain 76 milligrams of calcium. Not considered a "good" source of calcium but not too bad!

+ **Brazil nuts** are grown in the Amazon rainforest. Six Brazil nuts (1 ounce) contain 544 micrograms of *selenium.* One ounce of Brazil nuts is about 990% the Daily Value (DV) for selenium. Selenium is a trace mineral, only needed in small amounts. Most of the other nuts contain trace amounts of selenium. Only eat Brazil nuts occasionally. Brazil nuts are good sources of thiamine (B1), phosphorus, and manganese. They are excellent sources of magnesium, copper, and, of course, huge amounts of selenium.

+ **Cashews** have the most carbohydrates and the most iron of all the nuts. They are excellent sources of magnesium and copper. They're good sources of *iron,* phosphorus, zinc and manganese. Have you ever seen a cashew shell? You probably won't. The inside of the shell has a poisonous resin, similar to poison ivy. The shells have to be carefully removed.

♦ **Hazelnuts** or filberts are members of the birch family. They're good sources of fiber and magnesium. Hazelnuts are an excellent source of vitamin E, copper, and *manganese*. An ounce of hazelnuts is almost 100% the Daily Value (DV) of manganese.

♦ **Macadamia nuts** are healthy snacks. They have the pleasure of being first place for the nut with the most calories. These nuts have the highest levels of *monounsaturated fats*, which is a good thing. Macadamia nuts are native to Australia. Eventually, they made it to Hawaii. The rest is history. Macadamia nuts are a good source of thiamine (B1). They are an excellent source of manganese.

♦ **Peanuts** have more *protein* than any other nut. They are a good source of folate, vitamin E, phosphorus, copper, and magnesium. Peanuts are an excellent source of niacin and manganese. Peanuts are rich in *arginine,* an amino acid important for maintaining healthy blood vessels. Peanuts contain the phytonutrients resveratrol, which is also found in red wine, and beta sitosterol. Beta sitosterol may inhibit cancer growth and protect against heart disease.

♦ **Pecans** are native to North America. Pecan is a Native American word for "hard-shelled nut." These nuts are a good source of fiber and excellent sources of copper and manganese. They contain the antioxidant *ellagic acid* to fight cancer.

♦ **Pine nuts** – Did you even know that they're a nut? I know that pine nuts and pesto sauce go hand in hand. Pine nuts are the seeds of pine cones. Gathering them is labor-intensive so these nuts tend to be expensive. Pine nuts are good sources of vitamin K, phosphorus, magnesium, and zinc. They are excellent sources of vitamin E, copper, and *manganese* (110% DV).

♦ **Pistachios** are one of the oldest nuts on earth. In China, pistachios are called the "happy nut" because the shells are half opened. In Iran, pistachios are called the "smiling nut." They definitely make me smile. Pistachios contain 329 micrograms of *lutein* + *zeaxanthin,* and 45 micrograms of beta carotene, which are all carotenoids — not even close to any other nut. Pistachios are good sources of fiber, thiamine (B1), manganese, and phosphorus. They are excellent sources of *vitamin B6* and copper.

- **Walnuts** contain the highest amounts *alpha linolenic acid* (ALA), the essential omega 3 fatty acid, and also the most *linoleic acid*, the essential omega 6 fatty acid (LA). One ounce of walnuts (1/4 cup) contains 2.6 grams of alpha linolenic acid (ALA). No other nut comes close to these amounts. Walnuts are a good source of magnesium and an excellent source of copper and manganese.

More on Peanuts ❦

There are several varieties of peanuts, such as Virginia, Runner, Spanish and Valencia. Most of the roasted-in-the-shell peanuts are Virginia. Most of the peanuts grown are Runner peanuts. Half of the Runners are used to make peanut butter. Spanish peanuts are small and have reddish skins. Their high oil content is good for making peanut oil. Valencia peanuts are small with bright red skins. They are sweet and usually sold roasted in the shell.

When you buy peanut butter, don't buy reduced-fat peanut butter. You will be missing out on the healthy monounsaturated fat. Instead of cream cheese, spread peanut butter on toast and bagels for more health benefits. Peanut butter is an excellent plant protein. There are about 8 grams of protein in 2 tablespoons of peanut butter without saturated fat and cholesterol.

Nuts and Food Allergies

Ninety percent of food allergies come from these eight foods: *milk, eggs, peanuts, tree nuts, soy, wheat, fish, and shellfish.* With food allergies, the body's immune system thinks a food, usually a protein, is a foreign invader. It fights back with antibodies. The effects could be swelling of the lips, tongue, or airways, stomach cramps, vomiting and diarrhea, skin rashes, hives, or itching. Some reactions can be severe and life-threatening. As a result, some schools have become peanut- and nut-free zones. If you have a food allergy, be sure to see a board-certified allergist.

When You Feel like a Nut

Below are ideas for incorporating nuts into your meals and snacks in different ways:

- Nuts are good by themselves.
- They can be added to muffins, bread, pastas, stir-fry dishes, yogurt, or cereal.
- Use smaller amounts of chicken or red meat and add nuts to main dishes.
- Chopped nuts can be used to coat chicken or fish.
- Add nuts to salads instead of high-fat croutons, bacon, or cheese.
- Tired of peanut butter? Put any nut in a food processor and whirl – instant nut butter of your choice!
- If nuts are too tempting, don't eat them out of the jar or can. Measure one-ounce portions and put them in bags. The seasoned nuts may be too good to resist going beyond targeted portions.
- Eat nuts unsalted to avoid overdoing it.
- Trail Mix made from nuts and dried fruit packs a big punch of nutrition.
- Replace animal protein with nuts for a more plant-based diet. Studies show that nut eaters have fewer heart attacks. Eating nuts is a good way to reduce your risk of heart disease, stroke, and cancer.

Freshness Tip: Since nuts contain oil and can go rancid, store them in the refrigerator or freezer to keep them fresh.

Don't Overlook Seeds

Pumpkin seeds. Sesame seeds. Sunflower seeds. Do you eat seeds? Seeds are included in the protein foods group. Throw some sesame seeds on beef and broccoli. Toss sunflower seeds in a salad. One ounce of sunflower seeds is 165 calories. Sunflower seeds are a good source of fiber, niacin (B3), vitamin B6, folate, magnesium, and zinc. They are excellent sources of alpha-tocopherol (vitamin E), pantothenic acid, phosphorus, selenium, copper, and manganese. Sunflower seeds are fun to grow. One flower can contain 2,000 seeds. Have you ever seen a field of sunflowers? Beautiful.

Be Wary of Foodborne Illnesses

Did you know that protein foods, such as hamburger, chicken, seafood, and eggs, as well as milk and soft cheeses, are prone to bringing on foodborne illnesses? Carbohydrates, fat, and protein contain carbon, hydrogen, and oxygen. Along with these compounds, protein also contains nitrogen. Nitrogen allows the rapid growth of bacteria.

Bacteria doesn't like acid. Mayonnaise is acidic. Despite what you may have heard, mayonnaise deters bacteria growth. I still wouldn't leave egg salad unrefrigerated for more than two hours. Bacteria can double and reach dangerous levels in that amount of time. Besides time, temperature is a factor. Bacteria multiplies the fastest in the Danger Zone of between 40 and 140 degrees, especially between 70-110 degrees. E. coli is killed at 155 degrees. Most bacteria are killed at 165 degrees. Don't take chances and eat dangerous bacteria. Bacteria can produce toxins. These toxins may not be killed by cooking.

Follow these **food safety tips for protein**:

♦ Buy meat, poultry, and eggs last. They will stay colder longer, until you get home.
♦ Defrost protein in the refrigerator — not on the counter at room temperature.
♦ Don't rinse meat or poultry before you cook it. The risk of rinsing is the splashing of bacteria on the sink, contaminating the surrounding area.
♦ Use a thermometer to ensure that the protein is cooked to a high enough temperature. For egg dishes, ground meat, or poultry, check the temperature in several places.
♦ Don't eat raw or undercooked meat and poultry.

- Refrigerate leftovers in shallow, covered containers within two hours.
- Store eggs in the original carton. Don't store eggs on the refrigerator door.

If you are making a *turkey with stuffing*, don't pack the stuffing tightly. Test the center of the stuffing with a thermometer. It should reach 165 degrees. If the stuffing contains raw eggs and it doesn't get hot enough, it may cause a problem. Better yet, cook the stuffing in a casserole dish to avoid foodborne illness.

If you are at a party, is the hot food hot? It should be 140 degrees or above. Reheated food should be at least 165 degrees and then maintained at 140 degrees or above. Is the cold food cold? It should be 40 degrees or colder. Are the perishable foods on ice? Does the host know about the Danger Zone? Has perishable food been sitting out for more than two hours? If it's 90 degrees or above, don't eat perishable food left out for more than an hour. Think about food temperatures at restaurant buffet tables, also.

Ruth's **Rule:** *Take measures to avoid food poisoning with protein foods, such as hamburger, chicken, seafood, and eggs, as well as milk and soft cheeses, as they are prone to bringing on foodborne illnesses.*

Track Protein with a Food Journal

It's common for my vegetarian clients to learn that they aren't eating enough protein. A diet high in rice, bread, pasta, and sweets may lack protein. Non-vegetarians can be consuming too many "non-lean" proteins, and the portion sizes of protein are often too large.

If you're unsure of where you stand with protein, keep a food journal to track the grams or ounces of the protein you're eating. Note the amounts and whether the source is lean or not. If the results show you need to make improvements, review this chapter for ideas.

Moderate amounts of lean protein are your new best friends.

$\mathcal{D}$ay 20 CHECK-IN ☑

What did you accomplish yesterday?

JF: I WENT HIKING AND HAVE BEEN FOR THE LAST FEW DAYS!! I thought I was going to die but I did it and plan to continue.

You: _____

_____

What is your goal for today?

(Keep track of the ounces of protein in a day.) (Count the grams of protein that you eat in a day.) (Buy and try a new type of "dried" bean.) (Have a canned salmon sandwich on whole wheat bread for lunch.) (Try herring.) (Buy a refrigerator thermometer.)

JF: To jump rope and work out indoors because it is raining outside.

You: _____

_____

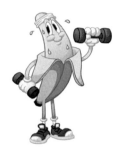

Day 21

All About Fats and Oils

*B*esides protein and carbohydrate, your body needs fat to function. Fat is a source of energy and essential fatty acids. Fat is needed to absorb the fat soluble vitamins A, D, E, and K, as well as the carotenoids. Fat supports cell growth, and it is needed to produce hormones. Fat also protects our organs. Some people have more protection than others!

We run into trouble with our weight and our health when we eat too much fat and the wrong kinds. Fat has more than twice the calories as protein and carbohydrate bite for bite. In the previous Food Guide Pyramid, the fat category sat in a tiny triangle at the top of the pyramid. In MyPyramid, it's a thin sliver running down the side of the pyramid. Fat is not included on the MyPlate icon. Food with a lot of fat can put on weight quickly and easily. You might have a good time eating it. The fun ends when it's time to get on the scale.

Recommended Intake

For adults, the daily allowance is a range of *5-7 teaspoons a day.* If you are physically active, you can consume more. Keep in mind that one tablespoon of vegetable oil equals three teaspoons or 14 grams. Two tablespoons of Italian dressing counts as 2 teaspoons of "oils." Ordering a salad with a generous scoop of Italian dressing could fulfill the fat allowance for the entire day.

For a MyPlate meal pattern of 1,800 calories, the daily amount for "oils" is 5 teaspoons. Do you think that you usually get this much or more?

JF: I am almost positive that I do not get that amount. But then again, there is all that oil in the fried chicken.

You: _____

_____

The National Academy of Medicine's Acceptable Macronutrient Distribution Range for adults is 20%-35% for fat. The recommendation for fat used to be 30% or less of the total calories. We are learning that we can eat more fat if it's healthy fat.

Let's look at the range of calories for fat. Based on 1,800 calories, 20% of the fat calories would be 360 calories or 40 grams. If you eat less than 20% fat, you might not get enough vitamin E or enough essential fatty acids. Thirty-five percent of the fat calories would be 630 calories or 70 grams. A reasonable 30% of calories from fat would be 540 calories or 60 grams. A lot of people eat more than 60 grams of fat a day. Hence, more "organ protection" (belly fat).

Continue keeping a food journal. Write down the number of grams of fat or the number of teaspoons of fat that you eat to get an idea of the total amount. You may be surprised to learn that you eat more fat than you think.

*R*uth's **Rule:** *It's important to stay aware of the amount of the fat that you consume, since 5-7 teaspoons a day isn't much.*

Know Your Fats

Not all fat is created equal. Here's a quick but important lesson on fat. There are different types of dietary fat.

Cholesterol

Cholesterol is a soft, waxy substance. Humans, animals, poultry, and fish make their own cholesterol and store it in their liver. Thus, animals, poultry, and fish are the foods that contain cholesterol. Egg yolks and organ meats (liver, kidney, heart, etc.) have a lot of cho-lesterol. Three ounces of cooked chicken liver has 479 milligrams of cholesterol. There seems to be confusion regarding whether or not foods contain cholesterol. Butter and lard come from animals so they contain cholesterol. If food comes from plants, it doesn't contain cholesterol. Coffee and tea would not contain cholesterol. Crackers would not contain cholesterol unless they were made with butter. When in doubt, look at the label for the amount of cholesterol.

Your body makes all the cholesterol that it needs. Depending on the individual, foods with cholesterol may or may not raise LDL (bad) cholesterol. However, where there's cholesterol, there may also be saturated fat. Be sure to look at the amounts of saturated fats on food labels. The average intake of dietary cholesterol is about 270 mg a day for Americans. As much as possible, limit foods with choles-terol.

Saturated Fats

Fat is composed of different chemical structures. The basic units or building blocks of fats and oils are called fatty acids. Saturated, monounsaturated, and polyunsaturated are the three main types of fatty acids.

Saturated fatty acids (SFA) (saturated fats) are unhealthy fats. They are solid at room temperature and are mostly found in foods that come from animals. Fatty meats (prime rib), poultry skin, butter, cheese, whole milk, cream, and lard contain a lot of saturated fat. Cheesecake and bologna are two foods with a lot of saturated fat. The tropical oils coconut, palm kernel, and palm are also high in saturated fat, even though they are plants. They should be considered solid fats. Saturated fat raises LDL cholesterol and may increase the risk of a heart attack, stroke, diabetes, and certain cancers.

Saturated fat is in a lot of tasty foods. If a food is "low saturated fat," it contains 1 gram or less per serving. One cup of shredded ched-dar cheese or one cup of premium ice cream is 22 grams of saturated fat, which is 2 grams over the limit for 1,800 calories. Have you ever ordered a rack of barbecued ribs for dinner? The serving size is enough for an entire family, not one person. The number of grams of saturated fat in a rack of ribs is enormous. Even half a rack contains more fat than you need. Have you ever seen and felt the white fat from a prime rib steak after it has cooled on your plate? This type of fat sticks to artery walls. To protect your heart, limit foods with saturated fat as much as possible.

Trans Fats

Trans fatty acids (TFA) (trans fats) are unsaturated fatty acids that receive a lot of attention. Trans fatty acids are formed by adding hydrogen to a liquid oil, thereby turning it into a solid fat. This process is called *hydrogenation.* To see if a food has trans fats, look for hydrogenated or partially hydrogenated vegetable oil on the ingredient list. Trans fats make food taste good and increase the shelf life. Stick margarine, vegetable shortening, French fries, donuts, and commercially made foods such as cakes, cookies, and crackers, *used* to contain trans fats.

It turns out that trans fats are just as bad for us as saturated fats. High intakes of trans fats increase the risk of heart disease. Trans fats raise LDL cholesterol and may decrease HDL (good) cholesterol. The FDA declared war on artificial trans fats. Manufacturers had a deadline to remove trans fats from their products.

Before the ban, the more processed foods with fat you ate, the more trans fats you ate. Depending on the oil, one glazed donut could contain 5 grams of trans fat, which is more than the recommended limit of 2-3 grams a day.

It was tricky. A label could say "no trans fats" or "0 trans fat," yet contain less than 0.5 gram of trans fat per serving. If you ate two servings, it could be almost 1 gram of trans fat. Always limit foods with artificial trans fats.

Small amounts of trans fats are found naturally in ruminant (cud-chewing) animals and include foods such as beef, pork, lamb, and dairy products. Natural trans fats may have positive health effects.

Healthy Fats – The MUFAS

Unsaturated fatty acids consist of monounsaturated fat and polyunsaturated fat. **Monounsaturated fatty acids** (monounsaturated fats) are healthy fats. In the "biz," we call them **MUFAs** (pronounced *MOO-fas*). Oils and foods containing high amounts of monounsaturated fats include *olive oil, canola oil, high oleic safflower oil, high oleic sunflower oil, peanut oil, peanut butter, nuts, avocados,* and *olives. Oleic acid* is a monounsaturated fatty acid.

When monounsaturated fat replaces saturated fat, the MUFAs lower LDL cholesterol. MUFAs decrease triglycerides and may increase HDL cholesterol. To eat more monounsaturated fat and less saturated fat, put a slice of avocado on your sandwich instead of cheese or grab a handful of macadamia nuts for a snack.

Most people used to cook with corn or vegetable oil. Then we discovered that people in the Mediterranean region of the world had lower rates of heart disease. They consumed a lot of olive oil (monounsaturated fat), among other healthy foods, for thousands of years. Research has confirmed that monounsaturated fat is good for our hearts. The National Cholesterol Education Program ATP III Expert Panel, 2002 reports that *up to 20% of the total calories can be monounsaturated fatty acids. Most of the fat in your diet should come from MUFAs.*

Polyunsaturated fatty acids (polyunsaturated fats), the **PUFAs** (pronounced *POO-fas*), are also healthy fats and include oils such as *corn, soybean, sunflower, cottonseed,* and *high linoleic safflower.* Polyunsaturated fats in place of saturated fats decrease LDL cholesterol.

Omega 3 fatty acids and *omega 6 fatty acids* are two types of polyunsaturated fatty acids. One of the omega 3 fatty acids and one of the omega 6 fatty acids are *essential fatty acids* (EFA). They are *alpha linolenic acid* (ALA) and *linoleic acid* (LA). Your body can't make them so you need to include them in your diet.

Linoleic acid (LA) is an omega 6 polyunsaturated essential fatty acid. *Corn oil, soybean oil, sunflower oil, high linoleic safflower,* and *cottonseed oil* are good sources of linoleic acid (LA). Linoleic acid (LA) is converted to *arachidonic acid* (AA), another omega 6 fatty acid. Although rare in the U.S., a deficiency of omega 6 PUFAs causes rough, scaly skin and dermatitis.

Alpha linolenic acid (ALA) is an omega 3 polyunsaturated essential fatty acid. Foods rich in alpha linolenic acid (ALA) are *flax seeds, flaxseed oil, walnuts, walnut oil, canola oil, soybean oil,* and *leafy green vegetables.* Whole flaxseeds must be broken down to access the omega 3s. Flaxseed meal can be added to anything from oatmeal to cookies.

Recommendations for Omega 6 Polyunsaturated Fatty Acids ℞

NAM's Acceptable Macronutrient Distribution Range for omega 6 polyunsaturated fatty acids is 5-10% of the total calories. Five percent meets the Adequate Intake for linoleic acid. An Adequate Intake (AI) of linoleic acid (LA) is 17 grams a day for adult men and 12 grams a day for adult women. Pregnant and lactating women need 13 grams a day.

Although rare in the U.S., a deficiency of alpha linolenic acid causes scaly and hemorrhagic dermatitis, slow wound healing, and reduced growth. Alpha linolenic acid (ALA) reduces the risk of heart disease through a handful of mechanisms.

Recommendations for Omega 3 Polyunsaturated Fatty Acids ℞

NAM's Acceptable Macronutrient Distribution Range for omega 3 polyunsaturated fatty acids is 0.6-1.2% of total calories. This 0.6% meets the Adequate Intake for alpha linolenic acid. The Adequate Intake (AI) of alpha linolenic acid (ALA) is 1.6 grams a day for men and 1.1 grams a day for women. A higher amount of ALA may offer more protection against heart disease.

Your body converts alpha linolenic acid (ALA), an omega 3 fatty acid, to *eicosapentanoic acid* (EPA) and *docosahexaenoic acid* (DHA), two longer chain omega 3 fatty acids. EPA and DHA are healthy omega 3 fatty acids found naturally in *fatty fish, their oil and eggs,* and *marine algae.* The fatty fish with the highest amounts of omega 3 fatty acids are cold water fish, such as *salmon, tuna, herring, trout, sardines, anchovies, Pacific oysters,* and *mackerel.*

A Closer Look at EPA and DHA

In the late 1970s, it was discovered that Eskimos had low rates of heart disease. Their diets contained a lot of fish with lots of EPA and DHA. *Now we know.* Consuming EPA and DHA, the omega 3 fatty acids in fish, twice a week decreases the risk of sudden cardiac death and coronary heart disease in adults. Sudden cardiac death means that you die within an hour of a heart attack.

Eating fatty fish (approximately 8 ounces) twice a week is the equivalent of getting approximately 250 mg of EPA and DHA a day or 1,750 mg per week. Besides reducing the risk of heart disease, omega 3s may be good for eye health, dementia, depression, arthritis, and other inflammatory diseases. Omega 3s may reduce the risk of cancer.

How much EPA and DHA do you need? NAM has not yet established an Adequate Intake amount for EPA and DHA, and there is no Upper Limit (UL) for ALA, EPA, and DHA. *The World Health Organization recommends 0.3-0.5 grams a day for EPA and DHA.*

What's for Dinner? Why Not Fish? ca

If you don't have a fish market nearby, frozen fish fillets and patties are easy to cook in the oven or microwave. Fish can be baked, grilled, broiled, or poached. To tell if fish is done, poke it with a knife. If it flakes apart, it is ready to eat.

- **To bake:** Cook fish at 400 degrees until tender and opaque (white, not clear). About 10-15 minutes.
- **To poach:** Simmer fish in broth, water, or wine in a covered pan about 10 minutes.
- **To grill/broil:** Marinate fish with olive oil and spices. Cook about 10 minutes.

The American Heart Association recommends that people without coronary heart disease should eat a variety of fish (preferably fatty fish) at least twice a week and include foods and oils rich in ALA. People with coronary heart disease should consume about 1 gram of EPA + DHA a day, preferably from fatty fish. People with elevated triglycerides should take 2-4 grams a day of EPA + DHA as capsules under a doctor's supervision. More than 3 grams a day of omega 3s could cause bleeding in some people.

Three ounces of cooked pink salmon, 2½ ounces of pickled herring, and 3½ ounces of cooked rainbow trout each provide about 1 gram of omega 3s. The amount of omega 3s can differ among fish.

Your body only converts a very small amount of ALA into EPA and DHA, so it's recommended that you get sources of EPA and DHA directly from fish. Consuming fatty fish twice a week will provide your body with enough EPA and DHA. More than two servings a week may protect your heart even more.

Most of the DHA in the human body is found in the brain and the eyes. Future research will determine the potential effects of DHA on macular degeneration and dementia. Do you want to take a chance and not get enough in your diet?

Yes, fish is good for us. Salmon looks like it has a lot of fat, but remember, it's the good kind of fat – omega 3s. Eating fish twice a week is easy. Eat salmon for dinner one night and eat a tuna sandwich for lunch once a week. There are many more possibilities. Let's bring back tuna casserole.

Fish Oil Supplements

If you don't eat fish or you're a vegetarian, consider taking a fish oil supplement. Fish oil provides EPA and DHA. Algal (from algae) oils provide EPA and DHA, as a vegetarian source. Flaxseed oil provides ALA (but hardly any ALA is converted to EPA and DHA).

Cod liver oil is fish oil that comes from the livers of cod. Cod liver oil is rich in vitamin A and vitamin D. There are 4,500 IUs of vitamin A in a teaspoon of cod liver oil. Five thousand IUs are 100% of the RDA for vitamin A. If you consume a lot of cod liver oil, it could be possible to attain toxic levels of vitamin A. Since the liver is a filter, cod liver oil may also contain contaminants.

Do some research before buying fish oil supplements. Choose a high-quality fish oil supplement without mercury or pollutants. Look for "USP" on the label. Check with your doctor before taking fish oil. Fish oil may increase the risk of bleeding for people taking blood-thinning drugs, such as Warfarin or aspirin. Ask questions, such as: *Is one capsule of fish oil enough? Are three too many? Is it safe? Will it interact with anything?*

So Far, So Good?

Unless you have heart disease, it seems easier to eat fish instead of taking a supplement. When you eat fish, you know what and how much you're eating. Fish is low in calories and saturated fat. Fish is a good source of protein, B vitamins, potassium, phosphorous, and selenium.

Omega 3s are being added to more and more foods and drinks. Read the label. What types of omega 3s? Is it ALA? You probably get enough ALA in your diet. So what's the point?

Balancing the Omega 3 and 6 You Consume ∞

To make things a little more confusing, there's talk that it's not healthy to consume too many omega 6 fatty acids in relation to omega 3 fatty acids. Some people say that *the current ratio is 10:1-15:1 or more.* Maybe the problem isn't the ratio. Maybe it's the lack of omega 3s. There are a lot of people who are lacking omega 3s in their diet because they don't eat fish. A desirable ratio of omega 6 to omega 3 is not known. For now, focus on getting more omega 3 fatty acids to reduce inflammation.

Heart disease is the leading cause of death in the United States. People who eat fish have a reduced death rate from heart disease. Are you making the connection? Choose to eat more foods with EPA and DHA. If you refuse to eat fish, add flax, chia, or hemp seeds, flaxseed oil, walnuts, and canola oil to your diet. *Maybe* the small amount of EPA and DHA converted from ALA will be enough.

Are you starting to understand what the following mean? An SFA and a TFA? A MUFA and a PUFA? An LA and an ALA? DHAs and EPAs?

JF: Yes, I am starting to understand that those acronyms are not from another language. If people had used these terms in regular conversation with me earlier, I would probably have felt offended!

You: _____

_____

Oils vs. Fats

Oils and fats contain different percentages of saturated fatty acids and unsaturated fatty acids, which include monounsaturated fatty acids and polyunsaturated fatty acids. Solid fats contain more saturated fats, cholesterol, and trans fats.

You wouldn't know by looking at fats and oils, but they are all different. Compare the percentages of fatty acids in a few oils and butter:

	MUFA	Saturated Fat	PUFA (LA) Omega 6	PUFA (ALA) Omega 3
Olive oil	75%	14%	10%	1%
Canola oil	65%	7%	19%	9%
Butterfat	27%	64%	3%	less than 1%
Coconut oil	7%	83%	2%	0%

Reference: USDA National Nutrient Database for Standard Reference, Release 28, 2016

What do you get when you crush olives? *Olive oil.* All types of olive oil contain the healthy monounsaturated fat, oleic acid. Extra virgin olive oil, olive oil, and light olive oil have the same amount of calories. Flavor, color, and fragrance depend on the grade or quality of the oil. More color means more flavor, but that's not always the case. The grading depends on how the oil was made and the acidity. Acidity affects taste and quality. Different grades of olive oil can have different uses.

How Olive Oil Is Graded

The International Olive Oil Council (IOOC) sets the standards for olive oil. There are three grades of virgin olive oil for human consumption:

- **Extra virgin olive oil** is the most expensive olive oil, with a superior fruity flavor. It cannot contain more than 0.8% oleic acid. EVOO (extra virgin olive oil) is the oil obtained from the first "cold pressing" of the olives. The oil is extracted using only pressure. It is made without chemicals or heat. Heat changes the oil's chemistry and reduces the flavor. Extra virgin olive oil is considered the highest quality olive oil, based on taste and smell. To make the most of its flavor, use extra virgin olive oil on salads, marinades, and for drizzling and dipping.
- **Virgin olive oil** is also a first-press oil, processed without chemicals. It has a good flavor but a slightly lower quality than extra virgin olive oil. This oil contains no more than 2% acidity.
- **Ordinary virgin olive oil** contains no more than 3.3% acidity. Olive oil with 3.3% acidity is considered inferior and is processed into refined oil. Refined oil is treated to neutralize the taste and the acidity. Refined oil has an acidity of less than 0.3%.

Extra virgin olive oil and virgin olive oil may contain more of the antioxidants called polyphenols. Virgin oils can only be obtained by physical or mechanical means, including washing, decanting, centrifuging, and filtering. They cannot contain refined oil.

- **Olive oil,** once called **pure olive oil** or **100% olive oil,** is a blend of refined olive oils with virgin or extra virgin olive oil added. The acidity is less than 1.5%. If you see the word "pure," it means that there are no other oils other than olive oil. This type of olive oil is good for grilling, stir-frying, and sautéing.
- **Light olive oil** is a blend of mostly refined olive oils. Light is a U.S. term. This type of oil has a lighter taste, color, and smell, not fewer calories. The refining process increases the smoke point, which makes it good for baking and frying.

Trivia question: How many olives does it take to make a quart of extra virgin olive oil?

JF: 1?   You:_____

Find the answer at the end of the chapter.

Other Oils to Consider

Canola oil is an excellent source of the essential omega 3 fatty acid, alpha linolenic acid (ALA). One tablespoon contains 1.3 grams of alpha linolenic acid. A tablespoon a day covers the requirement for women. One tablespoon of canola oil is 80% of the recommended daily intake for men. People used to be afraid of canola oil because they thought it came from the toxic rapeseed. Canola oil is not the same as rapeseed oil.

Oils can be modified to contain different types of fat. *Oleic safflower oil* contains mostly monounsaturated fat. This type of safflower oil is good for frying. *Linoleic safflower oil* is mostly polyunsaturated fat. This type of safflower oil is good for salad oils and soft margarines.

The Butter vs. Margarine Debate ℘

What's the answer to the age-old question: Which is better, butter or margarine? Butter is high in saturated fat, which raises LDL. Margarine is made from blends of soybean, canola, and sunflower oil, which are high in polyunsaturated and monounsaturated fats. Most soft margarines don't contain much, if any, trans fats anymore. *You be the judge.* It is okay to use soft margarine in place of hard stick margarine for baking and sautéing.

Tip:

All this talk about fat can make your head spin. For instance, what is a gram of fat? A gram is a measure of weight or mass. Because we live on earth and not the moon, we'll stick with it being a unit of weight. A paper clip weighs 1 gram. A pat (1 teaspoon) of butter or margarine weighs 4 grams. One tablespoon of margarine or butter weighs 12 grams. Fat is nine calories a gram. Therefore, a pat of butter is 36 calories (4 grams X 9 = 36). If you're thinking, "Wow. That's a lot of calories for a little pat of butter," you're right. Sometimes it's easier to understand a concept when you visualize it. **One gram of fat equals ¼ of a pat of butter.**

Fat in Milk?

Speaking of pats, have you ever thought about the fat content in milk? Whole milk is 3.25% fat. One cup of whole milk contains 8 grams of fat or two pats of butter. One cup of 2% milk contains about 5 grams of fat or a little over one pat of butter. One cup of 1% milk contains about 2 grams of fat or half a pat of butter. Fat-free milk contains no fat. Do you need the extra pats of fat? Switching from a cup of whole milk to fat-free milk saves 63 calories. Using fat-free milk versus whole milk or cream in coffee or tea saves a lot of calories over time.

*R*uth's **Rule:** *There is a surprising amount of fat in milk, so choose fat-free milk when you can to cut some calories.*

Eat Fat Wisely

Do you eat more fat than you need or should because you don't notice the fat?

JF: If I squint my eyes, cross my fingers, say a little prayer and envision Twinkies, I can usually enjoy fat-free or low-fat foods as much as I can foods with unaltered amounts of fat. New habits have to be learned; in my case, they have to be forced and coerced.

You: _____

_____

Fat is obvious when you spread butter on a roll. Potato chips leave a greasy residue on your fingers. However, what about the fat that you can't see? The hidden fat? It may not bother you to eat premium ice cream or a piece of cheese, especially because it tastes good. But the fat's there. It wouldn't be that difficult to eat a platter of greasy fried chicken and French fries with 150 grams of fat, which equals over 12 tablespoons of fat, which equals 1½ sticks of butter or margarine. Wow, that's an enormous amount!

The more unhealthy fat you eat, the more it accumulates in the blood. What foods with unhealthy fats could you be eating less often? What foods with healthy fats can you start eating?

JF: I can eliminate French fries or just eat less of them. It will require some therapy to get myself off them but worth the deprivation. I can eat more nuts, salmon, and other foods with good fat.

You: _____

_____

Eat fat. *Up to 35% of your diet can be fat. But eat healthy fat.* You can still eat sausage occasionally. Since saturated fat and cholesterol don't do anything to prevent disease, watch the frequency and the amount. If you eliminate high-fat foods, you'll be eating fewer calories and be able to eat more low-calorie foods – such as filling fruits and vegetables.

In goes the good air. Out goes the bad air. In go the MUFAs and PUFAs. Out go the saturated fat and trans fat. If you have a question about a product, read the ingredient list. Look for products made with canola oil, olive oil, sunflower oil, and soybean oil, rather than partially hydrogenated oils, coconut oil, or butter. Substitute vegetable oils for solid fats, as much as possible.

By the way, here's the answer to the trivia question: It takes *2,000 olives* to make a quart of extra virgin olive oil. Tell your friends. Dazzle them with your brilliance. Not only are you gorgeous, you're smart, too.

> *Moderate amounts of monounsaturated fat and polyunsaturated fat, especially omega 3 fatty acids, are your new best friends.*

End of Week 3

Congratulations! You're in the home stretch.

How is your new lifestyle going? What's working? What's still a challenge?

JF: I realize that I have to work out almost every day. As I get older, everything I eat stays with me. I've also learned that inches fall off me faster than pounds. So in order for me to adopt a healthy lifestyle for life as opposed to just a weekend, I have to move ... a lot.

You: _____

_____

It's time to weigh in.

_Weight:_____

You may have lost 1½-6 pounds. Keep making progress. Maybe you gained 2 pounds. You can only be you.

𝒟ay 21 CHECK-IN ☑

What did you accomplish yesterday?

JF: The rain stopped, and I went hiking with a girlfriend. I hear that the park where I hike is famous for mountain lions so I may get eaten. But besides the chance of death, I feel very proud of my new hiking routine.

You: _____

_____

What's your goal for today?

(Count the number of fat grams that you eat in a day.) (Buy extra virgin olive oil.) (Measure a tablespoon of oil.) (Try cod for dinner.)

JF: I will count how much fat I eat today. In other words, I will eat almost no fat today just to make this task easier and less painful.

You: _____

_____

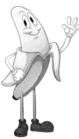

Jack Sprat could eat no fat.
His wife could eat no lean.
And so between the two of them,
They licked the platter clean!

*Better to eat the right kinds of fat
in the recommended amounts,
than to go to either extreme!*

Day 22

Rethinking Special Occasions

*T*reats used to be limited. Now we live in the Land of Special Occasions. On Mondays, Tuesdays, Sundays. More days besides birthdays and holidays have become special times to celebrate and a chance to eat out of our routine – and probably overeat.

Unless you're burning calories like crazy while training for the Ironman Triathlon World Championship, you're likely to slowly accumulate weight over time from the abundance of celebrations involving food.

Do you eat or drink more than your share? At work celebrations? After-work happy hours? Parties? Holidays? Vacations? Sporting events? Concerts? Plays? Conferences? Daylight Saving Time Day?

JF: I've been sneaky about eating my third or fourth piece of cake at an office party. I have no control when it comes to sweets. I've been an attendee at many an office party when I had no idea who the party was for. As long as there is cake involved, does it really matter why?

You: _____

_____

Of course, I'm not saying that you can never leave home. I'm saying *plan ahead* and be aware of what you're eating. The human body was not made for so many special occasions. How many tailgating parties did cavemen attend?

*R*uth's Rule: *It's time we enter special occasions with awareness, recognizing that it doesn't necessarily mean we have to put on extra pounds.*

Increasing Frequency, Widening Waistlines

When I grew up, treats were few and far between. That's just the way it was in those days. No one felt deprived. It was the norm. For a treat, we had a bottle of soda Saturday night. Halloween was the big day of the year to eat too much candy. And on the last day of school, students got a coupon for a box of Cracker Jacks and an ice cream bar. We had to wait to redeem it on the 4th of July. It was a big deal. Things are different these days. There is a profusion of treats available year-round. If you want, you can get sick from candy every day.

Years ago, it was difficult to get people to attend meetings – either for work or volunteering. At some point, someone came up with the brilliant idea to serve donuts to entice people to attend boring meetings, instead of only turning on the coffee pot. The idea spread like wildfire. I can remember thinking, "I don't want to go but at least I'll get a donut." From donuts, it expanded to other sweet snacks in massive amounts. After a while, I think that people became accustomed to getting something sweet as a reward. More meetings and events meant more treats and thus more calories. Today, work can be a minefield of high-calorie snacks. You never know when a co-worker will surprise everyone with goodies.

Eventually, adult-size treats began showing up at children's events and schools. Good grades and good behavior were rewarded with donut and pizza parties. Candy was given to students for doing their homework. The former "good job" or gold star wasn't good enough. Showing love and appreciation with food has become the norm. The current generation doesn't know the way it used to be. Kids these days have learned to "eat and be happy." The extra calories from treats have spun out of control, and now we have an obesity epidemic.

Let's see how we can handle these "special occasions" one by one.

Happy Birthdays

Everyone has a birthday. How do you celebrate?

JF: I usually have a gathering at a restaurant or nightclub. I have a cake made and available for everyone. Since it's my birthday, I get the most cake and probably a lot of free alcohol. So far, I'm not seeing how any of this is bad. My not seeing how this is bad for my waistline is probably part of my problem.

You: _____

Your birthday is one day. Many of my clients have week-long celebrations. First, they have a family get-together. Sometimes they go out on a separate night with in-laws. Co-workers take them out to lunch. They also have friends who want to take them to dinner. Eating out and celebrating numerous times throughout the week is not conducive to losing weight. There will be a net gain.

If you celebrate your birthday for more than one day, you need to carefully watch your intake. If you have a lot of family members and a lot of friends' birthdays to celebrate, there may be many occasions to overeat in a month. It will be difficult to lose weight unless you really streamline your calories. Clients get very sad when they see the scale go up after their birthdays.

Holiday Festivities

Holidays are a great excuse to "go off your diet." What's the use? There's so much food around. A big Thanksgiving meal with all of the trimmings can be 4,000 calories. There are 3,500 calories in a pound. If you normally eat 2,000 calories in a day, an extra 2,000 calories will cause a gain in weight. At 100 calories a mile, you would have to walk 20 miles to burn off the extra 2,000 calories. Does the pecan pie with whipped cream still look good? Fortunately, for most people, Thanksgiving doesn't cause too much damage because it's only one day.

If you're making a large holiday meal, downsize it. There are many healthy, yet delicious, side dishes. Serve more vegetables. Yams, cranberries, and green beans are colorful and full of nutrients. Make vegetables without butter and cream sauces. Add more celery, onions, and carrots to the stuffing. If you're serving dressing and mashed potatoes, you don't need bread. Use fat-free milk in mashed potatoes. Use fat-free sour cream, fat-free cream cheese, low-fat soup, low-calorie margarine, and fat-free whipped cream.

Thanksgiving is the start of the "holiday season." After Thanksgiving, some people start celebrating and don't look back until January 1st. And then, it's "Oh oh. What have I done?" It can take months to get back on track, if they haven't given up entirely.

For some people, the holiday season starts with Halloween. Halloween gets the ball rolling for candy that you had been able to resist. Eating Halloween candy is like sticking your toes in a swimming pool. By the time Thanksgiving rolls around, you have been splashing around for a while. By January, it's time to get out of the pool, only you're having too much fun and don't want to leave.

Are the holidays a problem for you? Relatives? Stress? Special foods? Do you eat too much? Do you drink too much alcohol? Do you get lots of food gifts? Do you go to a lot of parties? Do you forget about getting physical activity? Do you usually gain weight?

JF: I actually decided this year to stay home for the holidays rather than travel to see my parents, because all I do from the time the plane lands to when I leave is eat. The eggnog, cake, sauces, and all the animals on the farm stuffed with homemade dressing make going home a bad idea, at least until I get a grasp on my new lifestyle. So the answer is yes, the holidays are a problem for me and all the clothes I cannot fit back into January 2.

Parties are a mandatory part of my celebrating the holidays, or just to celebrate the fact that it is Tuesday. I usually gain close to 5 or 6 pounds every year during the holidays.

You: _____

_____

Strategies for a Svelte Holiday

Here are some tips for maintaining weight, not gaining it, during the holiday season:

- **Go in with a plan.** Is your goal to lose or maintain? If you have a busy holiday season and choose to maintain over the holidays, stop eating when you feel "just right." Or do you want to keep losing? Then you'll have to be more careful about what you eat. You will probably have to leave a party feeling like you could eat more, but be glad you didn't. Carrots and celery are your friends now, not chocolate mousse and crème brûlée.

- **Reduce stress eating.** If you don't have enough time to get everything done, don't worry about it. Decide where to cut back. Order gifts online. Give cash. Cut back on the decorations. Skip the baking. Visualizing a pleasant outcome will help you stay calm, cool, and collected.

- **Do you have to buy gifts for a lot of people and end up rewarding yourself with treats while you're at the mall?** Make a rule to not eat at the mall. Bring a fruit or some nuts with you for energy. Buy a low-calorie caffeine drink for some pep. Or when you get home, enjoy a cup of sugar-free hot cocoa.

- **If you love to make holiday treats, make one batch of cookies or candy instead of five or six.** Get used to not licking the bowl clean. It takes willpower in the beginning to skip this bowl ritual, but afterward you will have a feeling of superiority.

- **If you might eat or drink too much, plan on exercising before and/or after an event.** Nothing burns calories like exercise. Actually, it's the only thing. Make physical activity a priority with extra gym time or walking. Take advantage of holiday dancing.

- **If you're going to eat a big meal, do you need appetizers?** The rest of the meal will most likely be more than enough.

- **If you only eat a certain food once a year, enjoy it. Watch the portion size.** Next year is another year. Your special food will be back.

- **When trying to lose weight, aim at limiting extra calories to around 170 a day and stick with that exercising-more plan.**

It's conceivable that a person could eat 650 calories a day of sweets, fatty foods, or alcohol.

♦ **Watch the calories from beverages.** The calories from eggnog, punch, and after-dinner coffee drinks all count. Do you need the extra calories from whipped cream on that latte? Be careful of calories from alcohol.

♦ **Don't go to a party starving.** You'll quickly eat too much of the wrong foods. Have you ever felt like a Tasmanian devil whirling around the chips and dip until they are devoured? Unhealthy foods can taste heavenly. Take the edge off your hunger and eat a small yogurt before you leave home.

♦ **Watch out for hosts who are offended if you don't look like you're bursting at the seams.** If a host pushes food, take the food but don't eat it. Hold on to it and offer lots of compliments. If you're the host, don't pressure your guests to stuff themselves. Make less food and modify recipes, using less fat and sugar to reduce the calories.

♦ **Be warned that grabbing random bites is dangerous.** All of those bites can be enough calories for a complete meal. It's better to put all of the food you're going to eat on one plate. Then you know how much you're getting.

♦ **Are you nervous at parties and eat to give your hands something to do?** Hold a glass of spring or sparkling water in your hand. Be the life of the party and mingle. Start a Conga line and wind your way through the crowd.

♦ **Are there a lot of delicious foods that you can't resist? Take small portions and enjoy one bite of each food.** You can savor everything but still feel good about not over-indulging.

♦ **If you really like desserts, eat them first.** Then cut back on the other foods to avoid eating too much overall.

Do you eat desserts because they look too yummy to resist?

JF: Would "Hell, yes" be too dramatic or unprofessional an answer? I can't look at sweets or sit around and talk about recipes for desserts without having erotic fantasies about being smothered in buttercream frosting and then covered in sprinkles. I watch the Food Network to get my jollies.

At the holidays, there's bound to be more temptations than usual. Watch your portions. Eat one Buffalo wing, not six or seven. It's hard to eat perfectly every day, especially at parties. The people buying or making the food often aren't thinking about you or other people trying to lose weight. There are some outrageous foods out there these days. Avoid eating too much earlier in the day so that you still have calories to spare.

However Busy, Give Yourself the Gift of Exercise ❧

One of the biggest obstacles during the holidays is forgetting or not having time to exercise. People are busier than usual during the holidays. Days go by. Weeks go by. Exercise may be the first thing eliminated. Exercise should be a priority for your body and mind.

Stuffeth, Puffeth ... Or Succeed?

It has been reported that people typically gain 5-10 pounds during the holiday season. Other reports say that it's 1-2 pounds. It probably depends on the person. Almost everyone agrees that once people gain weight, most don't lose it. One or two extra pounds every holiday season can add up over the years.

Even if you try to keep the holidays as simple as possible, any extra activity can cause stress. Do what you can to relax and not let things get to you. Tai chi, yoga, and meditation can be relaxing. Make sure that you're getting enough sleep. If you're sleeping, you won't be stress-nibbling on fruitcake.

You know what they say ...

"If you indulge, you will bulge."
"Taste makes waist."
"He who stuffeth, puffeth."

I say, "If at first you don't succeed, diet, diet again."

*R*uth's Rule: *At holidays, load yourself up with winning strategies rather than excessive calories and weight gain.*

Vacation Indulgences

Do you usually gain weight on vacations?

JF: Yes, I gain weight whenever I step out of my regular routine. I have yet to master the art of carrying good habits and a workout routine to different parts of the country or world. I essentially look at a vacation as a vacation from all responsibility.

You: _____

_____

After working hard all year, you deserve to relax. Of course, there is the potential for a lot of extra eating on vacations. You're out of your usual routine. You see special treats that usually aren't available. You could put on an extra five pounds. *Is it worth it?*

Vacations are not the time to deprive yourself, especially if you're visiting a new place. The fun of a vacation is going to new areas and experiencing new things, including food. However, most people don't go on vacations by themselves. Buy one food and share it. Everyone gets a taste. Or buy a few different foods and share them. Children are small and need fewer calories. They don't need a large-size *anything*. In most cases, adults don't need a large size either.

Going on a cruise is one of the most difficult times to not gain weight. I've helped many clients enjoy cruises. They came back pleasantly surprised, actually thrilled, about not gaining weight.

Here are some **tips to manage your weight on a cruise:**

+ **Set a goal.** Do you want to maintain your weight or set a limit of gaining no more than 2-3 pounds? Setting a goal *to lose weight* may not be realistic. Weigh yourself before you leave and immediately after you return to assess any damages.
+ **On board the ship, always take the stairs – even if you're exhausted. Give it all you've got.** By the end of the week, your leg muscles will be stronger, and it will become easier. Of course,

some people have physical problems that limit their ability to take stairs. Most cruise ships are huge. Walk as much as you can on the ship and on land.

- **Take advantage of physical activity opportunities, such as the ship's gym, whenever possible.** Play ping pong. Find fun things to do. Stay active. You might find a new physical activity that you enjoy.
- **Prioritize where you want to eat and what.** There will be many restaurants and many food choices. If you feel out of control around so much food, the dining room might be better for you than the all-you-can-eat buffets.
- **Fill up on fruits and vegetables first.** They are lower in calories and filling.
- **Be especially careful of salad dressings, sauces, and cream soups.** They are sneaky, high-calorie foods.
- **If you're trying more than one entree, eat about ¼ cup or less of each.** When you're done, have the dishes taken away or get up from the table.
- **Watch the alcohol.** Food plus excess alcohol calories can easily push you over the top.
- **Don't feel like you have to finish *anything*.** There will be more food than any human can eat.
- **Do you like desserts? Take one bite and only one bite of each dessert.** All of the bites will equal one regular dessert.
- **Stay hydrated.** Flying to your destination and being on an air-conditioned ship can be dehydrating. It may be hot and humid outside. Drink plenty of water and other non-caloric beverages. A glass of sparkling water with a slice of lime is very refreshing.
- **After you get home, weigh yourself. By some miracle, you maintained your weight.** *Caution.* You will be going back to your usual routine, which may not be physically active. However, you may still be in the cruise eating mode. If your appetite doesn't slow down, but you do, you'll gain weight *after* you get home. Surprise!! It happens. When you get home, eat less than you were eating on the cruise.

+ **If you gained weight on the cruise, immediately cut back on portions.** Lose the weight ASAP. Don't wait until tomorrow.

Fad Diets to the Rescue?

Let's say that your glorious vacation is over. You're relaxed and calm, and Monday morning it's back to the salt mines. You happen to mention to a co-worker that your clothes are a little snug. She has a fantastic diet for you to try.

I'm glad that there are specialists in the world. Attorneys specialize in law. Mechanics specialize in fixing cars. There are doctors who specialize in brain surgery. These days buying a new television requires a special technician to set it up. Every occupation has a particular knowledge and special talent to get the job done. We need these people.

Meanwhile, everyone seems to have the right answer, regardless of their education and expertise, when it comes to losing weight. I am not fond of the "Food Combining Diet" to get you back to your pre-vacation weight. According to the diet, it's okay to combine protein with vegetables but not okay to combine protein with fruit. And don't combine different types of melons, such as cantaloupe with watermelon. These types of diets get copied and passed around to fellow employees. Amazingly, the accompanying explanation makes sense to people, and they're willing to try it for a few days.

It's no wonder there are so many nutrition myths and so much nutrition misinformation to confuse people. There are so many expert opinions. People are willing to accept whatever they are told. Luckily, most people who try these types of diets don't usually stick to it for more than a few days. It takes too much effort.

The next time a diet appears on your desk, be a skeptic. Did anything strange happen to you the last time you ate fruit salad? Use common sense to evaluate diets. Ask a real expert. See a registered dietitian nutritionist for your nutrition needs.

Enjoy More than the Food

Gaining weight is easy. Losing weight is hard. Prevention is the best option. Focus on the people and the occasion, not just eating. Enjoy and try everything in moderation. If you aren't eating as healthfully as you could, at least eat smaller portions. Show some restraint. No matter what the situation, only eat if hungry and try to stick to your usual intake of food. *Scan and plan.* There will always be another day, another holiday and another vacation.

How might you handle special occasion eating differently now?

JF: Now I would work out in the morning to rev up my metabolism. I would pick foods that were delicious but not detrimental to my goals.

You: _____

_____

Treat every day like it is January 1st. Keep working on your New Year's resolutions on May 1st, even October 1st. *It's a lifestyle.*

You can't undo one or two weeks' worth of vacation overeating in a day or two. It may take two or three times as long to lose the extra pounds. Losing weight and maintaining is always a process. Keep working on it. Feel good about yourself and be a winner. *You can do it.*

A "take it easy" celebration is your new best friend.

WEEKLY REMINDER
Your Reasons for Losing Weight
Are you reminding yourself *every day* why you want to lose weight? If not, this is your weekly reminder.

Why do you want to lose weight? Are you starting to notice some of those results showing up in your life?

JF: My new lifestyle is challenging, with all the traveling and being in different places. I am a work in progress.

You: _____

_____

*D*ay 22 CHECK-IN ☑

What did you accomplish yesterday?

JF: I worked out. Sorry, not very exciting. However, I have to learn to start to celebrate the basics so that they become more a part of my life.

You: _____

_____

What is your goal for today?

(Have you been physically active? Keep an exercise journal.) (Write down a plan for the next holiday. How are you going to avoid emotional eating?) (Set eating and activity goals for your next vacation.) (Bring your own snacks to the mall instead of buying a 1,000-calorie cinnamon bun.) (Decide to buy gifts, not candy, for Valentine's Day and other holidays.) (Don't listen to the self-proclaimed nutritionist at work.) (Give yourself a big hug.)

JF: My goal is to keep moving. When I move every day, my body is less likely to sabotage my new lifestyle.

You: _____

_____

Day 23

The Extras (aka Empty Calories)
(aka SoFAS – Solid Fats, Added Sugars)

*B*rownies, hot apple pie, mint chocolate-chip ice cream … these are a few of my favorite things. Chili cheese fries, gravy, Alfredo sauce … these are a few more of my favorite things. Not to mention gin and tonic, coffee liqueur and cream, and chardonnay wine.

What do all of these wonderful foods have in common?

JF: All of these foods are reasons to get out of bed every morning.

You: _____

_____

If you answered, "They are *extra calories*," you are correct. What about 1% milk, 2% milk, canned fruit packed in syrup, and fruit-flavored low-fat yogurt? *Yes.* They also contain extra calories. Healthy eating is lean and somewhat mean to people who are trying to lose weight. This chapter will help you find some balance in making your dietary changes.

Empty vs. Essential Calories

Essential calories are the calories required to meet the recommended nutrient needs. Those calories are very lean, low fat, and do not have added sugars. They are the foods that are used to calculate MyPlate meal patterns. Essential calories are nutrient-rich (lots of vitamins and minerals) and low-energy (low in calories), in contrast to nutrient-poor (little or no nutrients) and energy-dense (lots of calories).

Essential calories come from:

1. Fat-free milk
2. Very lean meat
3. Grains without added sugars or added fats
4. Vegetables without added fats
5. Fruits without added sugars
6. Oils and trans-fat-free soft margarines (meets vitamin E and essential fatty acid needs)

Empty calories or the "extras" are the balance of calories left from the estimated daily calorie allowance after nutrient needs have been met with essential calories.

Empty calories are allocated to:

1. *Higher caloric forms* of food in the basic food groups that contain added solid fats and added sugars (2% milk, cheese, sausage, sweetened yogurt, sweetened cereal)
2. Foods with solid fats, added sugars, and alcohol (candy, soda, butter, sauces, wine)

The calories in that second group of empty or *extra* calories are found mostly in fat, sugar, or alcohol. Alcohol doesn't contain solid fats or added sugars, but it counts as extra calories. Your body doesn't need these foods, even if you think it does. You can still eat them, just not too much.

Extra Calories in Foods

All of the calories from the following foods would be considered extra calories.

1 can (12 ounces) regular soda	136
1 bottle (20 ounces) regular soda	192
1½ ounces distilled spirits (80 proof)	96
5 ounces wine	121

1 can (12 ounce) of beer	155

Some of the calories from these foods count as extra calories.

1 teaspoon butter	33
1 tablespoon cream cheese	36
1 tablespoon heavy whipping cream	45
1 cup 1% milk	18
1 cup 2% milk	37
1 cup whole milk	63
1 cup low-fat chocolate milk	64
1½ ounces cheddar cheese	113
8 ounces fruit-flavored low-fat yogurt	152
1 cup vanilla ice cream	210
3 ounces 80% lean regular ground beef	64
3 fried chicken wings with skin	382
1 (2 ounce) medium croissant	111*
1 medium order French fries	185

*Note: One hundred and twenty calories from a medium croissant count as grain calories. However, the additional 111 calories from the croissant count toward extra calories, for a total of 231 calories.

Source: www.ChooseMyPlate.gov/foodgroups/emptycalories

Essential calories are low in fat and low in sugar. The energy expenditure food patterns for MyPlate are calculated using fat-free milk. The extra 18 calories from 1% milk count toward the extra calories. Are you still buying 2% milk?

If you're aiming for 1,800 calories a day, a cup of coffee with two dollops of whipped cream and two pumps of flavored syrup use up most of the 170 extra calories for the day.

Since most people use their extra calories for sweet foods, let's spend time in this chapter understanding more about sugar and other sweeteners.

*R*uth's **Rule:** *Allowing yourself a small amount of daily extra calories can help you feel less deprived as you begin to make healthier choices.*

Technical Terms for Sugar

Monosaccharides are the building blocks of carbohydrates. *Glucose, galactose,* and *fructose* are monosaccharides. Monosaccharides are known as "simple sugars." They are not digested. They are immediately absorbed into the body.

Disaccharides are two monosaccharides linked together. *Sucrose, lactose,* and *maltose* are disaccharides.

- **Sucrose** (table sugar) is glucose + fructose.
- **Lactose** (natural sugar in milk) is glucose + galactose.
- **Maltose** (malt sugar) is glucose + glucose.

A Spoonful of Sugar

Humans are born with a sweet tooth. Human milk is sweet. At an early age, humans learn that sweet means survival.

Sugar is a simple carbohydrate. A little sugar gives you an energy boost. A teaspoon of sugar has four grams of carbohydrate. A gram of carbohydrate also has four calories.

Sugar has many functions besides adding a sweet flavor. Sugar adds bulk, texture, and structure to food, retains moisture, acts as a preservative, provides fermentation, and adds color. If foods have sugar or syrups added to them during preparation and processing, they are foods with "added sugars," not the "naturally occurring sugars" found in fruits, vegetables, and milk.

Eating sugar does not cause diabetes. Most diabetes is determined by a combination of genetics and excess weight. If most of the excess weight is from eating foods with sugar, then sugar could indirectly be a factor. Sugar can increase the risk of dental caries, too.

Have you been to a restaurant recently and looked at the dessert menu? *Yikes.* So much temptation. Plus, the portions are *gigantic.* And the desserts these days aren't just good. They're great. In fact, they're incredible. It takes willpower to not eat too much. Actually, if you're eating out, you probably exceeded your calorie allotment for the day even before dessert.

Remember that a sugar by any other name is still sugar. All of the following are names for sugar:

- White sugar
- Sucrose
- Turbinado
- Honey
- Glucose
- Dextrose
- Invert sugar
- Maltose
- Malt syrup
- Corn syrup
- High fructose corn syrup
- Raw sugar
- Brown sugar
- Powdered sugar
- Fructose
- Levulose
- Fruit juice concentrate
- Lactose
- Brown rice syrup
- Corn sweetener
- Maple syrup
- Molasses

Sweets for the Sweet

Nutritive sweeteners contain calories, provide energy, and add sweetness. Let's become more familiar with the different types of sugar.

Table sugar is made from sugar cane or sugar beets. It is half glucose and half fructose. A packet of sugar has 11 calories. One teaspoon of sugar has 16 calories. Adding a teaspoon of sugar to the water in a bouquet of cut flowers will make them last longer.

Actual *raw sugar* has impurities and is not available for consumer use. It is a tan, coarse granulated sugar made from sugar cane juice.

Turbinado sugar is raw sugar that has been partially refined for consumer use. It has coarse grains, and the light tan color is from molasses. Most of the "raw sugar" you see on the market falls into this category.

Powdered sugar (confectioner's sugar) is white sugar that is ground into a powder. Cornstarch can be added to prevent caking.

Brown sugar contains sugar and molasses syrup; the syrup gives it more flavor and a brown color. One teaspoon of unpacked brown sugar is 11 calories. One teaspoon of packed brown sugar is 17 calories.

Fructose (levulose) is a simple sugar found naturally in fruits, some vegetables, and honey. Fructose does not raise blood sugar as quickly as table sugar but it may increase triglyceride levels. Crystalline fructose is pure fructose that is made from corn syrup or sugar and allowed to crystallize. Crystalline fructose is used in place of sugar in drinks, ice cream, breakfast cereals, cookies, etc. Crystalline fructose is about 1.2 times sweeter than table sugar, so less is needed.

Losing Weight on Sugar? ଓ

In the late 1970s, there was the Fructose Diet. "Lose fourteen pounds in two weeks" was the claim. *Not bad.* Protein was required at every meal (specifically lots of eggs and liver), and it included a small salad at lunch and dinner. Fructose drinks were required at every meal, and fructose tablets or fructose drinks were required as snacks three times a day for a total of 38-42 grams of fructose, or only 152-168 calories from carbs. They claimed that the fructose stopped the cravings for sugar. It stated that some of the 10-15 pounds of weight loss in the first two weeks were from unwanted fluid. *Ahhh. The '70s.* I would call this the potentially dangerous Ketosis Diet.

Dextrose is crystalline glucose made from cornstarch, sugar cane, or sugar beets. Dextrose is used in baked products, snacks, and as a filler in packets of artificial sweeteners.

Maltodextrins are short chains of (dextrose) glucose molecules. It could be made from starches, such as corn, rice, or potatoes. It is not sweet. It is used to add bulk and texture, often to packets of artificial sweeteners.

Molasses is the thick residue left from the sugar-refining process. Molasses has 19 calories per teaspoon. Blackstrap molasses (dark, thick and bitter) is the last step in sugar refining. It is known as a health food for its calcium, iron, and potassium.

Invert sugar is sugar that is broken down into glucose and fructose. The liquid contains equal amounts of glucose and fructose. It is sweeter than sugar and is used in candy and baked products.

Corn syrup is the sugar extracted from cornstarch. It has 21 calories per teaspoon. Commercial corn syrups can be from 20-98% glucose.

Corn syrup could be called glucose syrup. This type of sugar is a little less sweet than dextrose.

High fructose corn syrup (HFCS) is made from corn. From cornstarch, it is broken down and converted to a mixture of fructose and glucose. It has been a commonly used sweetener since the '70s. HFCS can be found in products ranging from soft drinks to salad dressings to cheese spreads to hot dogs.

Close-Up on HFCS ℞

If you have an opportunity, conduct a taste test with a cola sweetened with sugar and one sweetened with high fructose corn syrup (HFCS). There *is* a difference in taste. You may or may not have a preference.

Here are some facts about high fructose corn syrup:

- HFCS is either 42% or 55% fructose, and the rest is glucose. FYI: Table sugar is 50% fructose and 50% glucose. Without the water, honey is 49% fructose and 43% glucose.
- HFCS contains 4 calories per gram, the same as sugar.
- HFCS-55 is used in soft drinks and has the same sweetness as sugar.
- High fructose corn syrup has FDA's GRAS (Generally Recognized as Safe) status.

HFCS is controversial and gets a lot of media attention. Can we blame obesity on high fructose corn syrup? Or do we blame the excess calories consumed in products sweetened with high fructose corn syrup? The controversy continues.

JF: While I don't really believe high fructose corn syrup is the cause for obesity, it is easier (and personally preferred) to blame it for the fact that my thighs are such very close friends and want to literally "stick" together.

You: _____

Maple syrup comes from the sap of maple trees. It has 17 calories per teaspoon.

Fruit juice concentrates are often made from grapes and pears. The water, fiber, flavor, and color are removed from the fruit juice. The remaining sugar is used to sweeten products.

Agave syrup (nectar) comes from the agave plant, a succulent which is also used to make tequila. This syrup can contain from 55-90% fructose. It has 20 calories per teaspoon.

Honey starts with the nectar found in flowers. Bees turn the nectar into honey. This sweetener has 21 calories per teaspoon. The flavor depends on the source of the nectar. Honey is a type of sugar, and so it raises blood sugar. It contains antioxidants. *Honey should not be given to infants less than 12 months old because of the chance of ingesting bacterial spores of Clostridium botulinum.*

Start looking at the different types of sugar on the ingredient lists of foods. You might see sugar in products where you wouldn't expect it, such as ketchup or spaghetti sauce.

Sugar Guidelines

The DGA 2015-2020 recommends limiting daily calories from *added sugars* to less than 10%. The new Dietary Guidelines put the *extra* calories, which includes added sugars, in the category called *Limit on Calories for Other Uses*. Based on 1,800 calories, 10% of added sugars would be 45 grams or 180 calories or 11 teaspoons of sugar a day.

Eleven teaspoons seems like a lot but it can add up quickly. Some 20-fluid-ounce bottles of soda contain over 16 teaspoons of sugar. A king-size chocolate candy bar can have 10 teaspoons of sugar. A cup of sweetened cereal can have 3 teaspoons of sugar. One half cup of sherbet has 4.5 teaspoons of sugar. One tablespoon of jam has 2.5 teaspoons of sugar.

Do visions of sugar plums dance in your head? Maybe it's donuts, cookies, cake, pie, ice cream, soda, pastries, or candy. It's fun and easy to succumb to a warm brownie topped with vanilla ice cream topped with hot fudge sauce.

Do you like to binge on sugary foods? What? How much?

JF: If I had a choice between an expensive steak dinner and a few cupcakes, I would take the cupcakes. Help me!

You: _____

_____

By itself, sugar doesn't cause obesity. Not caring about your weight and eating too many sugar calories will make your weight go up. Eating when you're not hungry will increase weight. Eating for emotional comfort will also add weight. We can't blame sugar. It has been around a lot longer than our current obesity epidemic.

*ℛ*uth's **Rule:** *Watch your sugar intake, as the calories add up quickly.*

One Way to Stop a Binge ℛ

The next time you feel that you might binge on something sweet, calculate the teaspoons of sugar in the food. It might act as a deterrent. To find the amount of sugar, look at the label. Multiply the grams of added sugars *per serving* by 4. That's the total number of sugar calories. Divide that number by 16 to get the number of teaspoons of sugar (there are 16 calories in a teaspoon). For 8 ounces of fruited fat-free yogurt: 15 grams of added sugars x 4 divided by 16 = 3.75. *So, 8 ounces of fruited fat-free yogurt could have 4 teaspoons of sugar!*

What the Heck Is a "Sugar Alcohol"?

Sugar alcohols, also known as *polyols*, are being used in processed foods. They sweeten foods and also add bulk and texture. While sugar alcohols have been around for some time, you may not have noticed.

Can you get drunk from sugar alcohols? No. They are neither sugar nor alcohol. They are a group of low-calorie carbohydrates. Sugar alcohols are found naturally in fruits and vegetables but are commercially made from cornstarch, sugar, and whey. They are sweet but contain about half the calories of regular carbohydrates. They average about 2.5 calories per gram. Sugar alcohols are slowly metabolized and don't raise blood sugar as much as table sugar. There's no promotion of tooth decay from this type of sweetener.

Sugar alcohols are only partially absorbed by the body. When consumed in large amounts, they may give some people gas, bloating, and cramping. Large amounts (more than 20 grams a day of mannitol or more than 50 grams a day of sorbitol) may have a laxative effect on some people.

Here are the names of approved sugar alcohols and calories per gram:

Erythritol	0.2 calories per gram
Mannitol	1.6 calories per gram
Isomalt	2.0 calories per gram
Lactitol	2.0 calories per gram
Maltitol	2.1 calories per gram
Xylitol	2.4 calories per gram
Sorbitol	2.6 calories per gram
Hydrogenated Starch Hydrolysates (polyglycitols)	3.0 calories per gram

As you can see, there are fewer calories in sugar alcohols than sugar's 4 calories per gram. You will often see sugar alcohols in sugar-free and reduced-sugar foods. What's the powder on chewing gum? It could be mannitol.

Sugar alcohols are listed on the ingredient list either by their specific names or as sugar alcohols. Once you're familiar with the names, you'll notice them in candy, cookies, baked goods, ice cream, jam, gum, mouthwashes, toothpaste, and cough syrups.

Artificial Sweeteners - Friend or Foe?

Nonnutritive sweeteners (low-calorie sweeteners, sugar substitutes, artificial sweeteners, intense sweeteners, alternative sweeteners) replace sugar in food and beverages and provide few or no calories and no energy.

Consuming artificial sweeteners is not necessary to lose weight. In the 1950s, artificial sweeteners were not readily available, and excess weight for most people wasn't an issue.

Low-fat and fat-free versions of foods (such as fat-free milk) were also not available. Today, most Americans are overweight and hundreds of millions of people use artificial sweeteners. Therefore, do artificial sweeteners help reduce weight? On the other hand, would the obesity epidemic be worse without them?? Artificial sweeteners are definitely an option for diabetics who want to eat something sweet without raising their blood sugar.

Sugar substitutes can save calories, and theoretically help people control their weight. They can be a useful tool for people to use. Nutritive-sweetened foods can be substituted with artificially sweetened foods to decrease the number of calories. There will be fewer calories, resulting in weight loss. They are not a magic potion for losing weight. You cannot expect to eat foods with artificial sweeteners, and then eat whatever you want.

If you save calories by eating foods with artificial sweeteners, do you think that you can eat more calories from other foods?

JF: Actually, I have learned that foods that are naturally sweetened, such as fruit, are a great alternative to the sugary snacks I've been addicted to most of my life.

You: _____

Artificial sweeteners offer sweetness without the calories. They sweeten more than coffee and tea. Artificial sweeteners are in many products, including breakfast cereal, yogurt, diet sodas, energy drinks, ice cream, syrup, juice, and jams – to name a few. They are also in chewing gum, breath mints, chewable multivitamin/mineral supplements, and cough drops. Artificial sweeteners do not cause dental caries. Most artificial sweeteners are not metabolized and pass through the body unchanged.

Nutritive and nonnutritive sweeteners are regulated by the FDA either as *GRAS ingredients* or as *food additives*. The 1958 Food Additives Amendment to the Federal Food, Drug and Cosmetic Act requires the FDA to approve new food additives, unless the products contain GRAS ingredients. Manufacturers must prove that an additive is safe.

The GRAS status was created in 1958 when the Food Additives Amendment was modified. A product with GRAS status does not need FDA approval. If an additive had been used for many years and proven safe before 1958, it was exempt and considered GRAS. Either it had a long history of safe use in foods, or it had been determined to be safe based on proven science. If new evidence suggests that a GRAS substance may no longer be safe, the FDA can stop its use or require further studies. The FDA approves new additives, including artificial sweeteners, after a comprehensive analysis of extensive science-based studies.

The *Acceptable Daily Intake* (ADI) is a conservative estimate of the maximum amount that a person can safely consume *every day over a lifetime*. The FDA determines a safe intake based on average consumption. If you occasionally go over the amount, it is not a toxic dose. The ADI is intended to be about 100 times less than the maximum amount found to be safe in animal studies.

Acceptable Daily Intake (ADI) of Current U.S. Artificial Sweeteners

Saccharin	15 mg/kg of body weight/day
Sucralose	5 mg/kg of body weight/day
Acesulfame-K	15 mg/kg of body weight/day
Neotame	.3 mg/kg of body weight/day
Aspartame	50 mg/kg of body weight/day

As an example, an adult (150 pounds) would have to drink 17 12-ounce cans of diet soda sweetened only with aspartame or 97 packets of Equal a day to meet the daily ADI for aspartame. A 50-pound child would have to drink 6 cans of diet soda or 32 packets of Equal a day to meet the ADI for aspartame. According to the Calorie Control Council, 9 out of 10 people consume less than 10% of the ADI for aspartame.

Different organizations around the world have established their own Acceptable Daily Intake recommendations. Not all of their values for artificial sweeteners are consistent with the FDA's ADI values.

Individual packets of artificial sweeteners weigh 1 gram. The amount of artificial sweetener in a packet can range from 10-40 milligrams, depending on the sweetener. The rest of the packet contains fillers for bulk. The milligrams of artificial sweetener are not listed on the label but can occasionally be found on company websites. There is a wide range of amounts of artificial sweeteners in diet sodas. Some diet sodas contain only one artificial sweetener. Other diet sodas contain varying amounts of several artificial sweeteners.

Background on Artificial Sweeteners

Many people identify their favorite artificial sweetener by the color of the packet:

- Aspartame: Equal (*blue packet*), NutraSweet
- Saccharin: Sweet'N Low (*pink packet*), Sugar Twin, Necta Sweet
- Sucralose: Splenda (*yellow packet*)
- Acesulfame potassium: Sunett, Sweet One
- Neotame: Newtame
- Stevia: Truvia, PureVia, Enliten

Saccharin is 200-700 times sweeter than sugar and doesn't contain any calories. It's not metabolized and passes through the body unchanged. Saccharin has been around for a long time. It was discovered in 1879 and was used in World War I and World War II, when there were sugar shortages. Pink packets of Sweet'N Low have been around since 1957. Saccharin had FDA's GRAS (generally recognized as safe) status until it was taken off the GRAS list in 1972. Subsequent studies found that saccharin did not cause cancer in humans. In 2001, the warning label was removed. Saccharin has been around for over a century and is consumed in over 100 countries.

Aspartame was discovered in 1965 and was approved by the FDA in 1981. It is 200 times sweeter than sugar. Aspartame has 4 calories a gram, and since it's so sweet, only a little of it is needed. Over 100 countries have found aspartame to be safe. It's digested as protein. The body breaks down aspartame into small amounts of methanol and two amino acids, aspartic acid and phenylalanine. People with phenylketonuria (PKU), a rare genetic disorder, cannot metabolize phenylalanine. Phenylketonuria builds up in the blood, so aspartame should be avoided in people with PKU. More than 6,000 products are sweetened with aspartame.

Acesulfame potassium (also known as Acesulfame K or Ace-K) was discovered in 1967. It is 200 times sweeter than sugar and doesn't contain any calories. It isn't metabolized and goes through the body unchanged. The FDA approved Acesulfame-K in 1988, and it has been determined to be safe in over 100 countries. Many people don't know that Ace-K is an artificial sweetener. It's used as a sweetener in more than 4,000 products. It is often blended with other artificial sweeteners to make a product sweeter.

Sucralose was discovered in 1976. It is 600 times sweeter than sugar. To put that into perspective, the Calorie Control Council states that a 12-ounce can of diet soda requires about 70 *milligrams* of sucralose to make it sweet, compared to 40 *grams* of sugar. *That's a big difference.* The FDA approved sucralose in 1998. Sucralose passes through the body unchanged, so it doesn't add any calories. This is the only sweetener made from sugar. It is chemically modified by replacing the hydrogen-oxygen groups with chlorine atoms. The result is a sweet flavor without the calories. Some people are concerned about the chlorine. The chlorine does not separate from the sucralose molecule. Sucralose is approved in over 80 countries.

Neotame is a relatively new artificial sweetener. The FDA approved Neotame in 2002. It is 7,000 to 13,000 times sweeter than sugar and doesn't contain any calories. The structure of neotame is similar to aspartame. It is metabolized as a protein and eliminated. There doesn't have to be a warning for people with phenylketonuria. Neotame has been approved in over 20 countries.

Stevia is a South American shrub that has been used as a natural sweetener for centuries in Paraguay. Stevia is 300 times sweeter than sugar. Stevia extracts have been available as a dietary supplement in America, but it was not approved as a sweetener by the FDA until 2008. A purified form of stevia (Rebaudioside A or rebiana) has received GRAS status. Reb A is used to sweeten beverages, desserts, and other foods.

Most of the artificial sweeteners leave the body the same way they went in. Even after years of worldwide review and approval by the U.S. Food and Drug Administration, the Scientific Committee on Food (SCF) of the European Commission, and the Joint Expert Committee on Food Additives (JECFA) administered by the Food and Agriculture Organization of the United Nations (FAO) and the World Health Organization (WHO), do you think that artificial sweeteners are safe?

JF: Yup, I have no problem with artificial sweeteners. They save me from putting 12 teaspoons of sugar in my tea to give it taste. I thank God for aspartame.

You: _____

More time will tell. Hundreds of millions of people around the world have been consuming artificially sweetened food and beverages for many years. If problems show up in the future, it will affect a lot of people worldwide.

If you want to be the person who says, "I told you so," you can always go natural. Sixteen calories for a teaspoon of sugar isn't much. A sugar cube is 9 calories. Moderation is eating a small amount of foods sweetened with table sugar. You can lose weight without using artificial sweeteners.

*R*uth's Rule: *If you're worried about using artificial sweeteners, you can choose to eat a moderate amount of sugar-sweetened foods instead.*

Understanding the Glycemic Index

The *glycemic index* was developed in 1981 by David Jenkins at the University of Toronto to help diabetics manage blood sugar. This index ranks 50-gram portions of carbohydrate foods by how much they raise blood sugar levels compared to the same amount of the ingested reference food (white bread or glucose). For diabetics, the lower the number, the lower the impact on glucose levels. Since low GI foods are absorbed at a slower rate, this could make people feel full for a longer amount of time.

Low glycemic foods tend to be most fruits, vegetables, beans, and whole grains (such as oatmeal and barley). *That's good.* Carrots, watermelon, and baked potatoes are healthy foods but have a high GI. Some people may avoid healthy foods because they have a high GI value. Some unhealthy foods have a low GI.

The GI value for a food can vary greatly depending on the variety, ripeness, or the way it's cooked. A food consumed alone will have a different value than if it is part of a meal. Physical activity may lower the GI value of a food. Also, individuals could have different responses to the same food. All of these factors prevent consistency.

More research is needed to determine the effectiveness of using the Glycemic Index.

What Are Your Favorite Things?

As mentioned earlier in this chapter, many people like to use their extra calories on foods that taste sweet; perhaps this is because there are so many choices. However, there's more to life than sugar. Other folks use their extra calories on alcohol. Every person spends their extra calories in different ways.

Avoid eating too many calories by following MyPlate meal patterns. Then after all of the basic nutrients have been met, there will be an extra 170 calories a day to use for splurging. See the chart on the next page for the extra calorie allowance for other daily calorie targets.

One can of soda is around 140 calories. If you drink a can of soda, you only have 30 calories left to spend on sugar, fat, or alcohol. According to prior Dietary Guidelines, the average American consumes nearly 800 calories a day from solid fats and added sugars. You can see why most people in America are overweight.

Total Calories:	1200	1400	1600	1800	2000	2200	2400
Extra Calories:	100	110	130	170	270	280	350

Special Note: *The extra calorie allowance is a part of the total amount of calories, not in addition to the total amount. If you eat 1,800 calories, 1,630 calories are essential and 170 are extra. These amounts of extra calories are for people who get less than 30 minutes of moderate physical activity most days.*

Knowledge Is Power

Losing weight doesn't mean deprivation. If you're only eating 1,600 calories a day, you can still eat an extra 130 calories of anything that meets your fancy. It may not be a lot or as much as you want, but it's better than nothing. *Live lean. Make healthy choices. Choose foods without solid fats and added sugars.*

Some people need to control their "sweet tooth." Others need to control their "fat tooth," "carbohydrate tooth," "salt tooth" or "alcohol tooth." *What "tooth" do you need to control?*

JF: My sweet tooth is my nemesis. Some days, I need someone to take my car keys so my sweet tooth doesn't have a ride to Baskin-Robbins. By my "fat tooth," do you mean my fat booty needs to get control of its cravings or do you mean my affinity for "fatty" foods? Either way, my entire mouth of teeth needs to be controlled.

You: _____

Extra Calories, Be Selective

Here are some strategies for maintaining an optimal weight. Limit nutrient-poor foods (e.g., specialty coffee drinks) and energy-dense foods (e.g., anything fried). Go to www.myfoodapedia.gov to identify the number of calories from added sugars and solid fats in foods. Focus on eating essential calories to get the recommended nutrients. Stick to the nutrient-rich, low-energy foods, such as fruits, vegetables, grains, lean protein, and fat-free milk. If you want to eat more, get more physical activity.

A greater awareness of extra calories can have a tremendous impact on America's excess weight problem. Be particular and selective about your extra calorie friends, especially when losing weight.

One hundred seventy or less extra calories a day are your new best friends.

*D*ay 23 CHECK-IN ☑

What did you accomplish yesterday?

JF: I exercised yesterday. Not exciting once again, but day after day of exercise in a row is remarkable for me.

You: _____

_____

What is your goal for today?

(Limit extra calories to 170 calories a day.) (Go a day without or continue to eliminate: sweets, alcohol, or fried foods.) (Eat only essential calories.) (If you eat more than 170 extra calories, walk a mile for every extra 100 calories to burn it off.) (Look at the ingredients of your favorite treat.)

JF: My goal is to watch what goes into my mouth at non-meal times. I tend to nibble all day long and not realize that all that food can sabotage an awesome cycling class.

You: _____

_____

338

Day 24

Chug-a-Lug – Drink Up!

Are you a drinker? How many cups of fluid do you drink in a day, including coffee, tea, juice, milk, soda, and water? What is your best estimation?

JF: I grew up on Hi-C fruit punch and other delicious sugary drinks and soda. Then as I got older, I started drinking a lot of diet soda. Now I drink diet soda in moderation and mostly just water. To be honest, my body craves drinks with flavor but I have learned to enjoy water with lemon. I also have a cup of tea every morning as opposed to expensive flavored coffee and fancy beverages.

You: _____

_____

When you don't drink enough fluids, you feel thirsty. Eventually, you will become dehydrated. You don't really think about it, but water is one of the most important nutrients. Water regulates body temperature, cushions joints, transports nutrients, helps digest food, and assists in eliminating waste products, such as protein and excess electrolytes. Water is needed in large amounts. Think about your blood. It's mostly water. Muscle is about 75% water. The more muscle you have, the higher percent of fluid you have in your body. The human body is over half water. In fact, we carry around 10-12 gallons of water in our body.

Getting enough fluids *is essential*. Water leaves the body through sweat, breathing, urine, and bowel movements. Water has to be replaced *every day*. You can't go for more than 3-5 days without water. If it's hot, you wouldn't survive even a few days.

Do you often feel tired or constipated?

JF: Around that time of the month, I do get fatigued often. I am never, ever constipated. Most of the food I eat daily moves out of me quickly or within a few hours. If there is anything in life I need to be grateful for when I can't think of anything else, it is that I am extremely regular. My ability to poop should be on my resume, it is so amazing.

You: _____

_____

If you answered "yes," there's a good chance that you're dehydrated. *I'm not kidding.* You may not even realize that you need more fluids. Being just *a little* dehydrated makes you feel tired. Feel like you need a little sugar in the afternoon? Maybe a chocolate bar? Down a cup of water. You'll perk right up, just like a droopy plant. Feeling constipated? Eat more fiber. If you eat a lot of fiber, you'll need more fluid to bulk it up and move it out. Elimination will be quick and easy. Go for *whoosh*.

How to Be Well-Hydrated

Every person has different hydration needs. It depends on the air temperature and what you're doing throughout the day. An older person, who sits in an air-conditioned living room for hours, doesn't need as much fluid as a young man running ten miles on a warm day. The more you sweat, whether it's from a high outside temperature or physical activity, the more fluids you need. Some people with heart or kidney problems need to restrict their fluids.

Your body loses a lot of fluids *every day*. How much do you need? One easy way is to check your urine. Kidneys filter out waste from blood. The kidneys need enough water to flush out the waste. Be on the lookout for clear, light or pale yellow in color urine, not yellow or dark yellow. Of course, medications and vitamins can color urine. To keep your kidneys healthy, go for a light color.

The National Academy of Medicine's 2005 Adequate Intake (AI) recommendation for daily fluid intake for healthy men 19-70 years in temperate climates is 13 cups from beverages, with another 3 cups of fluid from food. For the average woman 19-70 years, the Adequate Intake is 9 cups from beverages, with another 2.5 cups of fluid from food. The fluid derived from food is 20% of the daily total fluid intake. Fruits like peaches and watermelon contain mostly fluid. Even meat and bread contain fluid. Otherwise, they would be beef jerky and croutons.

The NAM's recommended amounts were made to prevent dehydration. It is not a requirement. Individuals can be adequately hydrated at levels above or below these amounts. A person's needs depend on their thirst, usual drinking behavior, heat, and vigorous activity. People who eat lots of fruits and vegetables have more fluid from food than people who eat meat and crackers. Let thirst be your guide, but keep an eye on your urine.

Fluids come in many forms. Coffee, tea, milk, juice, soda, water, soup, fruits, vegetables, even popsicles and ice cream. Your body will use anything with fluid to replenish itself. Some fluids provide important nutrients, such as protein and calcium. The fluid recommendation is cups of "fluid," not strictly cups of water.

Beverages and Weight Loss ℭ

As far as losing weight or maintaining weight goes, it is essential to consider the calories in the beverages that you're drinking. People don't often think about the calories in liquids, especially when they're at a restaurant or drinking alcohol with friends. To fill up your stomach and get more fluids, chug-a-lug a small cup of water before every meal.

Water - Back to Basics

Are you a water drinker? How many cups do you drink in a day? Or are you one of those people who doesn't like to drink water?

JF: I have learned to love water. I now drink it with most meals and try to drink water several times a day so as to avoid eating when I know I'm not hungry.

You: _____

_____

If you're not a water drinker, keep trying until you get used to it. Water doesn't have any calories. If you don't like the flavor, add a squirt of lemon juice or a slice of lime. It's very refreshing. Cucumber slices, fresh ginger slices or sprigs of mint are also refreshing in water. A splash of 100% juice can add a bit of delicious flavor. If you like cold liquids, add ice.

Tap water is safe to drink. It is regulated by the EPA (Environmental Protection Agency). Some people don't realize that you can drink water from the kitchen faucet. If it wasn't safe, people would get sick. To feel comfortable drinking tap water, get your water checked. Lead in the pipes may be an issue. Some people don't like the taste of chlorine. Look into attaching a reverse osmosis system to your sink. Occasionally, tap water gets contaminated, but bottled water has also been found to be contaminated.

There are many choices of H_2O. These days bottled water is popular. Bottled water is regulated by the FDA (Food and Drug Administration). It is bottled from springs, wells, or purified water. (Purified water begins its journey as tap water.) If you like bubbles, drink sparkling water. Bottled water can be expensive. Many people are going green and drinking water from environmentally friendly bottles.

Consider these other tips:

♦ Water fortified with vitamins and minerals is an expensive way to drink water. Do you really need small amounts of a few vitamins in your water?

♦ Adding herbal supplements and caffeine to bottled water also increases the price.

♦ There are many flavored waters on the market to quench thirst. Flavored water may be more palatable than plain water for non-water drinkers. Besides the flavor, they may contain added sugars (calories) or artificial sweeteners.

- Read the label on seltzer and club soda for the milligrams of sodium.
- Sometimes the sweetness in artificially sweetened drinks triggers cravings for sweet foods (with calories) in some people. Natural water is a safe alternative without the cravings kickback.
- Clients have told me that they order regular soda at restaurants because they don't want to drink the water. News flash: Many restaurants hook up the soda syrup to tap water.
- Need a good night's sleep? Don't drink too much fluid a couple of hours before you go to sleep. Keep a glass of water by your bed and as soon as you wake up, drink it to start your day energized.
- Some people reduce their fluid intake because they retain water and swell. It's the sodium, not too much fluid, that causes puffiness. If you have hypertension, keep drinking water and reduce the amount of salt in your diet.

Water is a refreshing, calorie-free beverage.

*R*uth's Rule: *It may take a while before you get into the swing of drinking enough water. Adding a slice of lemon or lime, a sprig of mint, a slice of cucumber, ginger or watermelon can help.*

Increase Water Intake in Cold Weather ଔ

When it's cold, it's hard for some people to drink cold water. *Try this* … Fill a mug of water almost to the top and heat it in the microwave for a minute. Then add ½ ounce of cranberry juice. It is hot and hydrating.

When More Water Is Needed

There are certain conditions that increase the need to drink more water, besides sweating in high temperatures or exercising. Humid weather makes people sweat more than usual. High altitudes, circulated air on planes, and indoor heating during the winter increase the need for fluid. Fluid is lost from fever, vomiting, and diarrhea. Pregnancy and breastfeeding require more fluids than usual. Take into consideration that older adults may have a decreased sense of thirst. Yet their need for fluids is still there. Some diabetics with high blood sugars feel thirsty all of the time and drink *a lot.* If you retain fluid and feel puffy, see a doctor.

Are You Prepared for an Emergency? ☯

It seems that you only need it when you don't have it. Do you have a gallon of bottled water per day for each person for a week? Store water in a cool, dry place away from sunlight and replace every six months.

The Scoop on Water and Athletes

Water is the most important nutrient for athletes. You can't do your best without proper hydration. A 2% loss of body weight from sweat can decrease blood volume. The heart has to work harder to move blood through the body. To avoid dehydration, find your "sweat rate." Weigh yourself before and after a workout. For every pound lost in sweat, replace it with 2-3 cups of water.

Don't be happy about losing weight after exercise. As soon as you drink something, it will come back. Anyway, you want to lose *fat weight,* not water weight. If you weigh more than when you started, you drank more than necessary.

There's such a thing as *acute water toxicity* from drinking large quantities of water in a short amount of time. Occasionally, people running or walking marathons get into trouble because they drink too much water. It's called *hyponatremia.* Too much water dilutes the sodium in the blood, causing the brain to swell. It can lead to seizures and death. To avoid this problem, drink sports drinks to replace the sodium that's lost in sweat for physical activity lasting more than an hour. You can drink a lot of water throughout the day, but not a lot in a short amount of time.

The Goods on Sports Drinks

What are your thoughts on sweating? A lot of people don't like to exercise because they hate to sweat, or they don't want sweat to affect their hair.

JF: I am unfortunately one of those women who doesn't like to sweat because of what it does to my hair. But I realize that I have to make a decision to either be chubby with a gorgeous head of hair or be healthy and deal with the occasional frizz. I choose frizz.

You: _____

_____

Regardless of your situation, sports drinks provide fluid, some carbohydrates for energy, and key electrolytes. Remember, if you're vigorously active for more than an hour, choose a sports drink. The sodium also helps fluid stay in the body longer.

As a hydrating beverage, sports drinks contain calories. They don't have as many calories as soda, but think about whether or not you need to replace electrolytes. Some bottles are large. Check the number of servings per container for the total number of calories in a bottle. If you aren't hungry or you're not working out for more than an hour, there are other fluid choices without calories.

Do children need to drink sports drinks? They could provide unnecessary calories for a child. If your child plays the position of forward in soccer and sweats a lot on a hot summer day, a sports drink would be a good choice. If your child has extra weight, plays goalie, and doesn't see much action, a sports drink probably isn't necessary. In this case, water would be a better choice.

Coffee: America's Favorite Beverage

Coffee comes from plants so it contains antioxidants. Antioxidants prevent cells from getting damaged. *That's a good thing.*

Coffee tidbits:

♦ Store coffee beans in the freezer to keep them fresh.

♦ It has been said that Americans get more of their antioxidants from coffee than from fruits and vegetables. I'm not sure *that* is a good thing.

If you drink coffee, it counts as fluid. It may be a mild diuretic, but caffeinated beverages (coffee, tea, and caffeinated soft drinks) count toward your daily intake of fluid. A lot of people drink coffee and tea for the caffeine. It gets them to work. It keeps them awake. It makes them work harder. They feel that they can't function without it.

Some people don't drink any beverages with caffeine because it increases their heart rate. For other people, caffeine doesn't seem to affect them negatively. They can drink a cup of coffee and go to sleep. Everyone reacts differently to caffeine.

Caffeine: Info You Should Know

Caffeine is a mild stimulant. It occurs naturally in coffee and cocoa beans, tea leaves, kola nuts, and guarana berries. There is a wide range of caffeine content in drinks and no consistency of the amounts in the literature.

Here are some ballpark caffeine figures:

CAFFEINE		
	Average milligrams	Range in milligrams
Brewed coffee (8 ounces)	100	60-200
Instant coffee (8 ounces)	60	30-170
Black tea (8 ounces)	50	20-120
Green tea (8 ounces)	30	20-50
Espresso (1 ounce)	40	30-90
Energy drinks (8 ounces)		40-300
Soft drinks (12 ounces)		22-71
Bottled tea (12 ounces)		8-32
Decaffeinated coffee (8 ounces)	5	2-10
Dark chocolate (1 ounce)	23	
Milk chocolate (1 ounce)	9	

To find the caffeine content of a specific product, check the company's website. Amounts of caffeine on food labels would be helpful. The caffeine content in coffee depends on the type of bean, the brewing time, and how it is prepared. Lower quality Robusta coffee beans have twice the amount of caffeine than the higher quality Arabica coffee beans. The caffeine content in tea depends on the brewing time and the type of tea.

Coffee and tea provide more than caffeine, antioxidants, and fluid. Moderate amounts of caffeine can increase physical endurance, improve alertness and mood, and relieve painful headaches. Coffee and tea can be comfort foods. They can be warm and soothing to people. Drinking coffee and tea can be a ritual. Look at all the coffee shops that have sprung up. Meeting for coffee and tea is great for social gatherings.

There have been hundreds of studies over the last few decades blaming coffee for heart disease, cancer, and many other problems. Actually, it may inhibit disease. Recent research is showing more and more benefits from the antioxidants.

Limit caffeine to less than 400 milligrams a day to avoid adverse health effects. Three hundred milligrams of caffeine is about three cups of coffee or four to six cups of tea. To undo caffeine's effects to bones from calcium loss, add two tablespoons of milk to coffee or tea. A café latte is half coffee and half milk. This drink adds fluid, protein, and calcium to your diet. A cappuccino has less milk than a latte.

Specialty Coffee Drinks: An Eye-Opening Look

In the old days, a cup of coffee held about 7 ounces. People would add a splash of cream or a packet of sugar for about 30 calories. Today's delicious, high-calorie specialty drinks can be hard to resist.

Basic Coffee Calories

Coffee (8 ounces)	2 calories
Café latte, whole milk (8 ounces)	130 calories
Café latte, fat-free milk (8 ounces)	80 calories
Cappuccino, whole milk (8 ounces)	75 calories
Cappuccino, fat-free milk (8 ounces)	50 calories

Extra Coffee Calories

Whipping cream	51 calories/tablespoon and 5½ grams of fat
Half and half	20 calories/tablespoon
Powdered cream substitute	33 calories/tablespoon
Flavored liquid cream substitute	38 calories/tablespoon
Liquid cream substitute	20 calories/tablespoon
Whole milk	9 calories/tablespoon
Fat-free milk	6 calories/tablespoon
Sugar	48 calories/tablespoon
Artificial sweeteners	0 calories
Chocolate syrup	50 calories/tablespoon
Flavoring syrups	30 calories/tablespoon (20 calories a pump)
Sugar-free syrups	0 calories

People run into trouble — *big* trouble — regarding calories when they add whole milk, sugar, syrups, and whipped cream to their coffee consumption. The calories from a coffee drink can add up to that of a small meal. Some 12-ounce drinks (1½ cups) can be over 600 calories and contain 24 grams of saturated fat. Two hundred calories for a donut is reasonable. Would you believe 480 calories for a 12-ounce iced coffee? Two hundred and forty calories from a 20-ounce bottle of soda seems like a lot, but 600 calories from a coffee drink is outrageous. A mere 50 extra calories a day over time put on weight. *Drink responsibly.*

Are you on a first-name basis with your barista (an expert in making coffee drinks)? Are coffee drinks a source of hydration for you? Is it the flavor? The caffeine? Are they a snack? Are they a meal? Do they contribute to excess weight? What modifications can you make so that they have fewer calories?

JF: I usually stay the heck out of the expensive coffee shops. I manage to maybe buy one expensive drink a week or flirt my way into having a man buy me a cup. The allure is the environment, ambiance, fancy names, status, music in the store, cute single men who hang out there, and the friendly service. All those components can make the $7 lattes very enticing.

You: _____

Coffee can be a healthy, low-calorie beverage. To keep the calories under control, keep your coffee simple, whether it's hot or cold. Instead of whipping cream, whole milk, sugar, and syrups, drink coffee fat-free and sugar-free. It's easy to save 100-400 calories or more. Calorie counts are available online from chain establishments. If you order a coffee drink with too many calories, order a small size and make it a special treat.

*R*uth's Rule: *Specialty coffee drinks can be a source of many additional calories over the course of a week or even a day. Count them as part of your empty calories, and don't overdo it.*

Tea Time

Tea has been around for thousands of years. Besides water, tea is the most commonly consumed beverage in the world. Tea comes from the Camellia sinensis plant. It has about half the caffeine of a typical cup of coffee. Black tea leaves are dried and fermented for more flavor. Green tea is unfermented and has a little less caffeine than black tea.

Green tea has gained popularity in recent years. It contains flavonoids with powerful antioxidant properties that may reduce the risk of heart disease and cancer. It's important to note that black tea and green tea contain about the same amounts of flavonoids. It is not necessary to drink only green tea to receive health benefits. *Both* are good for you. Decaffeinated black and green tea also contain flavonoids. Processing tea to make powdered instant tea decreases the antioxidant content.

Bottled or instant tea is convenient but it may not have the same amount of flavonoids. It's very easy to brew a pot of black or green tea. When the tea cools down, put it in the refrigerator and add ice for a refreshing glass of iced tea. A squeeze of lemon adds a little more flavor and no calories.

Black tea has about 50 milligrams of caffeine. Green tea has around 30 milligrams of caffeine. If you're sensitive to caffeine, you can increase your fluid intake by choosing decaffeinated coffee, tea, or herbal tea.

Herbal teas are a great way to increase fluids, especially on cold winter nights. Over ice, herbal tea becomes a refreshing and delicious drink on a hot summer day. These teas come from the leaves, roots, flowers, herbs, or fruit of various plants, not from the Camellia sinensis plant. Technically, they aren't really tea. Herbal teas add flavor to your fluids without the caffeine. There's a wide variety of herbal tea flavors.

Be Savvy about Soda

What can I say? The ingredients in regular soda are sugar, artificial flavors, and artificial colors. Measure out 10 teaspoons of sugar. That's about the amount of sugar in a can of soda. All of the calories from soda come from sugar, without any nutrients. Restaurant servings of soda can be bigger than 12-ounce cans. The sugar in soda is not good for teeth.

Diet soda doesn't contain calories. Diet soda will not make you gain weight or raise blood sugar. If you want caffeine, choose a caffeinated diet soda for some pep without the calories.

Eliminating regular soda is an easy way to cut calories. If you drink sodas, count them as your extra calories. Diet sodas or other beverages sweetened with artificial sweeteners are a good way to hydrate without calories.

Energy Drinks: A Good Choice for a Boost?

Do you need energy? The logical answer might be to guzzle an energy drink. There are many choices of energy drinks. You might see caffeine, sugar, vitamins, minerals, amino acids, and herbs listed on the label. If you see guarana or yerba mate on the label, the drink contains caffeine. Vitamins, amino acids, and herbs do not give you mental or physical energy. Energy drinks are expensive sodas containing additional ingredients. Some energy drinks have a hefty dose of caffeine added to them. The benefits of some of these ingredients are questionable.

Above all, read the label for calories. "Energy" has consequences. If you want a low-calorie lift, drink a cup of coffee or tea (hot or cold) sweetened with a little sugar. The caffeine and the sugar will give you a boost. How about a banana or an orange for some energy?

Juice, Within Reason

Juice is occasionally considered the black sheep of the fruit family. Large amounts of juice can provide unwanted calories. Juice may be low in fiber yet high in nutrients. Orange juice and grapefruit juice are loaded with vitamin C, potassium, and folic acid. Fortified juice is a way to get extra calcium and vitamin D in the diet. Sometimes juice tastes too sweet. It's okay to dilute it with water. Diluted juice means more fluid and less calories.

How about some other juices?

- **Grape juice** is a good way to get the color purple into your diet. It contains the same antioxidants found in red wine.
- **Cranberry juice** is a good way to get the color red into your diet. Cranberries have diuretic properties and may protect against kidney and bladder infections.
- **Prune juice** is a good juice for added fiber.
- **Vegetable juice** can provide 100% DV of vitamin A and vitamin C. If necessary, watch the sodium on some vegetable juices.
- **Fruit drinks, nectars, and punch** contain extra sugar and may contain artificial ingredients.

Some kids drink two to four servings of juice or punch a day. They may be "drinking" excess weight. Fruit smoothies are another way to get into serious calorie trouble. If it's made from 100% juice, it seems healthy. But how big is it? Some smoothies can be 600 calories or more.

Don't think of juice as just a sugary drink. Juice contains powerful phytonutrients to reduce the risk of heart disease and cancer. Moderation is the key to control calories from juice. If you're diabetic, juice raises blood sugar quickly. In this case, eat whole fruits to get nutrients and drink water for some of your fluids. When you're really hungry, drink a half cup of juice and wait 15-30 minutes until your blood sugar rises. You won't have the appetite of King Kong.

Food - A Surprising Source of Fluids

You don't usually think of eating food as a way to supply fluid, but it is. Consider the following data from the USDA's National Database for Standard Reference.

Obviously, water is 100% water. Beverages, such as tea, coffee, and sports drinks, are mostly water. Milk, juice, and soda are about 90% water. Most fruits and vegetables are about 90% water. Cooked rice and pasta are about 70% water. Cooked beef, chicken, and pork are about 60% water. Fish contains more water at about 75%. Bread and bagels are about 40% water. Would you believe most cheese is about 40% water? Even nuts contain about 4% water. Pretzels and crackers are only about 3% water.

Don't try to get 100% of your fluid requirement from food. It would not be a good use of calories.

"Adult" Beverages

People have been getting drunk for thousands of years. These days, they're doing it with more calories. Wouldn't the Romans love a banana split martini with the rim of the glass coated with chocolate?

Ethanol or ethyl alcohol is found in beer, wine, and liquor. Fermented yeast, sugars, and starches produce alcohol, which has an intoxicating effect on humans.

Do you drink alcohol? What do you drink? How much? How often?

JF: Okay, I was wondering when these questions would get to cocktails. I'd say that I consume alcohol about once per week in clubs and bars, and, if I have a bottle of wine at home, that bottle is gone within three days. Is that the first sign of a problem? I hope not.

You: _____

Beware. Alcohol has seven calories a gram. It has almost the same amount of calories as fat. Alcohol is liquid calories, and it goes down *quickly.* According to the Dietary Guidelines for Americans, ***moderation is up to one drink a day for women and up to two drinks a day for men.*** This amount refers to *one day.* It doesn't mean that a woman can save all seven drinks for one day or that a man can drink 14 beers in one night.

How many calories are in those drinks you're having? Check out the list below for the calories in the amount considered to be "one drink." Each drink below has .6 fluid ounces (14 grams) of pure alcohol.

- ♦ 5 ounces of wine = 120 calories
- ♦ 12 ounces of beer = 150 calories
- ♦ 12 ounces of light beer = 100 calories
- ♦ 1.5 ounces of 80-proof distilled spirits = 100 calories (Distilled spirits include vodka, rum, bourbon, whisky, brandy, and liqueurs.)
- ♦ 5 ounces of dessert wine = 235 calories

Alcohol is alcohol. It doesn't matter if it's wine, beer, or distilled spirits. It has the same effect (benefits and risks) on your body. It would be very difficult to lose weight and drink large amounts of alcoholic beverages. To drink alcohol and not take the chance of gaining weight, you would have to cut out food and lose vital nutrients.

Drink alcohol in moderation for your health and the calories.

Alcohol Consumption Risks

Alcohol is *not* an essential nutrient. *Heavy* drinking (8 or more drinks a week for women and 15 or more drinks a week for men) causes serious health problems.

- ♦ Too much alcohol causes a fatty liver, liver cirrhosis, or pancreatitis. Save your liver.
- ♦ Excessive alcohol can increase blood pressure and cause strokes.

- Heavy drinking can cause vitamin deficiencies, memory loss, stomach problems, and psychological disorders.
- Too much alcohol can cause traffic accidents, falls, drowning, firearm injuries, unwanted snake bites, violence, suicide, alcohol dependence, etc.
- If you take medications that interact with alcohol, don't drink. Alcohol can increase or decrease the effects of some prescription or over-the-counter medications. It can cause a range of side effects from nausea, vomiting, and drowsiness to trouble breathing, internal bleeding, heart problems, or death.
- Even a combination of alcohol and herbs such as chamomile and valerian can increase drowsiness.
- Don't drink while you're pregnant or breastfeeding. No amount of alcohol is safe during pregnancy.
- If you drink alcohol while you're breastfeeding, your baby drinks, too. Breast milk has about the same blood alcohol content as mom.
- Too much alcohol causes cancer. Alcohol increases the risk of mouth, throat, larynx, esophageal, liver, breast, stomach and colorectal cancer.
- A combination of drinking and smoking is a lot worse for your health than drinking or smoking by itself.

On the bright side, the ethanol and the phytonutrients in wine, beer, and distilled spirits may be beneficial to your heart. But only *in moderation*. One or two drinks a day may lower the risk of coronary heart disease and strokes, especially in women 55 and older, men 45 and over, and people at risk for heart disease. However, if you don't drink alcohol, my advice is *don't start to get the heart benefits.*

Milk, Anyone?

Milk is a forgotten fluid with lots of important nutrients. When was the last time you ordered milk with dinner at a restaurant?

JF: I am not lactose intolerant because I am fine with all other dairy products. I just think regular milk is gross by itself.

Three glasses of milk provide 90% DV for calcium and 60% DV for vitamin D. Choose 1% milk or fat-free milk for fewer calories. The number of people, especially women, not getting enough calcium and vitamin D in their diets and at risk of getting osteoporosis is alarming. Get into the habit of drinking milk to reduce your risk of osteoporosis.

You can get fluid and nutrients for your bones from shakes and malts but you also get lots of unhealthy calories from fat and sugar. Fast-food shakes made with regular ice cream, whole milk, and pieces of candy have tremendous amounts of calories. Would you believe over 1,000 calories for some fast-food 20-ounce shakes? *That's incredible.*

Drinking fat-free or 1% milk is a great way to get fluid and important nutrients.

Gulp

Your body needs fluids. *Get enough of them.* The amount of fluid that you need is different every day depending on your metabolism, the environment, and your activity. Use your thirst and the color of your urine as a guide. The first sign of dehydration is a dry mouth. If you cry and you don't have any tears, you're in trouble.

Take a look at your daily fluid intake. Are you feeling sluggish? Think about ways to get hydrated. Unless you're a camel and can store extra water in your body, drink throughout the day. If you produce 4-8 cups of urine a day, good job. You're not dehydrated. If things look or smell a little strange down there, did you take a vitamin with riboflavin (B2) or eat asparagus or beets? These factors can affect urine smell and color.

Drink mostly water, fat-free milk, and unsweetened coffee, tea, or iced tea. Limit amounts of 100% juice. Adult beverages are not necessary. If you drink alcoholic beverages, limit intake to no more than one drink a day for women and no more than two a day for men.

Fluids with little or no calories are your new best friends.

*D*ay 24 CHECK-IN ☑

What did you accomplish yesterday?

JF: I was on a movie set. When it was time to eat, I didn't get a piece of red velvet cake or a freshly baked chocolate chip cookie. I am still in shock over the self-control I exhibited.

You: _____

_____

What is your goal for today?

(Fill up and carry around a water bottle.) (Drink a glass of water before every meal.) (Limit alcohol to one drink on weekends.) (Measure 5 ounces of wine in a wine glass.) (Drink diet soda or unsweetened iced tea instead of regular soda.) (Drink coffee or tea with fat-free milk instead of half and half or coffee creamer.) (Weigh yourself before and after a workout. Replace lost fluid.) (Count up the number of cups of fluid for the day.)

JF: I plan to drink water deliberately all day. I also plan to stay on track with the elimination of sweets and alcohol in my diet until I grasp and master my new lifestyle.

You: _____

_____

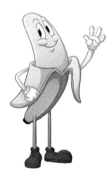

Day 25

Let Food Be Thy Medicine

"*L*et food be thy medicine and medicine be thy food," said Hippocrates two and a half thousand years ago. He practiced medical nutrition therapy a long time ago. Hippocrates was a registered dietitian nutritionist before his time.

Do you agree with Hippocrates? Can food be medicine? After 24 chapters of The Food Is My Friend Diet, do you believe that the best way to lose weight and prevent or delay health problems is to eat moderate amounts of healthy food and get physical activity?

JF: I would so not be a team player if I said no to this question. But of course TFIMFD has taught me that moderation and not complete deprivation is the way to a healthier life. Writing and reading for this book project has made me answer questions that I have never been asked or have been too ashamed to consider seriously.

In case you aren't totally convinced of food's benefits, this chapter will discuss vitamins, minerals, and some foods with special qualities, specifically foods with antioxidants, phytonutrients, and functional properties.

Those Oh-So-Important Vitamins and Minerals

The macronutrients are protein, carbohydrate, and fat. The micronutrients are **vitamins** and **minerals**. Let's review what they are:

- **Water-soluble vitamins:** *Vitamin C and the B vitamins.* Excess water-soluble vitamins are secreted in the urine.
- **Fat-soluble vitamins:** *Vitamins A, D, E, and K.* Fat-soluble vitamins attach to fat and are stored in the body.
- **Major minerals:** *Calcium, phosphorus, potassium, magnesium, sodium,* and *chlorine.*
- **Trace minerals:** *Iron, fluoride, chromium, iodine, selenium, zinc, cobalt, copper, manganese,* and *molybdenum.*

Your body needs varying amounts of vitamins and minerals every day for growth and development.

Gather up your collection of supplements providing vitamins and minerals. List all of the vitamins and minerals that you're taking. If your supplements contain the same nutrients, add up the total amount.

JF: I am taking fish oil, B12, a multivitamin, Vitamin C, St. John's Wort, Biotin, Ginkgo Biloba, and a green tea pill.

You: _____

_____

Look at the ingredients. Some people are sensitive to the fillers, colors, binders, and flavors in supplements. It's important to read labels, even on vitamins and mineral supplements.

Vitamins and minerals are not magic. They don't have the ability to melt away fat or cure diseases. Taking certain supplements can cause problems during surgery. Some supplements may interfere with chemotherapy. Vitamins and minerals cannot and should not replace prescription medicines.

Less Can Be More

Your body uses small amounts of vitamins and minerals. Taking too many minerals could offset the body's delicate physiological balance. If you're taking a vitamin/mineral supplement, you may not need more than 100% of the Recommended Dietary Allowance (RDA) for your age.

Excessive amounts could build up over time and increase the risk of adverse effects, such as liver toxicity. If you take megavitamin/mineral supplements and eat foods fortified with vitamins and minerals – such as breakfast cereals and energy bars or drinks – there might be overlapping nutrients.

The Dietary Reference Intakes (DRI) contains a category with 24 nutrients from vitamin A to zinc called the Tolerable Upper Intake Level (UL). The chart contains the highest daily amounts allowed that probably won't cause adverse effects. Compare your vitamin and mineral supplements to the Tolerable Upper Intake Levels (UL) at: http://www.nap.edu. Find any unsafe levels? Did you find overlapping amounts that may not be necessary?

JF: I sometimes wonder, since I am taking a multivitamin, if I need to take separate Vitamin C, Biotin, and B12 supplements, as the label lists these as part of the multivitamin. I figure if I take them all, then I will not only be healthy but will also have superhuman strength. My powers have not kicked in yet. I better check for overlapping amounts.

You: _____

_____

Go for the Food Sources

Remember when vitamin E was the rage? Studies showed that vitamin E was beneficial for heart health. Even doctors were popping vitamin E like candy. Recent studies have found that large amounts of vitamin E increase the risk of heart failure in some people. The Dietary Reference Intake for vitamin E is 22 IU a day. Typical soft-gel capsules are 400 IU. The Tolerable Upper Intake Level is 1,500 IU a day. Thirty years ago, we didn't dare take more than the recommended amounts – especially fat-soluble vitamins. Vitamin E supplements are not recommended to the general public to prevent heart disease anymore. Vitamin E doesn't appear to reduce the risk of cancer. Why not get your vitamin E naturally from foods by consuming vegetable oils, wheat germ, nuts, and seeds? You won't have to worry about excess amounts causing problems.

Should you take a bilberry supplement to improve night vision? Or should you add blueberries to your oatmeal? The chances of natural foods causing future health problems are slim.

Do you want to take 20 or 30 different vitamin and mineral tablets every day to cover all of the perceived benefits? In any case, the dozen or so vitamins and minerals in a multivitamin/mineral supplement cannot replace all of the nutrients in a plant-based diet.

Ruth's **Rule:** *Think about food options when you're looking to safely increase your intake of a particular vitamin or mineral.*

Know What You're Getting/Know What You Need

Regarding any supplement, don't automatically assume that it's safe for you or that it contains what is on the label. Some supplements contain too much or not enough of a nutrient. Some supplements are contaminated. *It happens.* Buy mainstream brands.

Red alert: If a person "tests" you for nutrient deficiencies and then tries to sell you a lot of expensive supplements that may or may not be related to the "proposed" deficiency, run away as fast as you can. Think about the way that the test is conducted. Does it sound plausible? Is the person an expert in nutrition? Maybe the person is a snake oil salesman in a nice person's clothing who is only trying to make money. Helping you may not be their primary interest.

Use common sense. Blood tested at your doctor's office or a hospital lab will determine nutrient deficiencies. If you're not getting enough calcium in your diet, there is no need to buy an expensive, unknown brand of calcium. There are many people spending a lot of money on vitamin and mineral supplements needlessly.

When Supplements Are Important

Certain people should consider taking a vitamin/mineral supplement because they need more nutrients than they can get through food. Certain medications can cause nutrient deficiencies. Eliminating food groups can result in nutrient deficiencies. Consider taking the necessary vitamin and mineral supplements if you're a vegetarian or vegan, an older adult, pregnant or breastfeeding, a smoker, drink excess amounts of alcohol, or have absorption problems. Supplements may fill the gaps.

If you're anemic, should you take an iron supplement? *Yes.* If Cheese Puffs are your idea of a source of calcium, should you take a calcium supplement? *Yes.* If you're like the typical postmenopausal woman and only get 600 milligrams of calcium a day, should you take a calcium supplement? *Yes.* People have different nutrient needs, depending on their situations.

If you're among the majority of Americans who don't follow My-Plate guidelines, it wouldn't hurt to take a 100% RDA mainstream vitamin/mineral supplement until you shape up your eating habits. Studies often find that people with certain diseases have low levels of various vitamins and minerals.

Beneficial or toxic? Sometimes it's difficult to know whether you should take certain supplements. As science evolves, what's good one year isn't necessarily good the next year. Check with a doctor or a registered dietitian nutritionist. Take vitamins and minerals responsibly. Base your decision on research over time, not one study.

The RDIs, the Dietary Guidelines for Americans, and MyPlate base their recommendations on a consolidation of current evidence-based science. It's important to remember that nutritional needs cannot be met by eating an unhealthy diet and relying on vitamin and mineral supplements. If you follow MyPlate guidelines every day, you may not need to take a multivitamin/mineral supplement.

Watch Out for "Diet Pills"

I hope that you've thrown away your diet pills by now. But just in case, watch out. At the end of 2008, the FDA issued a warning to consumers about tainted weight-loss pills. Even though the dietary supplements claimed to be "natural" and to be made of "herbal" ingredients, they contained potentially harmful ingredients that were not listed on the labels. More than 25 diet pills contained *undeclared* active pharmaceutical ingredients. Some of the diet pills contained high doses of *prescription* drugs. Others contained *carcinogens* and chemical solutions. Some of the drugs in the diet pills were not approved for marketing in the U.S. People died, and others got liver damage from these products. Not everyone got the memo that they could be harmful. I thought these types of problems were fixed, repeatedly, since the early 1900s. In my professional opinion, eating moderate amounts of healthy foods is a better way to lose weight than taking risky diet pills.

The Role of Antioxidants

Antioxidants are good for you. Antioxidants keep your body from "rusting." You should eat foods that contain antioxidants *every day*.

Your body needs oxygen to function. As a result of the cells in your body using oxygen, *free-radicals* can form. The free radicals wander through the human body and cause damage to healthy cells. Free radicals are also produced by alcohol, cigarette smoke, x-rays, ultraviolet light, and pollution.

Too many free radicals and the resulting oxidation to cells are linked to inflammation. Inflammation leads to aging and the start of diseases, such as heart disease, some forms of cancer, Alzheimer's disease, Parkinson's disease, cataracts, macular degeneration, and other chronic illnesses.

Antioxidants have a variety of tasks:

♦ Antioxidants reduce and neutralize the damage caused by free radicals.
♦ They promote vision and heart health.
♦ They protect the immune system and affect brain function.
♦ Basically, they protect the body's cells and tissue from oxidative damage, making skin, organs, and blood vessels stronger.

A strong body supported by antioxidants is vibrant and less prone to disease.

Antioxidants are found in fruits, vegetables, beans, whole grains, nuts, seeds, herbs, spices, coffee, and tea. They come from plants. Antioxidants include nutrients – such as *vitamin C, beta carotene, other carotenoids (lycopene, lutein, zeaxanthin, etc.), vitamin E,* and the trace mineral *selenium* – along with some other minerals and some phytonutrients.

Do Antioxidant Supplements Help? ∝

It's unknown whether taking antioxidant supplements produces the same health benefits as food. Vitamin E can interact with certain medications. Vitamin A and selenium are toxic at high levels. Too much vitamin C may cause diarrhea and increase the risk of urinary stones. Look at what high doses of beta carotene supplements did to smokers in the antioxidant studies. The study had to be stopped because the beta carotene supplements sped up lung cancer. Excess amounts of some antioxidants may decrease the absorption of other antioxidants. The long-term effect of taking antioxidant supplements is unknown. There's no evidence that people receive benefits from taking single antioxidants.

The best and safest way to get the most antioxidants is to include the recommended amounts of fruits, vegetables, and whole grains every day:

- **For vitamin C:** Citrus fruits (oranges, grapefruit, citrus juices), strawberries, blueberries, blackberries, raspberries, papayas, kiwis, cantaloupes, papayas, potatoes, broccoli, red peppers, and green peppers
- **For beta carotene and other carotenoids:** Yellow/orange/red fruits and vegetables (tomatoes, carrots, sweet potatoes, pumpkin, winter squash, cantaloupes, watermelon, apricots, mangoes, peaches) and dark green leafy vegetables (broccoli, romaine lettuce, spinach, kale). If the foods containing carotenoids are chopped or pureed and cooked in a small amount of oil, they will be absorbed better.
- **For vitamin E:** Vegetable oils, nuts, seeds, peanut butter, wheat germ, fortified whole grain breads and cereals, green leafy vegetables (spinach, broccoli), avocados

• **For selenium**: Brazil nuts (limit consumption), seafood, meat, poultry, eggs, whole grains, and enriched grains

If you follow a high-protein, low-carbohydrate, animal-based diet, do you think that you'll get enough health benefits? Would a high-protein diet provide enough antioxidants?

JF: Well, here's my answer. A pure protein diet is not enough. Variety will provide the nutrients I need. Any diet based on one component is not enough to get what my body needs overall.

You: _____

_____

Whenever you see foods with antioxidants, go for it. No particular food is superior. Keep adding healthy foods and eat fewer unhealthy foods. For instance, you could sprinkle cinnamon on your oatmeal for potentially more antioxidants.

Are you willing to eat a prune instead of a chocolate truffle?

JF: As a comedian, I so see a joke in this question. Kind of like asking would I have wanted to date Ernest Borgnine or his hot 6-foot son. I believe the truffle is the obvious preference, but for some reason I think the prune is the right answer.

You: _____

_____

A prune on a rice cake is tasty, crunchy, satisfying, low in calories, and healthy.

People who eat lots of fruits and vegetables get less cancer than people who don't eat many fruits and vegetables. Use food as thy medicine to help slow down your body's oxidation process. Eat something orange like a carrot or cantaloupe instead of nachos.

Don't Be Phytonutrient-Deficient

Do you have a few favorite foods that make you feel healthy?

JF: I really enjoy fresh spinach with little to no dressing. I feel like Popeye when I eat it and prefer every salad be made with spinach. I also enjoy vegetable juices. I have recently discovered that beets are scrumptious.

You: _____

_____

The term **phytonutrient** is relatively new to the health scene. "Phyto" means plant in Greek. Phytonutrients aren't vitamins or minerals. They don't have calories. Our bodies don't make them. They may provide color, smell, and taste to plant foods. As individual phytonutrients, none of them are magic but they possess extraordinary capabilities.

Phytonutrients (also called phytochemicals) are the substances made by plants that naturally protect the plants from viruses, bacteria, fungi, insects, and sunlight. When we eat foods with phytonutrients, they offer us protection from health problems, such as heart disease and cancer. There can be hundreds of different phytonutrients in every plant.

Phytonutrients are found in fruits, vegetables, beans, nuts, seeds, and whole grains. Don't forget about coffee and tea. Many of the active components found in functional foods (more on this later in the chapter) are phytonutrients.

Properties of the Amazing Phytonutrients ଔ

We've learned that many phytonutrients act as antioxidants and have anti-inflammatory properties. Phytonutrients are amazing. The phytonutrients in plants seem to act like drugs, in that they can lower blood pressure, prevent platelet aggregation, stabilize heart rhythm, enhance arterial flexibility, improve the immune system, repair or reduce free radicals, repair and protect DNA, stimulate enzymes to reduce carcinogens, slow down, shrink, or stop cancer cells from growing and dividing, and protect eyesight, to name a few. Not bad for a plant.

*R*uth's **Rule:** *To protect your body against disease, eat a variety of fruits, vegetables, whole grains, beans, nuts, seeds, herbs, and spices every day.*

Here are the common classes of phytonutrients:
- *Carotenoids*
- *Flavonoids (Polyphenols)* including *Isoflavones (Phytoestrogens)*
- *Isositol Phosphates (Phytates)*
- *Lignans (Phytoestrogens)*
- *Isothiocyanates* and *Indoles*
- *Phenols* and *Cyclic Compounds*
- *Saponins*
- *Sulfides* and *Thiols*
- *Terpenes*

Carotenoids

Let's take a closer look at **carotenoids**. There are more than 600 of them. *Alpha carotene, beta carotene, beta cryptoxanthin, lutein, zeaxanthin,* and *lycopene* are the most common carotenoids. Many people are familiar with lycopene in tomatoes. People with macular degeneration may be familiar with lutein.

Flavonoids

There are over 6,000 **flavonoids**. Here are a few: *flavonols, flavanols, flavones, flavanones, anthocyanidins,* and *isoflavones.* The isoflavones in soy are a commonly known phytonutrient. *Genistein, diadzein,* and *glycitein* are three types of isoflavones. The phytonutrient in tea may be referred to as a *flavanoid,* a *catechin* or *epigallocatechin gallate* (EGCG). Onions contains *quercetin.* It is a flavonoid, and its subclass is a flavonol. There are classes, subclasses, and subsubclasses of phytonutrients.

Many Other Phytonutrients

There may be 100,000 different phytonutrients. Once you become familiar with the names, you will notice them often. Here are the names (not even a drop in the bucket) of some phytonutrients or a subclass and a few food sources:

Allyl sulfide	Garlic, onions, leeks, chives, scallions
Anthocyanin	Red, blue, and purple berries, red and purple grapes, red wine, cherries
Apigenin	Parsley, celery hearts, rutabagas
Beta carotene	Carrots, pumpkin, sweet potatoes, dark green leafy vegetables, squash
Capasaicin	Chili peppers
Carnosol	Rosemary
Catechin	Tea, red wine, cocoa, dark chocolate, apples
Curcumin	Turmeric
Ellagic acid	Raspberries, strawberries, pomegranates, walnuts, pecans, cranberries
Epicatechin	Cocoa, tea, grapes, blueberries
Epigallocatechin gallate (ECGC)	Green tea
Flavanol	Cocoa, dark chocolate
Flavanone	Citrus fruits
Flavone	Parsley, thyme, celery, spinach, hot peppers
Flavonoid	Berries, beans, grapes, tea, red wine, citrus, apples, cherries, coffee
Flavonol	Onions, kale, cocoa, tea, apples, broccoli, berries
Gingerol	Ginger root
Glucosinolate	Brussels sprouts, mustard greens, turnips, kale, cabbage
Glutathione	Potatoes, asparagus, avocados
Indole & Isothiocyanate	Broccoli, cabbage, kale, Brussels sprouts, cauliflower, bok choy
Isoflavone	Soybeans, tofu, soy beverages
Lignan	Flaxseeds, sesame seeds

Limonoid	Oranges, grapefruits, tangerines, lemons, limes, citrus peels
Lutein & Zeaxanthin	Kale, spinach, collard greens, avocados, peas, corn, egg yolks
Lycopene	Tomatoes, tomato products, watermelon, pink grapefruit, guava
Oleocanthal	Extra virgin olive oil
Orthophenol	Whole wheat
Perillyl alcohol	Cherries, lavender
Phenethyl Isothiocyanate	Watercress
Phthalide & Polyacetylene	Carrots, celery, parsley, parsnips, cilantro
Phytate	Whole grains, beans
Phytoestrogen	Soy beans, soy milk, tofu, flaxseeds
Polyphenol	Onions, apples, tea, red wine, grapes, berries, coffee, walnuts
Proanthocyanidin (PAC)	Cinnamon, cocoa, kidney beans, hazelnuts and skins, cranberries
Quercetin	Onions, tea, red wine, apple skins
Resveratrol	Green, red, and blue-black grapes, peanuts (skins, too), red wine
Saponin	Soy beans, peas, oatmeal, brown rice, legumes
Silymarin	Artichokes
Sulforaphane	Broccoli, Brussels sprouts, cabbage
Terpene	Carrots, spinach, tomatoes, citrus fruits, beans
Xanthohumol	Beer, hops

Do you see any foods that you don't normally eat? It would be a good idea to include more of them.

♦ **Some plant foods contain active components to fight disease, and they are referred to as "super foods." These foods include** apples (with the skin), pears, broccoli, berries, oranges, nuts (including the skin), cherries, prunes, carrots, artichokes, oregano, potatoes (with the skin), garlic, onions, cranberries, oatmeal, cinnamon, beans, chili peppers, spinach, and tomatoes.

- **Super foods are not super expensive or exotic. They are everyday foods.** Take a few bites of good health. They taste good. Don't just eat them. Enjoy them. Enjoy them often.

- **Do you see why it's important to eat apple skins, potato skins, even almond skins?** The skins contain high levels of phytonutrients.

- **Pick any plant, and there will be benefits from the phytonutrients.** Blueberries aren't better than raspberries. Each phytonutrient protects the body in slightly different ways. All of them are important.

- **You don't have to drink red wine to get the benefits of resveratrol.** This phytonutrient is found in the skins of all grapes. You'll get many health benefits from eating grapes of any color. Resveratrol is also found in peanuts.

- **When you cook, add garlic, basil, or ginger to your food to increase the amount of phytonutrients.** For convenience, they can be purchased in jars, already chopped.

- **For some extra oomph (health), grate the citrus peel from lemons, oranges, or other citrus fruits.** The zest will also add some flavor and provide health benefits.

- **Think color. Add yellow corn, red onion, and black beans to soups, salads, or main dishes.** You'll be very healthy. Instead of walking, you will bounce. It will seem like you have springs on your feet.

- **Half of your grains should be whole grains.** Why? There are hundreds of phytonutrients in whole wheat, oats, and other whole grains. Most of the phytonutrients are in the bran and germ of the grain. Refined grains are missing many beneficial phytonutrients. Shocking!

One of my favorite Indian dishes is aloo gobi. It's a curry dish made from potatoes and cauliflower. It is loaded with vitamins, minerals, and powerful phytonutrients. The combination of the phenethyl isothiocyanate in cauliflower and the curcumin in turmeric may have more health benefits than the vegetables or the spices by themselves. The combination of phytonutrients from herbs and spices with fruits and vegetables may work together to fight disease and promote health even better. It's all about teamwork.

Two Meals and Their Phytonutrient Content

We know that many people are not eating enough fruits and vegetables. Some people don't eat *any* fruits and vegetables. These people are missing out on important phytonutrients. Eating more fruits and vegetables is part of a healthy lifestyle. You cannot obtain the benefits of phytonutrients by eating vegetables only a couple of times a week.

Look at the differences between these meals.

Meal 1: A 16-ounce slab of prime rib. A half plate of French fries. A sprig of parsley on the plate. A white roll. An iceberg lettuce salad drenched in Thousand Island dressing. A martini.

Meal 2: A mixture of tofu cubes, broccoli florets, slices of red pepper, garlic, and onions stir-fried in oil, seasoned with fresh herbs and served with brown rice.

The first plate is a cry for help. It's saying that if you die young, you don't care. The sprig of parsley is the only ray of hope.

Meal makeover: Share the beef with three or four people on a special occasion. Order a baked potato instead of fries. Instead of sour cream and butter on the baked potato, ask for salsa or Italian dressing made with olive oil. Instead of a lettuce salad, ask for steamed vegetables. Choose a whole-grain roll. Skip the alcohol.

The second meal has oodles of phytonutients. It's saying that you want to live with vim and vigor. No saturated fat. Little or no sodium. No added sugar. It contains whole grains, a source of calcium, monounsaturated fat, and lots of vitamins, minerals, antioxidants, and phytonutrients.

Let's hear it for plants and phytonutrients. Power to the plants!

Variety Is the Herbs and Spices of Life

What are your favorite herbs and spices? Or do they take up space in your cupboard, unused and forgotten?

JF: I love onions and garlic. I use thyme when I cook and am getting to know cumin, curry, fennel, and other spices. So I am venturing into using spices more often, especially when I have no idea what they are.

You: _____

What are herbs and spices? Herbs are leaves. Spices, often dried, come from other parts of the plant (bark, berries, buds, roots, and seeds).

Herbs and spices are more than crushed or ground-up leaves and twigs. Do spices have any nutritional value? Should you eat them? *You betcha.* People have been using herbs and spices for thousands of years to heal wounds and treat health problems. Hippocrates used herbs and spices as medicinal remedies. Herbs and spices are functional foods because of their active components.

Researchers are taking a closer look at turmeric and other spices for the potential health benefits of preventing and fighting disease. Herbs and spices are concentrated sources of powerful antioxidants. They may lower cholesterol, lower blood pressure, boost immunity, have antimicrobial and anti-inflammatory properties, and be a digestive aid.

Many people don't think about using herbs and spices. Herbs and spices add different flavors to food, eliminating the need for added sugar, fat, and salt. Do you need the names of some herbs and spices? Try:

- Basil
- Chives
- Cinnamon
- Dill
- Ginger
- Marjoram
- Oregano
- Peppermint
- Chili powder
- Cilantro
- Cumin
- Garlic
- Lemongrass
- Parsley
- Pepper (black and red)
- Rosemary

- ◆ Sage
- ◆ Thyme
- ◆ Tarragon
- ◆ Turmeric

(However, don't cook with them all at once!)

Start adding herbs and spices to your foods instead of salt *before* your doctor tells you that you should limit your sodium intake. Experiment and find flavors that you enjoy. In case it's not love at first taste, try them a few times. Herbs and spices add great flavors to food and promote health without adding calories. This is good news for your waistline.

The Wonders of Turmeric ❧

People from India consume a lot of turmeric and have lower rates of certain cancers and Alzheimer's disease than people in America. This might be a reason to add turmeric, an anti-inflammatory spice, to more foods.

Understanding Functional Foods

Functional foods provide more than the basic amounts of protein, fat, carbohydrates, vitamins, and minerals necessary for growth, development, and survival. They go beyond meeting the minimum nutrient requirements and preventing deficiencies. The special properties in functional foods come from their *biologically active components*. Functional foods can provide therapeutic health effects.

The active components in functional foods can be **vitamins, minerals, fatty acids, fiber, probiotics, antioxidants,** or **phytonutrients**. They are foods, not drugs. Functional foods give 110% by going above and beyond what is required of them. Functional foods are foods with benefits.

Most natural foods act as functional foods in some capacity. Functional foods can be *whole foods and beverages*, such as fruits, vegetables, whole grains, fish, beans, and milk. Oatmeal, nuts, and garlic are whole functional foods. Functional foods can also be *modified foods* that are fortified, enriched, or enhanced with the active components. The active components can come from plants, animals, or bacteria.

There are hundreds of health components in food. New ones continue to be discovered, and more foods are being modified every day. It's common to see juice and other products *fortified* with calcium. Grains *enriched* with folic acid are functional foods. Eggs *enhanced* with omega 3 fatty acids are an example of a functional food.

Some functional foods have an *FDA health claim.* The claims must have sufficient scientific agreement among experts, not just be emerging evidence. The health claims must be truthful and not misleading. The foods may improve health, and they have the potential to reduce the risk of certain diseases. Currently, there are qualified health claims for osteoporosis, high blood pressure, heart disease, certain birth defects, dental cavities, and cancer.

Here are some health benefits to consider from functional foods:

- **There is a health claim for plant sterol/stanol esters to reduce the risk of coronary heart disease.** Plant sterols and stanols prevent cholesterol from being absorbed. According to the National Cholesterol Education Program, two grams of plant sterols or stanols a day may reduce LDL cholesterol 6-15%. It would be impossible to get 2 grams naturally from food. Eating functional foods enhanced with plant sterols or stanols or taking a supplement would be necessary. Sterols or stanols are being added to table spreads, juice, milk, and other qualifying products.

- **As a functional food, salmon is more than a source of protein. The omega 3 fatty acids in salmon and other fatty fish reduce inflammation and may decrease the risk of cancer.** EPA and DHA may prevent coronary heart disease by lowering triglycerides, blood pressure, and inflammation. Eating fatty fish two times a week provides enough EPA and DHA for heart health. If you eat plenty of fish, will you benefit from milk enhanced with EPA and DHA? Consider the cost of modified products and supplements.

- **As a functional food, cranberry juice inhibits bacteria from sticking to the walls of the bladder to prevent urinary infections.**

- **Yogurt is a functional food.** Probiotics (live bacteria) are added to qualifying products to improve digestive health, possibly preventing diarrhea, bacterial infections, and constipation.

♦ **Are you willing to eat kale, spinach, corn, and egg yolks for the lutein to maintain healthy vision and perhaps decrease the risk of macular degeneration?** How about a spinach and corn omelet for dinner? For heart health, add garlic and onions to get the benefits from the diallyl sulfides.

Many people don't think about their health until they have a problem. It's never too late to start eating healthier. Functional foods may appeal more to aging adults. For people who don't like to take supplements or drugs, who wouldn't want to eat natural foods to preserve memory and eyesight, reduce arthritis and bone fractures, and prevent heart disease and cancer? Staying well by eating healthy food sounds easy and appealing.

Functional foods have been providing health benefits for thousands of years. Over the centuries, food has been used as "medicine" to reduce health problems without people realizing it. For example, take Christopher Columbus. He was going for taste, but look at the functional foods he was eating: *"You will never eat anything more delicious than sweet potatoes soaked in the milk of almonds."* And healthy, too, Mr. Columbus. Loaded with antioxidants and phytonutrients!

Here's to a Banana or Orange for Your Health ଓ

Do you eat foods that provide health benefits? Do you eat a banana or an orange for a snack to maintain a healthy blood pressure, or do you grab a candy bar? If you have high blood pressure, eating a banana or an orange doesn't take the place of your medication, but it provides potassium. Good sources of potassium that are low in sodium may reduce the risk of high blood pressure.

The Future

Preventing disease is more complicated than simply eating an apple a day. The future of nutrition may involve *"nutrigenomics."* An individual's nutrient requirements may be determined by his or her genetic profile. Depending on a person's genes, eating a handful of almonds a day may prevent colon cancer. Eating quercetins – found in onions, apple skins, tea, and cranberries – may help some people fight Alzheimer's disease. In the future, individuals may have their own designer diet. Genetic engineering may be able to produce su-per-duper functional foods to reduce the risk of disease. The future of nutrition will be exciting.

As of yet, there are no functional foods that cause weight loss. We'll have to continue eating less food to lose weight. Maybe some-day there will be a designer food that can help us take off the extra pounds. Maybe someday we'll be able to eat as much food as we want and still lose weight. Never give up hope.

Scientists continue to find new components with functional quali-ties. Eating a variety of functional foods on a regular basis, along with daily physical activity and a healthy lifestyle, will increase the odds of staying healthy, thereby increasing the quality of life and reducing the risk of major diseases in the future.

To your health!

Functional foods are your new best friends.

✑ay 25 CHECK-IN ☑

What did you accomplish yesterday?

JF: I ate well and exercised ferociously. I am working out more. My stamina is increasing and I am less homicidal after an hour on the treadmill.

You: _____

_____

What is your goal for today?

(Eat a food with lycopene.) (Eat a food with beta carotene.) (Eat a food with lutein.) (Eat a food with isoflavone.) (Eat a food with omega 3 fatty acids.) (Eat a food with vitamin C.) (Eat a food with catechin.) (Eat a food with anthocyanin.) (Eat a food with allyl sulfide.) (Eat a food with curcumin.) (Eat a food with resveratrol.) (Eat a food with ellagic acid.) (Make a meal with spaghetti sauce.) (Drink orange juice fortified with calcium.) (Make a recipe with curry.) (Eat a handful of almonds with the skins.)

JF: Well, I'm starving as I write this, and I have to choose food that is good for me and filling. So as I type the last word for this chapter, I'm going to resist the urge to throw the laptop down and run toward a bag of chips. Wish me luck!

You: _____

_____

Day 26

The Truth About Carbs

*W*hy does everyone pick on the lowly carbohydrate? They're like the nerd at school that every one put down. One day the nerd grew up and found the cure for cancer. Now everyone wants to hang out with him.

Many people criticize and avoid carbs. Fad diets hate them. I'm not calling anyone a bully but carbo-phobics should get to know carbohydrates. They would end up looking up to carbs and appreciating them. Carbs deserve to be your friend. You'll love hanging out with them.

If you're not eating protein or fat, you're eating carbohydrates. Those are your three choices in macronutrients. Carbohydrates have 4 calories a gram. Protein has 4 calories a gram. Calorie for calorie, they are the same. In contrast, fat has 9 calories a gram.

What's your stand on carbohydrates? Do you love and perhaps overindulge in them? Or do you avoid them? Are you the person who eats a high-protein diet of 40% protein, 30% fat, and 30% carbohydrates?

JF: I don't believe in the extreme "cut out that entire food group" type of diets. Carbs rule!! In moderation. Freshly baked bread could end wars, in my opinion.

You: _____

_____

Carbs - The Energy Macronutrient

Carbs are not the enemy. Most foods are carbohydrates. Keep in mind that *two-thirds* of your meals should be plant-based (carbohydrates). That makes carbohydrates your hero. Carbohydrates include rice, bread, pasta, and cereal, as well as fruits and vegetables. The only place to get vitamin C and fiber is from carbs. Carbohydrates are also found in milk and milk products. *Combo carbs* (carbohydrates and protein) include beans and nuts. Plus, foods with added sugars – such as soda, cakes, candy, and other sweets – are also carbohydrates.

Let's put carbohydrates under a microscope. Carbohydrates contain a carbon atom with a molecule of water. Hence, carbo-hydrate (carbon with water). Since most carbohydrates are made by plants, they're produced through photosynthesis. A little water, plus some carbon dioxide from the air, plus some energy from the sun makes sugar (stored energy) and oxygen. Have you ever put a bean seed in a cup of dirt, watered it, and watched the seed grow into a plant? *It's a miracle.*

Carbohydrates are our main source of energy. We use carbohydrates *for fuel.* The brain and the central nervous system prefer to use carbohydrates as a source of glucose. If you do any type of physical activity, carbohydrates are a necessity. When we eat carbohydrates, our bodies break down the stored energy and use it for various functions. It seems healthier to eat living energy from fruits, vegetables, and grains compared to eating processed foods like crackers or cupcakes from a box. In the end, it's all broken down into glucose.

*R*uth's Rule: *Aim to make two-thirds of your diet carbohydrate, including fruits, vegetables, grains, and the combo carbs (carb and protein) of beans and nuts.*

Types of Carbohydrates

Carbohydrates are classified as **monosaccharides, disaccharides, oligosaccharides,** or **polysaccharides.** Monosaccharide means one sugar. Monosaccharides are single units of sugar (*glucose, fructose,* or *galactose*). Disaccharide means two sugars. Disaccharides are double units of sugar (*sucrose, lactose,* and *maltose*). Oligosaccharide means a few sugars. Oligosaccharides are short units of sugar (3-10). Polysaccharide means many sugars. Polysaccharides are many sugar units linked together, better known as *starch* and *fiber*. There may be thousands of sugar units in a starch.

There are **simple carbohydrates** and **complex carbohydrates**. Simple carbohydrates are sugars (*monosaccharides* and *disaccharides*). Simple carbohydrates are found in fruits, milk, and milk products. Simple carbohydrates include white and brown sugar, honey, molasses, fruit sugar, corn syrup, and candy. Complex carbohydrates are starches and fiber (*polysaccharides*). Complex carbohydrates are found in vegetables, whole fruits, potatoes, grains (wheat, corn, oats, barley, rice) and all types of legumes (beans, peas, and lentils).

Living at Peace with Carbs

A lot of my clients say that they could live on bread. Some say that they could live on white rice. Both are relatively low in calories. Unfortunately, they do not contain a lot of nutrients compared to fruits and vegetables. Although rice and bread don't contain a huge amount of calories, there are two problems with these types of carbohydrates:

1. Portion size
2. Stuff added to them

With bread and rice, some people need to eat a huge amount before they feel satisfied. Also, adding things like butter and creamy sauces takes up a lot of your empty calories. For losing or maintaining weight, these are both problems.

Has anyone ever told you to not eat potatoes? Are they too starchy or fattening?

JF: If by no potatoes you mean no McDonald's French fries, then yes, I have been told to stay away. Meanwhile, I must admit that the thought of a baked potato makes me yawn.

You: _____

Potatoes are healthy complex carbohydrates. A baked potato with the skin is relatively low in calories and loaded with nutrients and fiber. Before you shun a food, look at the whole picture. How many calories? Are there any nutrients? How much fiber? What is the fat content? Do you slather your baked potato with sour cream and butter? That makes a potato fattening.

What's your favorite carb? If you became allergic to your favorite carbohydrate (a carb that you say you couldn't live without), how would you survive?

JF: My favorite carb is bread. When I go to a restaurant and order the healthiest thing on the menu, I can botch up all of my efforts with breadsticks, garlic bread, or freshly baked rolls.

You: _____

_____

If a particular food is preventing you from losing or maintaining weight, you may have to "bite the bullet" and move ahead without it.

Carbs and Enzymes

Put a piece of bread in your mouth. It will immediately begin to dissolve and disintegrate. Did you know that you have enzymes in your saliva? *Don't worry.* They're supposed to be there. The enzyme *amylase* in your mouth starts the digestion process by breaking down starch. Protein and fat do not break down in the mouth.

Enzymes end in –ase. Amylase breaks down amylose (a starch). *Sucrase* breaks down sucrose into glucose and fructose. *Lactase* breaks down lactose into glucose and galactose. Individuals with digestive problems might have a deficiency of a certain enzyme.

The Problem with Low-Carb Diets

The National Academy of Medicine recommends that adults and children consume at least 130 grams of carbohydrate a day to provide a minimum amount of glucose. That's 520 calories.

Low-carbohydrate diets may not contain enough carbohydrates to keep minds and bodies feeling perky and alert.

If you don't eat enough carbohydrates, your body will use protein and fat for energy. Ketosis is not a comfortable feeling for most people. Ketones build up in the blood. The brain may function less efficiently. Do you know anyone who needs more carbohydrates?

JF: I have some slim friends who stay away from bread and pasta. They do seem to be a little less quick than others, but don't tell them I said that.

You: _____

_____

A long-term diet low in carbohydrates is very restrictive, may result in bone loss, and may increase the risk of kidney stones. It may also affect the nervous system. To prevent ketosis, at least 50-100 grams of carbohydrates (200-400 calories) a day is necessary. Two hundred to four hundred calories isn't much in terms of carbohydrate. If you aren't eating carbohydrates, then you are eating more protein and fat (potentially more saturated fat).

Carbohydrates attract water. If you start eating more carbohydrates and notice a weight gain, it could be additional fluid weight. Some people say that they feel bloated after they eat carbs.

*R*uth's **Rule:** *Stay away from low-carb diets, as they don't supply all the carbohydrate that your body needs.*

Carbs - An Athlete's Ally ℞

Athletes don't eat steak and eggs for breakfast anymore. For energy and to meet their calorie requirements, athletes consume most of their calories (55-65%) from carbohydrates. The carbs are broken down to glucose and immediately used for energy. Or they are stored in the muscles and liver as glycogen and can be used for energy later, especially for endurance sports.

6-11 Servings - Seem Like a Lot?

Clients used to gasp when they saw the 6-11 servings of carbohydrate on the bottom row of the Food Guide Pyramid. Many people told me they couldn't possibly eat that many carbs! I think they interpreted that amount to mean they were supposed to eat 11 pieces of bread a day. Then we would look at the calories in a serving or we measured a serving size (1/2 cup). Afterwards, they could see that the average 6-7 servings of carbohydrate a day wasn't that much for their age and activity. Even 11 servings of carbohydrate for a young person or an active person is not excessive.

Have you ever measured ½ cup of pasta and put it on a plate? It's relatively easy for some people to eat 1½-2 cups of pasta at dinner along with two pieces of garlic bread. That's five or six carbohydrates (1 carb = ½ cup or one slice of bread) just for dinner. Such giant portions of carbohydrates are out of control! (Keep in mind that MyPlate does not use servings. To refresh your memory further on MyPlate and carbs, go to Day 3, and look under the Grain Group.)

Many processed carbohydrates are empty calories. They contain mostly white flour or sugar with few or no nutrients. Empty calories from processed carbohydrates include syrup, cakes, cookies, candy, brownies, soda, punch, jelly, and pies. Too many added sugars from processed, refined carbohydrates will add unnecessary calories and unwelcome weight.

Without enough healthy carbohydrates, your body may not get protective vitamins, minerals, fiber, antioxidants, and phytonutrients.

Grains - A Good Source of Complex Carbs

Let's take a closer look at a ready source of complex carbohydrates – *grains*. Known as the "staff of life," grains have contributed to the survival of humankind since ancient times. "Grains" are the *seeds* or *kernels* of grasses. An example of a grass would be wheat. The seeds (or kernels) of wheat are ground up and made into flour. Flour is used to make bread. Wheat, rice, oats, corn, and barley are examples of grains.

Whole Grains

What's a whole grain? Many people don't know. There are three parts in the seed (kernel) of a grain, which includes the *bran*, the *endosperm*, and the *germ*. A whole grain contains all three parts of the seed. (Note: All grains also have an outer, inedible *hull* to protect the seed.)

The *bran* is the outer shell of the seed. Bran provides fiber, B vitamins, trace minerals, and phytonutrients. The *endosperm* is the inner part of the seed. It provides carbohydrate, protein, and some B vitamins. The small *germ* (for sprouting) contains vitamin E, B vitamins (thiamin, riboflavin, niacin, folate), trace minerals (selenium, magnesium, zinc, iron, copper, calcium, phosphorous, potassium), lipids, antioxidants, and phytonutrients. All that good stuff in the tiny, little seeds protects our heart, thus reducing the chance of a heart attack. It's really amazing. These benefits start to appear when eating three or more whole grains a day.

Just because the label says multi-grain (more than one grain), 100% wheat (only contains wheat), stone-ground, seven-grain (seven types of grains), or "high in fiber" doesn't mean it's a "whole grain." Cereal and crackers are processed grains. They can still be whole grains, as long as all three parts of the grain kernel are included. Don't judge a whole grain by its color. Caramel coloring or molasses can be added to make grain products look more healthful.

Whole grains can be cracked, crushed, or flaked. Whole grains may or may not be a good source of fiber. If you aren't sure it's a whole grain, look for a whole grain stamp. Some products contain the Whole Grains Council stamp.

You can also look for the FDA-approved health claim for whole grains. To include the whole grain health claim on the package, whole grain foods must contain 51% or more whole grain ingredients by weight. The products must also be low in fat and cholesterol.

A food can look and taste healthy but that doesn't mean it's a whole grain. Look for the words "whole" or "whole grain" on the ingredient list. Whole grain should be the first ingredient. A food can contain a variety of whole grains – for example, "whole wheat," "whole oats," "whole grain corn." Any whole grain can be made into flour and used in products. Foods can have a mixture of whole and refined grains. Look for the word "whole."

There's more to whole grains than whole wheat. Whole grains include whole wheat, brown rice, popcorn, whole grain barley, oatmeal, bulgur (cracked wheat), wild rice, whole rye, whole cornmeal, and whole wheat couscous. Less popular whole grains include amaranth, buckwheat, quinoa, triticale, millet, and sorghum. *Try them.* You might like them.

Staple Grains

Different societies around the world have their own particular staple grain. It could be wheat, rice, or corn. It could be millet, rye, oats, or barley. Grains are an inexpensive way to get energy. Beans, legumes, potatoes, or cassavas are other starches that provide major sources of energy in different parts of the world.

Many people eat white rice. White rice starts off as brown rice. What's *brown rice?* Brown rice contains the bran, the endosperm, and the germ. White rice is only the endosperm. Brown rice has more color, flavor, and texture than white rice. How about sushi with brown rice?

Wheat

In the U.S., we are very familiar with wheat. Many of our basic foods – breads, pasta, crackers, and cookies – are made with it.

The wheat kernel is called a *wheat berry. Cracked wheat* is the wheat berry that has been broken into pieces. *Bulgur* is a popular whole grain in the Middle East. Bulgur comes from the wheat berry. It has a chewy texture. Tabbouleh is a healthy salad made with bulgur and parsley.

What's *wheat germ?* Wheat germ contains the *germ* portion of the wheat kernel. Wheat germ is chock full of nutrients. Keep the jar of wheat germ in the refrigerator, or it will go rancid.

If you bake, whole wheat flour can replace ¼ to ½ the amount of white flour to increase health benefits. *Graham flour* is coarser whole wheat flour. Since whole wheat flour contains the germ from the wheat kernel, store it in a moisture-proof bag in the refrigerator or freezer.

How About Some Oatmeal? ❧

Oatmeal is a healthy, whole-grain cereal. Do you prefer to eat steel-cut oatmeal, 5-minute oatmeal, 1-minute oatmeal, or instant oatmeal? The ancient Greeks were the first to make a hot oatmeal cereal. Oatmeal is produced by grinding oats, a type of cereal grain. Oat bran is the bran part of groats, hulled oat seeds.

To increase your intake of oatmeal, replace ¼ the amount of white flour with quick or old-fashioned oatmeal in baked goods. Add oatmeal instead of bread crumbs to meatloaf. Make your own parfaits with toasted oatmeal, yogurt, and fruit. (To toast oatmeal, spread 1 cup in a pan and bake at 325 degrees for 15 minutes.) Store the toasted oatmeal in the refrigerator to keep it from going rancid. Instead of gooey chocolate desserts, make fruit cobblers, crisps, or crumbles, topping them with toasted oatmeal. Also, don't forget to add 1/4 - 1/3 cup raw oatmeal to smoothies. Eat oatmeal often.

Other Typical and Not-So-Typical Grains

Popcorn is a whole grain, and it's a great source of fiber. The endosperm in popcorn is harder than in sweet corn. Pressure from steam builds inside the kernel and makes it "pop."

Look for hulled *barley*. The bran is polished off pearl barley. Barley is a good source of soluble fiber (beta glucan), which helps to stabilize blood sugar and lower cholesterol. This is an under utilized whole grain with many health benefits.

When was the last time you ate quinoa? Be honest.

JF: I read the definition below and I don't think I've ever seen Quinoa. I have a friend who is half Irish and half Quinoan but I don't think that is what is meant here.

Quinoa (KEEN-wah) is gaining popularity. It comes from the goosefoot plant. It is native to Peru, Chile, and Bolivia. It is considered a complete protein. How about a warm bowl of quinoa with raisins for breakfast? This grain is similar to couscous. Look for whole grain couscous for more nutrients.

Triticale (trit-ih-KAY-lee) is a hybrid of wheat and rye. It's similar to wheat.

Millet is a staple grain in parts of Africa and Asia. It has a mild flavor. In the U.S., you'll see it in birdseed.

Amaranth is from South America. It's a complete protein and high in iron and calcium. Amaranth is a good choice for gluten-free diets.

Buckwheat is high in protein and fiber. Buckwheat kasha is made from buckwheat groats.

Feels Familiar, But It's Different ℞

Looking for the flavor and color of white bread? Choose *whole wheat white bread*. The bread is made from an albino variety of wheat. It has the nutrients and fiber of whole grain wheat with a sweet flavor.

Refined Grains

White rice is a refined grain. Other examples of refined grains are white bread and pasta, which are made with refined flour. It's a little confusing. White bread and white rice are refined grains, but they are *complex* carbohydrates. (Complex carbohydrates include starches.)

Refined grains have been processed to remove the bran and the germ, leaving only the endosperm. Refined grains provide energy, but vitamins, minerals, phytonutrients, and fiber are lost during refining.

Refined grains are found in white bread, pizza, pastries, biscuits, cereals, pasta, cookies, and cakes. Sweetened grains, such as cinnamon toast or honey-nut waffles, contain refined grains. A whole-grain waffle would be a healthier choice.

Since the vitamins, minerals, fiber, and phytonutrients are taken out during milling, white flour is "enriched." That is, thiamin, riboflavin, niacin, iron, and folic acid are added back to the flour. Flour, rice, cornmeal, and other products were required to be enriched in the 1940s to prevent beriberi, pellagra, and anemia. These vitamin and mineral deficiencies were common during that time.

An advantage to refined grains is the folic acid content. There's another benefit to refined grains. Refining removes the oil found in the germ. The lack of oil increases the shelf life of refined grains.

Throughout time, man has ground up grains to make food. Why go to the trouble of separating the bran and the germ from grains? Why take away the nutrients, the fiber, and the phytonutrients? Because at some point in history, people decided that they liked the texture, flavor, and appearance of white bread and pasta. Many people have become used to eating refined grains.

Wheat Flour vs. White Flour ℃

Whole-grain wheat flour and white flour contain significant differences in nutrients. Here are some examples from the USDA National Nutrient Database for Standard Reference, Release 28, 2016. One cup of whole-grain flour has 12.8 grams of dietary fiber compared to 3.4 grams of dietary fiber in one cup of white, all-purpose, enriched unbleached wheat flour. Whole-grain flour has more protein, calcium, magnesium, potassium, zinc, manganese, selenium, choline, and lutein, not to mention the phytonutrients. There are 53 micrograms of folate in a cup of whole-grain wheat flour compared to 364 micrograms of folate in a cup of white, all-purpose, enriched, unbleached wheat flour, because it is enriched.

Switching to Whole Grains

Whole grains are interesting. They add a variety of flavors and textures to meals. Make a batch of whole grains and freeze the leftovers for another meal. Whole grains are versatile. Whole grains can be added to soup (beef and barley soup). A whole grain can be a side dish by itself. A whole grain, vegetables, and the protein of your choice make a good stir-fry or casserole main dish. Vegetables can be added to a whole grain to make a salad (tabbouleh). There are many spices (Thai, Chinese, Italian, Indian, Mexican) that can be added to grains to create different flavors. Whole grains can also be used to make desserts. Your imagination is the only thing stopping you.

Meanwhile, it's easy to not eat any whole grains. A bagel with cream cheese for breakfast. A burger with an enriched bun for lunch. Chips for snack. Pasta for dinner. Cake for dessert.

But would you believe that it's also easy to eat whole grains? A whole-grain cereal or whole-grain English muffin for breakfast. A turkey sandwich on whole wheat bread for lunch. Popcorn for snack. A chicken and vegetable stir-fry with brown rice for dinner. An oatmeal cookie for dessert.

It's just a different way of looking at things.

What Your Body Needs

MyPlate recommends making *half your grains whole*. Yet 9 out of 10 Americans don't do it. *All* of your grains don't have to be whole. Just half. The rest of your grains can be enriched grain products.

In MyPlate, 1 ounce of whole grains equals one piece of whole-grain bread, ½ a small whole-grain bagel or English muffin, ½ cup brown rice, whole-grain pasta, or cooked oatmeal, one cup of dry whole-grain cereal, five whole-grain crackers, three cups popcorn, or a six-inch whole-grain corn tortilla.

If you only ate white bread growing up, you may not like the taste of whole wheat bread. Whole-grain products have more flavor. Start getting used to eating them. Serve whole-grain products to your children. If that's all they know, they'll prefer them.

How many whole grains a day do you eat? Is there room for improvement? Are you eating too many refined grains? What whole-grain foods will you add to your meals?

JF: I gave up white bread a long time ago. I eat oatmeal regularly, but beyond that I don't have a lot of memory of grains in my diet. Now that I know what they are exactly and where to find them, I will definitely incorporate them into my diet.

You: _____

Choose "Whole Grain" Carbs

Whole grains can have as many or more antioxidants as fruits and vegetables. Taking individual nutrients in a supplement is not the same thing as eating whole-grain foods. It's like taking a vitamin versus eating a fruit. You're better off eating an orange than taking a vitamin C supplement. All of the individual components in a whole food work together as a team to promote health. Is that enough of a reason to make your grains whole?

People have been eating whole grains for ages. It's unfortunate that we started eating so many refined grains. White rice and pasta have been popular for a long time. It's time for a change. Eating whole grains is an inexpensive way to get nutrients. *Try something new.* You're now a whole-grain specialist. Go forth and eat them.

Whole-grain carbohydrates are your new best friends.

𝒟ay 26 CHECK-IN ☑

What did you accomplish yesterday?

JF: I tried on some size 10 skirts from my closet and didn't feel like an encased sausage. I am working on fitting into this size loosely.

You: _____

_____

What is your goal for today?

(Eat bran cereal for breakfast.) (Dissolve a piece of bread in your mouth.) (Make barley for dinner.) (Find a recipe for quinoa.) (Measure ½-cup portions of cooked rice or pasta.) (Keep track of the grams of whole grains that you eat.)

JF: I am going to research this quinoa thing you speak of and get to know bran beyond just an occasional bran muffin.

You: _____

_____

Day 27

Fabulous Fiber

Sugar is sugar. It's sweet. There's a lot more going on with fiber. Fiber is fabulous for your health.

How's your roughage (skins, husks, seeds, leaves, pulps, and peels)?

JF: I didn't think that any of those things above were types of foods we were supposed to eat. It kind of sounds like what you find in the garbage at a restaurant.

You: _____

_____

Americans aren't getting enough fiber or "roughage." Most people get around half (about 16 grams) the recommended amount of fiber every day. *That's not enough.* Most of our fiber comes from white flour and white potatoes. That's not saying a lot. Fiber reduces the risk of disease, specifically heart disease, diabetes, diverticulosis, and irritable bowel syndrome. It also helps lower blood pressure and cholesterol and increases mineral absorption. *That's right.* Let's hear it for fiber!

The Facts on Fiber

This complex carbohydrate is found in various edible parts of plants. It can also be commercially produced. Humans don't have the enzymes to break down fiber. As fiber goes through the body, it passes through undigested. (It is a nondigestible carbohydrate.) Fiber isn't absorbed in the small intestine. It's not converted into glucose. Fiber can be found naturally in fruits, vegetables, whole grains, legumes (beans, peas and lentils), nuts, seeds, and soy.

Cereal fiber is found in the bran portion of a grain's kernel. Some kinds of fiber are like a plant's little skeleton. In celery, the strings are fiber. The fiber helps celery stand up straight. Other types of fiber are more subtle. For example, the pulp of a plum is a type of fiber.

The hull – the hard outer covering of the grain that occasionally gets stuck in your teeth – is often thought of as fiber. It's not. It's inedible.

Fiber has strange names. If you see one of these words on an ingredient list, you'll know that the food has fiber: *Beta-glucan, cellulose, chitin, chitosan, fructans, fructooligosaccharides, gums, hemicellulose, indigestible dextrins, inulin, lignin, mucilage, oligofructose, oligosaccharides, pectin, polydextrose, psyllium* and *resistant starch*.

Fiber's Classifications

The FDA has a new, official definition for "dietary fiber" to be used on the Nutrition Facts label: "Non-digestible soluble and insoluble carbohydrates and lignin that are intrinsic and intact in plants; isolated or synthetic non-digestible carbohydrates determined by FDA to have physiological effects that are beneficial to human health."

Intrinsic and intact means the natural occurring fiber in whole foods, such as fruits, vegetables and whole grains. Lignin is not a carbohydrate, but it is found in cell walls of woody plants.

Fibers that have been added to foods by isolating or synthesizing them have to demonstrate that they have health benefits.

Different fibers have different properties. Different properties come with different terms.

Soluble fiber dissolves in water. It is known for its fat- and glucose-lowering properties. However, *some* soluble fibers don't have an effect on cholesterol and blood glucose.

Getting Your Quota of Soluble Fiber ∞

The National Cholesterol Education Program (NCEP) recommends consuming 10-25 grams of viscous (soluble) fiber a day as a part of the Therapeutic Lifestyle Changes (TLC) diet to lower cholesterol.

Insoluble fiber doesn't dissolve in water. Insoluble fiber, known as roughage to many people, comes from the skins, seeds, and husks of plants. Wheat bran and whole grains have *a lot* of insoluble fiber. This type of fiber attracts water and increases bulk to waste material, which helps it move through the intestine with ease. Insoluble fiber promotes regularity by acting like a broom. It tidies up the intestines. In nonmedical terms, it's "swish," "swish" and *"whoosh."*

All plants contain soluble and insoluble fiber in varying amounts.

Feeling "Bran" New

What's bran cereal? Bran cereal contains mostly the *bran* portion of the wheat kernel. It's not a "whole" grain. It is missing the germ and the endosperm. Some people are sensitive to fiber. They run to the bathroom after eating a pea. Other people require larger daily amounts of insoluble fiber for regularity.

If you only have three or fewer bowel movements a week, you're constipated. If "number 2" looks like it came out of a rabbit, you're constipated. You might feel bloated and uncomfortable, possibly resulting in pain and difficult elimination. As bowel movements move through the intestinal tract, water is removed. The longer the waste material stays in the colon, the more water is taken out. A small, hard stool means that it has been in the colon for a while. Certainly not five years, though! If you're constipated, you need more fiber, more fluid, or both. Keep adding one or the other until you get results.

High-fiber diets are standard treatment for softening stools and relieving diverticulosis and hemorrhoids. Moving fecal material at a swift pace through the colon may reduce the risk of colon and rectal cancer. And don't forget about exercise to get things moving.

If your "laxation" needs improvement, fiber (cellulose and psyllium) is the way to go. Add a couple tablespoons of unprocessed wheat bran to cereal or sprinkle bran in yogurt.

Viscous and Nonviscous Fiber

Viscous fiber, rather than soluble fiber, is a more accurate term for the kind of fiber that lowers LDL cholesterol and stabilizes blood glucose levels. It forms a gel in water. Viscous fiber then soaks up cholesterol like a tiny sponge and carries it out of the body. Apples (*pectin*), beans, peas and lentils (resistant starch), oatmeal, oat bran, barley, and psyllium seed husk are a few fiber foods that lower cholesterol levels. Viscous fiber also delays gastric emptying, perhaps creating a sense of fullness.

For some people, foods with fiber fill them up. They feel full after eating a bowl of oatmeal versus not feeling full after a bowl of corn flakes. If you feel full, you won't eat as much.

Fiber and Emotional Eating ∞

High-fiber carbohydrates are filling and low in calories. *That's good news for losing weight.* If you feel full, you'll stop eating (in theory). However, feeling full doesn't stop emotional eaters from eating. Full or not, emotional eaters eat. Take control of your emotions so that you can respond to physical hunger cues. Your goal is to stop eating when you feel "just right."

Viscous fiber includes beta glucans (oats and barley), gums (guar gum), mucilages (psyllium) and pectins (citrus peels, apples, and berries). The fiber found in cereal fiber and pectins lowers coronary heart disease. How about a bowl of oatmeal with apple slices for breakfast?

Nonviscous fiber doesn't form a gel. Nonviscous fiber is cellulose, some hemicelluloses, and lignin. Cellulose is found in wheat bran and cereal. Again, lignin is cellular material from woody plants.

The terms soluble and insoluble fiber are used more than viscous and nonviscous fiber. They are often used interchangeably, but they are different.

The Fermentability Factor

Fiber has varying degrees of **fermentability**. When some types of fiber reach the colon, they are fermented or partially fermented by bacteria. This action results in short-chain fatty acids and *gases*. (You may have noticed.) The short-chain fatty acids have health-promoting benefits. Other kinds of fiber pass through unfermented.

Beta glucan, guar gum, inulin (chicory, onions, and Jerusalem artichokes), oligofructose, pectin, and resistant starch are very fermentable. Fermentable fiber can be found in fruits, vegetables, barley, and oats. Cellulose, found in wheat bran and lignin, is not very fermentable.

Let's think about this for a minute. Since most people only get half the recommended amount of fiber each day, they may be choosing high-calorie, low-fiber foods. It's often easier, and maybe a bit more appealing, to eat two pieces of fudge (no fiber) rather than two apples (8.8 grams fiber). To lose weight, train yourself to fill your stomach with low-calorie, high-fiber foods.

Would you prefer eating two pieces of fudge over the apples?

JF: The answer to this question is another obvious yes. I love apples but they would have to go head-to-head in a death match for me to pick apples as the winner over fudge. But now that I know better, I wouldn't encourage the violence and I'd just eat the apples.

You: _____

Becoming Fiber-Fabulous

The recommended amount of fiber is based on the amount needed to decrease the risk of coronary heart disease. Is 25-38 grams a day a lot? Keep in mind that 28 grams equals 1 ounce. One ounce is not that much. The Adequate Intake (AI) level is 14 grams of dietary fiber per 1,000 calories, and it also applies for children and older adults. Nothing says you care like a bran muffin with a candle for a loved one's birthday.

The amount of dietary fiber is listed on the label. Look at the % Daily Value. Twenty percent or more is high in fiber. The food label uses 28 grams of dietary fiber a day for 2,000 calories as a goal. Look for the words "excellent source of fiber," "rich in fiber," or "high in fiber" on packages.

Good source of fiber 2.5-4.9 grams per serving
High fiber 5 grams or more per serving
More or added fiber: At least 2.5 grams or more per serving than the traditional food

Some people don't have any idea how many grams of carbohydrate or fiber are in foods.

Let's clue you in and dispel the mystery:

Serving Size and Food	Grams carbohydrate	Grams fiber
Cereals and grains		
1 cup corn flakes	24	.9
3/4 cup bran cereal	24	5.5
1 cup cooked oatmeal	28	4.0
1 cup cooked oat bran	25	5.7
1 slice white bread	12	.6
1 slice whole wheat bread (varies)	14	1.9
1 cup cooked white rice	45	1.2
1 cup cooked brown rice	46	3.5
1 cup cooked pearled barley	44	6.0
1 ounce pretzels	23	1.0
1 ounce popcorn	22	4.1
Vegetables		
1 medium cooked artichoke	14	6.8
1 cup cooked broccoli	11	5.2
1 cup cooked Brussels sprouts	11	4.0
1 cup cooked cabbage	8	2.8
1 cup cooked cauliflower	6	4.9
1 serving candy corn (22 pieces)	36	0
1 cup cooked corn	41	4.2
1 cup cooked okra	7	4.0

Serving Size and Food	Grams carbohydrate	Grams fiber
1 cup cooked green peas	25	8.8
1 medium baked potato with skin	37	4.0
1 boiled white potato with skin	27	2.7
1 medium baked sweet potato	24	3.8
1 cup frozen spinach, cooked	9	7.0
Fruit		
1 cup unsweetened applesauce	28	2.7
1 medium apple	25	4.4
1 medium banana	27	3.1
1 cup blueberries	21	3.6
1 large fig	12	1.9
1 cup orange juice	26	.5
1 medium orange	18	3.1
1 medium pear	27	5.5
4 prunes	24	2.8
1 cup raspberries	15	8.0
1 cup strawberries	11	2.9
Legumes		
½ cup canned garbanzo beans	16	5.3
½ cup canned kidney beans	18.5	5.5
½ cup canned navy beans	27	6.7
½ cup canned pinto beans	18	5.5
½ cup cooked lentils	20	7.8
½ cup hummus	17.5	7.4
½ cup roasted, salted soybeans	26	15.2
Nuts & Seeds		
1 ounce almonds	6	3.5
1 ounce peanuts	5	2.4
1 ounce walnuts	4	1.9
1 tablespoon ground flaxseed	2.5	2.0
1 ounce sunflower seeds	6.5	3.0
Miscellaneous		
1 cup cooked chicken	0	0
1 chocolate cupcake with frosting	29	1.8

Serving Size and Food	Grams carbohydrate	Grams fiber
1 tablespoon jelly	15	.2
1 cup fat-free milk	12	0
1 tablespoon olive oil	0	0
1 12-ounce can of soda	38	0

USDA National Nutrient Database for Standard Reference, Release 28, 2016

Most foods from plants provide fiber. To get more fiber, eat fruits and vegetables with their skin (apples and potatoes). Fruits with seeds have more fiber (strawberries, figs, kiwis). For more fiber, eat beans and lentils as a side dish instead of rice or pasta. They're loaded with fiber. Look for bread with 3 grams of fiber per serving. A cold cereal with 5 or more grams of fiber per serving is high in fiber.

To increase your daily intake of fiber:

♦ Choose more whole fruits and less juice.
♦ Eat lots of vegetables.
♦ Eat plenty of beans.
♦ Eat whole grains (at least 3 ounce equivalents a day).
♦ Eat fewer foods and beverages with added sugars and fill up with fiber.

Ruth's **Rule:** *Once you "up" your fiber awareness, you'll realize that there are countless foods that can serve as fiber sources.*

To Supplement Fiber ... or Not? ଔ

Are fiber supplements effective? Taking supplements is a way to "supplement" the diet. They are not intended to replace foods. The whole is greater than the sum of its parts. A purified fiber by itself in a supplement, powder or added to foods may or may not be as protective as eating the whole food. Taking a lot of pills and powders is no way to live. But it may be necessary, depending on the situation.

The Good Guys: Probiotics and Prebiotics

Good bacteria are the champions in our intestinal tract. Consuming **probiotic bacteria** seems like an easy way to keep healthy. They fight the harmful bacteria. If there's not enough good bacteria, the bad bacteria will win, causing infection, disease, and possibly cancer.

Probiotic bacteria are found in cultured milk products and fermented foods, such as yogurt, kefir (fermented milk drink), cottage cheese, buttermilk, fresh sauerkraut, tempeh (fermented soybean cake), kimchi (fermented cabbage), and miso (fermented soybean paste). The two most common types of probiotic bacteria are *Lactobacillus* and *Bifidobacterium*. We don't live in a perfect world, and I will tell you why. Bacteria are used to ferment certain foods. However, the fermented foods may not end up with live cultures. Pasteurizing, baking, and processing can kill the bacteria. The actual amount of bacteria in products is unknown. Probiotics may not be safe for all people, especially people with immune system problems.

Probiotics with the most live and active bacteria are found in fermented dairy foods, such as yogurt and kefir. In yogurt, the acidity is right, and the cold temperature keeps the probiotics alive. Whenever you hear about people living to 110 years of age, many of them say that they eat a lot of yogurt. Maybe it's the probiotics.

As consumers, we don't know for sure if the bacteria in active cultured foods or supplements are still "alive." Check expiration dates. Nothing lives forever, including bacteria. Does the supplement match what's on the label? There's no guarantee that every brand of supplement is effective. The health benefits depend on the number of bacteria and the specific strain of bacteria. Certain types of bacteria work on certain conditions. Get a variety of good bacteria.

When you take antibiotics, the good bacteria are killed along with the bad bacteria. Too many bad bacteria will result in diarrhea. An unhealthy diet may not generate enough good bacteria. For better health, it seems logical to increase the number of good bacteria. To keep the good bacteria happy, give them what they want (prebiotics).

Prebiotics are "food" for the probiotics. They stimulate the growth of good bacteria. Prebiotics are nondigestible (not digested) carbohydrates. A lot of the prebiotics are fermentable fiber and are classified as functional fibers. Prebiotics are fermented in the colon by good bacteria, resulting in short-chain fatty acids. This creates an acidic environment in the colon that reduces the bad bacteria. *Go fiber!* Specific prebiotics stimulate the growth of specific probiotics. Not all fermentable foods are prebiotics. Good bacteria are particular about what's on the menu.

Prebiotics are found naturally in foods. They can also be isolated from foods, or they can be synthesized. Two common prebiotics are *inulin* and *oligofructose* (soluble fibers). Inulin and oligofructose contain chains of fructose. They are found naturally in plants (bananas, chicory, garlic, onions, and wheat), extracted from chicory roots, or made from sucrose.

Some other prebiotics include *fructooligosaccharides* (FOS), *resistant starch* (aka resistant cornstarch, maltodextrin, modified food starch), *oligosaccharides, galactooligosaccharides, lactulose, tagatose, polydextrose,* and *lactitol.*

Resistant starch "resists" digestion. It travels to the colon where it is fermented. Resistant starch can be naturally occurring (unripe bananas), made by modifying starch, or manufactured. Cooking and cooling potatoes produces resistant starch (potato salad). About one-third of the starch in legumes is resistant starch, therefore not digested. It produces gases and acts as a prebiotic.

Prebiotics can be found in grains (barley, rye, oatmeal, wheat), soy, Jerusalem artichokes, legumes, bananas, berries, asparagus, leafy greens, chicory root, honey, onions, leeks, and garlic. Prebiotics have other purposes, besides being prebiotics. Inulin and oligofructose add fiber, provide bulk and texture to food, and can be used as fat and carbohydrate substitutes. Prebiotics increase the absorption of calcium.

Prebiotic and probiotic science is evolving. Be on the lookout for food products and beverages containing prebiotics and probiotics. These foods have the potential to reduce the risk of disease and positively promote health. Food, beverages, and supplements containing prebiotics and probiotics are called **symbiotics**. An example would be fiber added to yogurt with active cultures (inulin and bifidobacterim). Keep in mind that eating real food is a healthier lifestyle than taking an arsenal of pills and powders.

Let's hear it for the *several pounds* of microorganisms (mostly bacteria) in your intestine. The potential of prebiotics and probiotics is exciting. For now, we have to rely on what's available. It seems that yogurt and other fermented foods have worked for others in the past. Do what you can to increase your good bacteria.

*R*uth's **Rule:** *Fermented dairy foods, like yogurt and kefir, are among the best sources for beneficial bacteria known as probiotics.*

Getting It Right

Fiber is an essential component to your diet. Men and women who consume the recommended amount of fiber have fewer heart attacks. Besides reducing heart disease and diabetes, fiber may reduce the risk of cancer and help with weight loss. Considering all of the important health benefits, it's amazing that less than 10% of Americans get enough fiber. Now that you know, I hope you will eat enough foods with different types of fiber. You'll quickly become fiber-fabulous!

Getting enough fiber isn't rocket science. Review this chapter and consider the following:

Benefits of Probiotics ଓ

Here are some documented health effects of good bacteria (probiotics), as well as some potential claims:

- Decreases diarrhea.
- Improves lactose intolerance.
- Makes vitamin K and biotin.
- Prevents tooth decay.
- Improves irritable bowel syndrome.
- Decreases pathogenic bacteria.
- Controls intestinal inflammation.
- Speeds up digestion.
- Reduces allergy symptoms.
- Decreases stomach infections.
- Prevents eczema.
- Prevents vaginitis.
- Suppresses colon cancer.
- Boosts the immune system.
- Keeps healthy people healthy.

Eat more

Whole grain cereal and oatmeal

Brown rice, barley, and wild rice

Whole wheat pasta

Eat less

Rice and corn cereal

White rice

Enriched pasta

Whole wheat bread, rolls, and crackers	White bread, rolls, and crackers
Whole wheat flour	White flour
Whole wheat bagels and English muffins	Enriched bagels, muffins, and donuts
Whole wheat tortillas and pitas	Flour tortillas and pita bread
Bulgur or buckwheat	Grits and couscous
Polenta and cornbread from whole cornmeal	Polenta and cornbread
Vegetables and beans	White rice, pasta, and bread
Nuts or sunflower seeds	Candy
Popcorn	Pretzels
Fruit	Cakes, cookies, pies, and chocolate
Oatmeal cookies	Chocolate chip cookies

Feel the love. Welcome moderate amounts of healthy fiber into your diet.

Fiber-rich foods are your new best friends.

ᗞay 27 CHECK-IN ☑

What did you accomplish yesterday?

JF: I've come to understand that meal replacement shakes are not so bad when I am on the go and cannot fix a proper high-fiber breakfast. They have extra fiber shakes that curb my appetite.

You: _____

_____

What is your goal for today?

(Keep track of the grams of fiber that you eat.) (Look at a label and identify the types of fiber.) (Find different ways to add oatmeal to your diet.) (Add another fiber-rich food to your routine.) (Eat a snack high in fiber.) (Have a daily "whoosh.")

JF: I will add more fiber to my day and find the fiber or lack thereof on labels. I may make a few more trips to the bathroom but it's all in the name of good health.

You: _____

_____

Day 28

Stressed? Wanna Eat?

*H*ave you ever heard the expression, "Stressed is desserts spelled backwards"? Actually, being stressed and desserts were made for each other. What a dynamic duo! How could you deal with stress without desserts? (Actually, if you can't, that's why you're here.)

In case you haven't noticed, life can be stressful. If you let it, stress can affect your day and make you feel tired, depressed, frustrated, anxious, or angry. Do you have stress? Are there others around you who are experiencing stress?

Do any of these scenarios sound familiar? A single parent? A dangerous job? A long commute in heavy traffic? Fearing foreclosure? Working two to three jobs? A psycho boss or co-worker? Job insecurity? Running late? Going through a divorce? Experiencing abuse? Health problems? Taking care of a loved one? Car won't start? Have to give a speech or a presentation? Too many bills? Neighborhood unsafe? Relationship problems? Afraid to step outside of your comfort zone?

The list of stressors is endless. At times, life seems overwhelming. Stress is *everywhere,* whether you want it or not. Stress can happen at a moment's notice. Sometimes there's nothing we can do about it. There are stress givers and stress receivers. Where there's yin, there's yang. Some people get stressed from worrying about stuff that *could* happen. And believe it or not, some people cause their own problems. *Phew!*

There are different types of stress. There's the annoying short-lived stress, such as a bad hair day. There's also more intense stress, such as when a loved one is involved in a tragic accident. Both types of stress can take a toll on a person's health.

Stress isn't fun. It can cause headaches, muscle tightness, insomnia, fatigue, even elevated blood sugar. Stress is a major factor affecting some people's weight. There are people who lose their appetite and can't eat because of stress. But others use food as a *distraction*. They start nibbling and may try to find relief from a favorite food. If you react to stress by eating, it can keep you from losing or maintaining weight. *Who needs it!*

Eating for Stress

Life is full of ups and downs. Life can also be full of pounds.

What stressful things are happening to you right now? What bothers you? Big and small.

JF: I am stressed by my profession as a comedian and actress. Everything's going great. However, with great comes the need to stay great, to always develop, and to always be seeking out the next project. I'm in a constant state of not knowing and that sometimes creates a lot of anxiety.

You: _____

_____

Which of these stressors causes you to eat?

JF: The not knowing what's in store from day to day creates the need to eat my favorite comfort foods. I know the foods will taste great and provide some solace when I'm not sure about much else. But then I need to watch the amounts or I gain weight.

You: _____

_____

Which problems or situations can you do something about?

JF: I can talk to a friend, when I feel anxious and when I feel like eating, I can exercise. Usually when I am involved in a workout regimen,

I don't have the desire to eat. I can cope better with the feeling of not knowing and just accept that when I need to know, I will.

You: _____

_____

Which ones are out of your control?

JF: "Not knowing" is out of my control. But I can work on accepting that one is not meant to understand every moment of every day and that is okay.

You: _____

_____

It may be necessary to let go of the problems or situations that are out of your control. If there's nothing you can do about it, set it free. Close your eyes. Put the problem in an imagery boat. Untie the boat from the dock and let the problem drift away. *Gone!*

Is there something causing you stress that you can fix? Make a list and pick one thing. (*Look for a new job. Finish the taxes. Get a physical exam.*) One by one, work on the problems that you can change. It will free your mind. You'll be able to get more done and feel less stressed.

*R*uth's **Rule:** *Next time you're stressed, consider whether or not the stressor is something you can control. If not, let it go. If it could be under your control, take action!*

A Common Habit

If you eat for stress, you're not alone. Here are 30 reasons people gave me for why they eat for stress:

Susan	Rude, inconsiderate customers and a mean spouse
Maria	Health problems
Christina	Not being organized and a temperamental boss
David	A long day at work
Terry	Two-year-old screaming and work deadlines
Kendra	School, family drama, and dating
Mary Ann	Too many jobs

Marsha	Relationship problems
Roseanne	Not enough money
Eliza	Financial problems and family
Flaviano	Overwhelmed with too much work
Eloise	Pressure from boss
Louise	Work deadlines
Jessica	Problems with friends
Clarissa	Brainstorming with co-workers under work pressure
Catalina	Grandkids and health problems
Garen	Irritated by stupidity of self or others
Claudia	Bills
Alissa	Three kids
Mauricio	Work pressure deadlines
Fred	Never enough money
Alicia	Social life
Elaine	Not respected or appreciated at work
Claudine	Too much paperwork – work pressure
Marissa	Work load
Maggie	Husband trouble
Susie	Chasing baby
Mary	Not in control of a new situation
Cheryl	Pressure from not enough time
Fannery	Co-workers and work pressure – too much, too fast

These reasons cause these people to eat for stress. Some people eat for small, annoying problems. Some people eat for major problems. Some people react to every situation by eating. It's interesting to see that work is a prevalent reason for stress eating.

When I asked people to tell me what situations cause them to eat for stress, many people were reluctant to talk about it. At first, they denied eating for stress. When I asked folks to tell me their comfort foods for Day 11, it was a different story. They could have gone on for days talking about their comfort foods and what it meant to them.

The results of my survey are not based on randomized, placebo-controlled clinical trials or epidemiologic studies. But since work stress is common, it seems logical to me that worksite wellness programs – which could include nutritional education, weight loss info, physical activity, and stress reduction – would benefit the employee and ultimately the employer.

Learning New Ways to Cope

We are all unique. A troublesome problem to you may not be an issue for others. If there are people who aren't bothered by things that drive *you* crazy, try to let it go. If a problem doesn't bother them, don't let it bother you. If being stuck in traffic raises your blood pressure and causes you to reach for the bag of chips in the back seat, do what other people do: Turn on music or listen to a recorded book to pass the time. They have found a way to make driving in traffic productive and relaxing.

Many people have comfort foods and turn to them during stress. If comfort foods are high in fat or sugar, the extra calories will gradually (or quickly) put on weight. Eating or drinking excess calories creates other issues.

Do you ever get mad at yourself for gaining weight after you ate too much? Did eating make the problem go away?

JF: In all honesty, eating comfort foods feels great while you're eating them but the problem is usually there after the last spoonful. I don't always feel guilty because I try to control the binge eating. It is hard work to find something to replace the feeling fattening foods give you, but this is all a work in progress.

You: _____

_____

Stress doesn't have to be about eating comfort food. Turning to comfort food is a learned activity. Substitute comfort foods with comfort activities or comfort places. Many people jog to reduce stress. Other people like to watch waves at the ocean or a lake. Water is calming. The sound of gurgling water from an indoor fountain brings the ocean to you. It's important to find healthy ways to relieve stress.

A healthy lifestyle copes with stress naturally. Being relaxed is the opposite of being stressed. When you're stressed, it makes sense to relax. Hopefully, you can't be stressed and relaxed at the same time. At least, try to be more in control of the situation. Different things upset different people, so it's logical that the same ways to relax won't be effective for everyone. Try some of these ideas. See what works for you.

*R*uth's **Rule:** *Turning to food when stressed is a learned behavior. Learn something new!*

Avoid Overdoing Alcohol When Stressed ≪

Many people reduce tension with alcohol. Excess alcohol is *not* a healthy solution. More than one drink a day for women or more than two drinks a day for men increases the risk of cancer. This fact could cause stress for some people. For a reminder of other dangers from alcohol, see the Alcohol Consumption Risks in Day 24.

Breathing for Relaxation

Since everyone breathes, try deep breathing. Trying it once or twice is not enough. You have to practice it over and over. In a stressful situation, start deep breathing. It will help you feel better.

Try this …

+ Close your eyes. Breathe in and out slowly and naturally. Think about a past or present person, place, or thing that makes you feel happy or relaxed. Were you walking along the beach barefoot, holding hands with someone, listening to the birds, smelling the fresh air, feeling the warmth of the sun and the cool breeze from the water? Re-live the calm, peaceful feeling. You can also look at a favorite picture to relax.

+ Sit in a chair with your feet grounded to the earth. Close your eyes. Slowly breathe in through your nose and exhale through your mouth. Focus only on breathing. Close out the rest of the world. Listen to the air going into your nose. Feel the air fill your lungs. Expand your chest. Exhale a little longer and louder than you inhaled. Listen to the air leave your mouth. Continue deep breathing for a few minutes. If your mind starts to drift and you think about anything besides breathing, refocus. Forget about what's going on in your life. The only thing that matters right now is listening to the air going into your nose and the air going out of your mouth.

♦ Another type of deep breathing is abdominal breathing. Practice while you're sitting or lying down. Place your hands on your abdominal area. As you inhale, push your abdominal area up. As you exhale, blow out the air from your mouth. Tighten and make your abdominal area go down. Breathe slowly and deeply for a minute or two. Blow the tension out of your body. Practice abdominal breathing several times a day.

♦ Meditate. Drop your jaw. Close your eyes and relax. While you're slowly breathing in and out from the abdominal area, repeat a word in your mind that is "special" to you over and over again as you exhale. *Om* is a popular mantra sound. Do you like the of sound *thin*? Practice 10 minutes a day. Concentrate only on the word.

♦ When you're tired, take a deep breath. Fill your lungs with as much air as you can. Hold it for a few seconds. Blow the air out through your mouth. Do it two or three times. It's energizing. While you inhale, raise your arms over your head.

♦ If you "don't have time" to breathe, take one minute to "breathe" before you fall asleep at night and one minute when you wake up. Take baby steps. *Every little bit helps.*

Breathing exercises can be refreshing and rejuvenating. If you really focus on breathing and not the stressful situation, you'll forget about the problem and feel relaxed. Find peace for your mind so that eating food doesn't become the focus. Take care of your mind, or your body will be affected.

It's important to practice deep breathing. When you need it, it becomes second nature.

15 Ways to Reduce Stress

1. **Getting a massage is relaxing for some people.** When there isn't time for a massage, increase the circulation in your head

by lightly tapping the fingertips of both hands around your face and head.

2. **Drink more water.** Dehydration can cause fatigue and make you feel drained.

3. **Watch the sunset.**

4. **Pray.**

5. **Increase muscle mass by lifting weights.** Muscle mass gives you strength and energy. Muscles are empowering. Muscles give you a "Yes I can" attitude.

6. **Slowly count to 30 once or twice a day.** Concentrate on counting. When stress hits, count to 30 slowly. If you have done it enough times, your mind focuses on counting. Your mind will be distracted, and you will relax. Or count backward from 50.

7. **Look in a mirror and smile.** Smile at other people. When you smile, try smiling with your eyes, as well as your mouth.

8. **Give yourself a compliment.** If you feel happy, you won't be stressed. Give someone else a compliment, a pat on the back, or a friendly hug. They might be stressed, too. They will be nice to you, and you'll feel better.

9. **Stop and take a break.** Could it be worse? Take a 20-minute power nap.

10. **Take a tai-chi or yoga class to relax.** It really works.

11. **Do you have a favorite perfume or cologne? Smelling good can put you in a good mood.** Give yourself a splash. To relax, take a whiff of lavender. Also, the smell of lemon is uplifting.

12. **Play your favorite music.** Dance or sing along.

13. **Make the world go away for a while.** Let your mind go blank. People have told me that this is easy for them.

14. **Light a scented candle.** Turn off the lights and focus on the flame.

15. **Laugh a lot.** Watch a funny movie. Go to a comedy club. Be around upbeat, supportive people.

Try Some Muscle Relaxation

Relaxing your muscles can reduce the tension in your mind. Try this relaxation method lying down. Tense each muscle group for a few seconds. Then relax. Wait ten seconds before tensing the next muscle group. Raise forehead and relax. Grit teeth and relax. Shrug shoulders and relax. Make a fist with both hands, flex biceps, and relax. Suck in stomach and relax. Squeeze the butt and relax. Tighten the thighs and relax. Point toes toward the air, tighten calves, and relax. Practice muscle relaxation to fall asleep. You'll likely be sleeping before you get to your toes.

Stre-e-e-e-e-etch

Five minutes of stretching does amazing things for your mind, body, and spirit. Here are a few easy stretches to do at home or at work.

- While sitting in a chair with your feet on the ground, bend over and rest your body on your thighs. Let your arms go loose in front of you. Feel the stretch in your back, neck, and shoulders. Relax for 10 seconds. Slowly sit up. Repeat a few times.
- While sitting, raise your arms above your head. Keep your arms straight and reach for the sky. Hold for 5 seconds. Then lower your arms. Do the stretch three times. Next, turn your head to the right and hold for 5 seconds. Return your head to the center. Turn your head to the left, and hold for 5 seconds. Repeat three times. Let go of any tension in your upper body.
- Stand. Lift one arm up at a time and bend to the side. Switch arms and bend to the other side. Repeat three times.
- Stretch your arms out to your sides. Do five *small* backward arm circles. Do five *large* backward arm circles. Repeat three times. Do five *small* forward arm circles. Do five *large* forward arm circles. Repeat three times.
- Stand in a doorway. Raise your arms and grab the molding of the door frame with your hands. Lean forward and hold. This stretches out your shoulders. Or sit and put your hands together behind you and stretch out your arms.

Do you ever get "stuck"? Have there been times when stress caused you to procrastinate, and you didn't seem to be able to get anything done, except go out to dinner?

JF: I get stuck daily. It's hard work when you work for yourself because your only motivator is you. Procrastination is always something I deal with because the to-do list is so overwhelming.

Going out to eat has been my problem. For some reason, knowing that a gigantic bowl of pasta dripping in Alfredo sauce is at the end of the rainbow makes an unproductive day worthwhile.

You: _____

_____

15 More Stress Reducers

To further support you, here are 15 more ways to let the stress go … *without* eating.

1. **With your eyes closed, trace the shape of the number eight lying in its side in your mind for about 5 minutes.** It can be a distracting, yet relaxing, way to pass time.

2. **Some people clean house to relax.** *To each his own.*

3. **Pets relieve stress.** Adopt a Fido or a Fluffy. They appreciate your love.

4. **Can't sit and do nothing?** *Take action.* Do what you can to solve the problem. Call someone. Write a letter. Get involved.

5. **Maybe vigorous activity is a better release for you.** Sign up for a boxing class. Work out at a gym for an hour. Take a spinning class.

6. **Short on time? March in place and swing your arms for three minutes.** Get your heart pumping to feel energized and relaxed.

7. **Nurture yourself with positive thinking.** Tell yourself, "Everything will work out for the best." Being negative takes too much energy. When one door closes, a new and better door will open.

8. **Don't let little things bother you.** Is it really that important in the scheme of life? Sometimes little stresses are more irritating than big stresses, causing more emotional eating.

9. **Get busy.** Don't dwell on your problems. Volunteer your time to help others.

10. **Enjoy the small things in life.** I found $1 bottles of nail polish. Five little bottles of nail polish kept me happy for weeks.

11. **Go to a sporting event or a concert.** Being a fan and vocalizing your support can be relaxing.

12. **If you're in over your head, it's okay to say "no."** Otherwise, your circuits will overload. Avoid putting too much on your plate, so to speak, or you'll end up putting too much on your dinner plate. The world will survive.

13. **When the going gets rough, feel better by getting something accomplished.** Set measurable goals for yourself. (Example: Bike three times a week.) Focus on the process, not the outcome. If you only bike one day, you might quit. Give yourself something to believe in.

14. **Don't keep stress inside. Talk to a friend.** Stress over time can become issues. Deal with it as it happens. Is it worth getting crazy?

15. **If you can't deal with stress on your own, get help.** Make an appointment to see a mental health professional.

Now, instead of eating to cope, reduce the tension. *Relax.* You'll feel energized and be free to enjoy life without the need to eat.

Name three things that you will do to relax:

JF: This is a family book so I'll refrain from dirty but fun answers. I'll just go with exercise. Although the other answer is great for stress release, too.

You: _____

_____

It helps to write down and post your favorite ways to relax. When you need an idea, you'll see it. Empower yourself before you reach the end of your rope. Did you notice that eating a hot fudge sundae is not listed as a way to relax?

Trading Boredom for Stress

Stress is the new boredom. Twenty years ago, most of my clients said that they ate out of boredom. Now most of them say that they eat because of stress. If you usually escape with food, don't underestimate your ability to deal with stress.

Stress can make life difficult. In all likelihood, all stress cannot be eliminated from our lives. If you learned to eat for stress, unlearn it. Try not to rush through meals and end up eating too much. Don't go back to old habits and feel obligated to finish what's on your plate. Don't skip meals and risk overeating at the next meal. Catch yourself when you're eating without being hungry. If you're overdosing on food, listen to hunger cues. The name of the game is beating mental hunger.

Living Healthy

To prevent stress from taking a toll on you, practice a healthy life-style. Enjoy life. Let the little things go. Deal with the big things, as they happen. Eat healthy in moderation. Get daily physical activity. Get enough sleep. Don't smoke. Express your feelings. Be kind to yourself, your family, friends, and coworkers.

"Life is in the breath. He who half breathes, half lives."
~Yoga proverb.

Remember, deep breathing can help you get through a stressful situation. You don't have to be a Zen master to do it. It's quick and effective. Get in the habit of taking deep cleansing breaths throughout the day. It takes concentration and discipline. Learning discipline will help you turn down cupcakes more often.

Smile. Be happy. Let it go. *Repeat.* Smile! Be happy! Let it go! *One more time.* SMILE. BE HAPPY. LET IT GO! Work on not eating for stress. *Yuck.* Stress does not taste good.

Healthy stress reduction is your new best friend.

𝒟ay 28 CHECK-IN ☑

What did you accomplish yesterday?

JF: I tried almond butter for the first time and it was delicious. I also had a girlfriend make me dinner and she introduced me to quinoa. Funny how all the things I'm learning about in this book are coming to fruition.

You: _____

_____

What is your goal for today?

(Practice deep breathing for five minutes.) (Be aware of stress eating.) (Smile with your eyes.) (Tell yourself that everything will work out for the best.) (Do something that you enjoy for 30 minutes.) (Don't give anyone stress.) (Stretch for a couple of minutes.)

JF: I am going to work out for another consecutive day. The people at the gym are starting to know my name. That feels way better than the cashiers knowing my name at McDonald's.

You: _____

_____

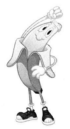

End of Week 4

Just two more days to go with the initial 30-day program!

It's time to weigh in.

Weight:_____

See you at Day 29!

Day 29

To Snack ... Or Not to Snack

A snack is a small meal that occurs between main meals. Snacks contain fewer calories than regular meals. Healthy snacks are low in sugar, unhealthy fat, and salt, and they are high in vitamins, minerals (such as calcium or potassium), fiber, antioxidants, phytonutrients, whole grains, lean protein, healthy fats, and even live and active cultures.

Do you snack? What are your unhealthy snacks? When you're being "good," what are your healthy snacks?

JF: My unhealthy snacks are usually full-fat Pringles potato chips or gummi bears. For some reason when I have long trips to take by car, I need a big bag of gummi bears to make the driving time not seem so long. I think gummi bears are my cigarettes. My so-called healthy snacks include veggie chips. The thing is that a snack is not healthy if you eat the entire bag or box in one sitting.

You: _____

_____

When and where do you usually snack? During trips to the mall? While watching movies or television at night? When attending concerts? When you're at sporting events? While waiting at the airport? At work? At the computer? In the car? At school?

JF: Yes to all of the above. I had a giant bag of popcorn at the movies the other day and justified it because there was no added butter or salt.

Never mind that is was a ginormous bag of popcorn.

You: _____

_____

Snacks can be confusing. Should you or shouldn't you? Let's take a look.

You Shouldn't Snack ...

Big portions of high-calorie snacks can thwart your efforts to lose weight. Even 200-300 additional calories a day can add extra baggage over the years.

Do you have a nervous habit of snacking all day long? Grazing on snacks all day may be the reason for excess weight. Boredom or stress can result in unconscious snacking. Keeping a food journal will increase your awareness of *what* and *how many* snacks you're having. If you're a grazer, limit yourself to one or two snacks a day. However, munching on broccoli and cauliflower all day is fine.

Maybe snacks are your comfort foods. If cake is your comfort food and you can't stop eating until it's gone, don't have this dessert around. You most likely have noticed that high-calorie comfort foods are counterproductive. If you choose to snack on baby carrots, you probably won't eat more than a couple of cups. *No harm. No foul.*

*R*uth's Rule: *Remember, comfort snacks do not solve problems. Let go of food as a solution. Go for a walk to burn off stress and think things out.*

You Should Snack ...

Snacks can have a positive effect on your overall diet. They're a good way to increase your intake of important nutrients. Snacks can be a source of energy. Carbohydrate snacks improve performance. To get the most out of your workout, have a carbohydrate snack (banana, yogurt) before you hit the gym.

Choosing low-calorie snacks rather than high-calorie snacks will help you lose weight and assist in preventing future weight gain. *Every calorie counts.*

Compare the calories of these snacks:

	Calories		Calories
Banana	100	Candy bar	300
Pickle	20	Ice cream drumstick	350
Mineral water	0	Can of soda	150
Bag of pretzels	110	Small fries	230

Snacks can *make or break* your efforts to lose weight. You might as well use them to your advantage.

*R*uth's Rule: *Eat small meals and eat snacks to take the edge off hunger between meals.*

In Pursuit of the Healthy Snack

Snacks don't have to be chips, soda, or brownies. My son's cat, Felix, loves snacks. When Felix wants a snack, he stands in front of the snack drawer and says, "Snaaack!" His snacks involve some type of fish or protein.

Here are a few healthy and relatively low-calorie snack ideas for us humans:

+ Any type of fresh, canned, or dried fruit
+ Any type of vegetable: baby carrots, cauliflower, sugar snap peas, red bell pepper, zucchini, radishes, broccoli, cucumber, edamame, cherry tomatoes
+ Whole wheat pretzels
+ A handful of any type of nut, including soy nuts or seeds (salted or unsalted)
+ String cheese and whole grain crackers
+ A carton of flavored yogurt or a cup of plain yogurt with fruit
+ Raw vegetables and hummus
+ Trail mix

- Cinnamon graham crackers, rice cakes, popcorn
- Small bran muffin
- Cashews and raisins mixed together
- Baked tortilla chips with salsa, guacamole, or bean dip
- Frozen grapes, cherries, blueberries, or banana slices
- Granola bar
- Frozen 100% juice bar
- A bowl of whole-grain cereal with 1% milk – could be sweetened whole-grain cereal or a packet of oatmeal
- A cold chicken drumstick – no skin
- Apple slices and peanut butter
- ½ sparkling mineral water and ½ 100% fruit juice
- Black or green olives
- Fat-free chocolate milk
- A hard-boiled egg
- Fat-free café latte
- Toasted whole-grain English muffin with peanut butter
- Canned tuna fish and low-fat mayo with crackers
- A baked potato or sweet potato
- A slice of vegetable pizza
- A scoop of low-fat cottage cheese and a small can of peaches

Snacks can fill the nutrient gap. Since most people don't get enough fiber or whole grains, choose a whole grain snack with fiber and "kill two birds with one stone." A snack containing fiber and some protein will help stabilize blood sugar levels. If you need more calcium for the day, choose yogurt, fat-free chocolate milk, or low-fat cheese. A snack with a little fat will keep you feeling satisfied longer. Most Americans don't eat enough fruits and vegetables. Bring a couple of bags of baby carrots to work. Keep fresh fruit in a bowl on the counter. Have cut-up vegetables ready to eat in the refrigerator. When you're ready to snack, the veggies will be ready to eat. Fruits, vegetables, and whole-grain snacks are low in calories and nutritious. They also protect your health while keeping off the extra pounds.

Before you choose a snack, think about what would taste good to you. Find healthy substitutions for high-calorie snacks. Celery is crunchy. Pretzels are salty. Fat-free chocolate milk is sweet.

Are most of your snacks processed? You won't find celery in a vending machine. Celery filled with peanut butter and sprinkled with raisins is a crunchy, creamy, chewy snack. Don't be naïve. If a snack is "made with real fruit" or "made with vegetables," ask tough questions. Is a cracker made with bits of carrot as nutritious as a real carrot?

What healthy snacks will you try?

JF: I will stock up on fruit and nuts, and I'll try the small bran muffin idea. Most of the alternatives listed above I eat now; I just don't incorporate them often enough to say I eat them the way I should. I noticed M&Ms are not on the list. What if they have peanuts in them? I know the answer; just thought I would try.

You: _____

*R*uth's **Rule:** *Remember, you've got lots of options when it comes to healthy snack food.*

Tread with Care: Your Extra Calories

If you eat healthy and control your calories, you can use your extra calories for an unhealthy snack. Just don't go overboard. Choose a donut hole instead of a donut. Instead of a two-scoop hot fudge sundae, choose a frozen 100-calorie ice cream bar. A snack means *moderation.* Eat one or two cookies, not half the package. Drink a 5-ounce glass of wine, not the entire bottle. Eat half a cupcake, not half a cake. You are downsizing and eating fewer calories.

Obviously, if you choose a 600-calorie coffee or juice drink and a 500-calorie muffin, it's more of a meal than a snack. If your snack is a mini-meal, your next meal should be a mini-meal. Everything needs to balance so that you don't end up eating too many calories for the day.

Finding a "Just Right" Snack Size

One-hundred-calorie snack packs are convenient. If you can't stop yourself from finishing the bag, at least it's only 100 calories. *Listen to your hunger cues.* Maybe 50 calories will be enough to satisfy your hunger.

Bag your snacks. It takes a little time, but this is definitely worth it. Making your own 100-calorie snack packs saves money and it's an education. You may be surprised to learn that 100 calories of your favorite snack looks rather small. Three cups of air-popped popcorn is only 100 calories. Now that's a good deal!

I had a client who ate a candy bar every afternoon for energy and comfort at her new job. This woman made an appointment with me because she didn't understand why she had gained 15 pounds in a year. She had no idea that a candy bar five days a week could cause her to gain weight. If you want chocolate, eat one or two mini candy bars instead of a large candy bar. A sweet and satisfying snack with no nutritional value is a handful of miniature marshmallows and chocolate chips. The small pieces are good for nibbling. They are bite-size so you can stop at any time. This type of snack is good if you want something sweet but can't stop eating a candy bar until it's gone.

Processed Snacks: A World of Whopping Calories ≪

Keep in mind that many processed snacks can have meal-size calories. If it's 100 calories, *no problem.* Two hundred calories? *Not the end of the world.* A large cinnamon bun with 1,000 calories far exceeds the calorie allowance of extra calories. *Before* you eat, check the calorie counts on huge cinnamon buns, large muffins, giant cookies, extra-large coffee drinks with whipped cream, large juice drinks, and oversized fries with ranch dressing. It will take your breath away. Unhealthy snacks should be a special occasion, rather than a daily occurrence. Share them with a few people.

Other People's Snack Foods

When you're trying to lose weight and be "good," do you eat lots of "bad" snacks and pretend that you didn't eat them? Do you not want to think about all those extra calories and how they will make you gain weight?

JF: The problem I have is the serving size. If I buy a bag of Oreo cookies, I can eat only two if someone takes the remainder and locks them in a high-security vault guarded by attack dogs and armed guards.

You: _____

_____

It happens. Sometimes you can't stop yourself, and you go into denial.

Just for fun, I asked random people to tell me their *usual* snack:

Sarah	Fruit (usually apples)
Louise	Bag of bite-size cookies
Jim	Peanut butter
Lona	Crackers with peanut butter and milk
Irene	Cheese and crackers
Jennie	Peanut M&Ms
Christina	Fiber One Oats and Chocolate Bars
Jackie	Homemade 100-calorie shakes made with milk, cocoa powder, and vanilla
Sharon	Wasa Crispbread
Amy	Hummus and baby carrots
Robert	32-ounce Pepsi
Elizabeth	Nonfat Greek yogurt with berries
Deanna	Starbucks Mocha Frappuccino light
Sue	Pretzels
Pat	Salt & vinegar chips
Josh	Charleston Chews
Michelle	String cheese
Rebecca	Sunflower seeds
Laura	Popcorn
Eric	Chips and salsa
Tawny	Bagel drowning in butter
John	Cashews
Jessica	M&M McFlurrie
Raquel	Cheetos
Hector	Yogurt with almonds
Rose	Chocolate

Eymard	Ice cream
Jeannette	Fries
Gordon	Maple pecan granola
Theresa	Cheese
Joy	Green grapes
Jeff	Jelly beans
Randy	Monster Energy drink

When I asked people to identify their usual snack, a lot of them answered, "When I'm being good or being bad?" Mood can determine whether people eat healthy snacks or unhealthy ones. If your emotions are talking to you, talk back by crunching on popcorn. It's better than eating an entire bag of potato chips. Keep unhealthy snacks (soda, candy, donuts, chips) out of the house. If it's not there, you can't eat it. When you're bored or anxious, having unhealthy snacks around is dangerous. You can run, but you can't hide. *They will find you.*

Or only have one "bad" snack to eat. Otherwise, you could bounce back and forth and go from one unhealthy snack to another. First you feel like something sweet. Then you feel like something salty. Look deeper for an unresolved emotion.

A handful of people told me that they don't snack. It's okay to not eat snacks. Some people do fine with two or three meals a day. Snacks aren't mandatory. However, make sure that you don't wait too long to eat and then end up eating too much at the meal.

Practice "The Rules of Snack Time"

Make rules for snacking. *No eating in the grocery store. You're there to watch a movie, not eat snacks. Don't eat while you watch TV. Don't eat in the car. You're at the game to see your team win, not drown yourself in snacks.* Eat snacks at certain times. 10-11 a.m. 3-4 p.m. Keep to a schedule. If embarrassment and guilt stop you from eating badly or too much, eat in front of other people. It may prevent you from sneaking down to the vending machine for a candy bar a couple of times a day.

Do you wolf down snacks? Do you load up your fork or spoon with food while you're still chewing the previous bite?

424

JF: I don't necessarily wolf down snacks. I am a lady when I am stuffing my fat face with yummy crap.

You: _____

_____

Here's another rule to add: *Always eat slowly, no matter what you're eating.* Taste and enjoy every calorie.

Nighttime Snacking Wisdom ❧

Snacking after dinner may be the easiest habit to give up, and it can be a pain-free way to eliminate unnecessary calories. An after-dinner snack is usually a habit. Most people aren't hungry for a snack because dinner was only a few hours ago. If you ate a small dinner and you are hungry and can't sleep, have a snack. A handful of nuts or a glass of fat-free milk and a graham cracker are nice bedtime snacks. Sleeping does not require many calories. Do you really need to eat at midnight? If you take medication and have to eat something, plan for it. Eat less at dinner. Eating 100 calories every night, when you're not hungry, will add 10 pounds in a year.

Tips for Children's Snacks

What do your kids eat for snacks? If your kids feel content after eating a healthy breakfast, an unhealthy snack at 10 a.m. will not be appealing. Some kids buy delicious cookies warm from the oven every day at school. After they graduate, they'll find a replacement food out of habit. The excess calories will be the beginning of an unwanted journey toward excess weight and unhealthy eating habits.

Children need nutrients to grow and be healthy. If you have kids to feed, start them off on the right foot. Get them used to eating healthy food and healthy snacks.

Consider these tips:

+ Cupcakes and chips don't belong in a lunch box.
+ Give your children fruit to eat for a snack after school. Kids walk by my office on their way home from school. Many of

them carry bottles of regular soda (not cans) and big bags of chips.

♦ Buying donuts on Saturday mornings doesn't promote healthy habits.

♦ Candy and cookies are not healthy snacks after games, practices, or extracurricular events. Talk to other parents, teachers, coaches, and anyone else who provides snacks to your children.

♦ Children shouldn't get the same size snack as an adult. For special treats, buy mini-muffins and bite-size cookies.

♦ Slice up fruit so that it's easier for kids to eat.

The apple doesn't fall far from the tree. If you're not used to eating healthy snacks, prepare them together as a family. It will be fun for everyone to learn together. Later in life, your kids will appreciate your concern for their health.

Workplace Temptations

Sometimes co-workers bring unhealthy food to work because they want to get rid of it. Have a response ready. *"No thanks. I'm not hungry."* Or *"Chocolate before noon gives me a stomachache."* Or *"It looks great but I had a big lunch."* Some clients tell me that they lie to get out of eating. They tell co-workers that they have diabetes and can't eat sweets. For them, it's easier than saying they're trying to lose weight. Keep some healthy snacks in your desk so that you can resist persuasive co-workers. Some school wellness policies specify that the staff should be role models. They don't allow candy on desks. This helps employees who are trying to eat healthy but give in to temptation.

Here are some further ideas:

♦ Get everyone to agree that if they're going to bring food to work, it should be healthy.

♦ For work parties, balance the unhealthy food with nutritious food. One cake is enough for a treat. Additional cookies and candy are not necessary.

♦ If you feel sluggish in the afternoon, think about whether you're tired or hungry. A few stretches or walking in place for a few minutes may take away the need to eat.

- If you're tired, a caffeinated beverage may hit the spot instead of a comforting, high-sugar snack with a lot of calories.
- Maybe you're thirsty, not hungry. Have an iced tea with lemon instead of a granola bar.
- If you're around people who are snacking, treat yourself to an herbal tea, a flavored water, or a sugar-free hot chocolate. Don't give in to peer pressure and overeat.

Just like meals, plan your snacks. Grabbing whatever might be available at the office, convenience store, or coffee shop is not usually calorie-friendly.

Become a Creative Snack Chef ❧

If you like to cook, make spinach dip and serve it with whole grain crackers for a snack. Or make low-fat pumpkin muffins for healthy snacks. You could mix together whole grain cereal, nuts, and dried cranberries for a filling and nutritious snack. A bowl of strawberries, sliced pears, or other fruit with a splash of chocolate syrup is a delicious treat. It's low in calories compared to a slice of cheesecake. The possibilities are endless!

Yes, You Can Snack Healthfully

If you're very hungry and can't wait until the next meal, eat a snack. Healthy snacks can be filling, taste good, and be energizing. Maybe just a cup of crushed ice would be satisfying. After you get used to eating healthy snacks, greasy chips and sugary sweets will not appeal to you. Think about what you need and keep empty calories to a minimum.

- *Am I unconsciously eating because of an emotion?*
- *Is it hunger or a habit? Am I social eating?*
- *Am I lacking any nutrients? Do I need more calcium? More fiber? More protein?*
- *Can I spare a few calories and splurge on a snack without nutrients?*
- *Will a snack help me eat less at the next meal?*

A healthy snack is your new best friend.

WEEKLY REMINDER ◆

Your Reasons for Losing Weight

You know the drill by now …

Why do you want to lose weight?

JF: Good health and stamina so I can fit into the clothes I am passionate about and be a better performer. Overall I just want to be healthy. With good health comes the trimmer waistline. Oh, and to look extra hot. I am hot already but there is always room for more hotness.

You: _____

_____

𝒟ay 29 CHECK-IN ☑

What did you accomplish yesterday?

JF: I am working on not eating after a certain time so as to not feel: (1) guilty and (2) like a fat walrus when I lay myself down to sleep.

You: _____

_____

What is your goal for today?

(Bring a bag of apples and a jar of peanut butter to work.) (Take all the unhealthy treats out of your house.) (Buy or make mini bran muffins.) (Buy 100-calorie bags of pretzels.) (Make small bags of trail mix.) (Brush your teeth after dinner. You're done eating for the night.)

JF: Snacking is a huge part of my challenge and I am determined to eat peanuts that are not surrounded by chocolate and a hard candy shell.

You: _____

_____

Day 30

Never Give Up!

*C*ongratulations! You've reached the finish line. You've lived and breathed 30 DAYS of *The Food Is My Friend Diet.* You have begun the process of changing your habits and developing a healthy lifestyle.

This book is all about *you* and what's best for you. Your health is a priority, but looking and feeling good count too. I hope that the experience was fruitful for you. Stay motivated with your reasons for losing weight. This is a lifestyle, not a fad diet. Fad diets put your health at risk. Think of this book as a 4th of July fireworks celebration. Each chapter has been full of "oohs" and "aahs." The last chapter is the grand finale.

Do you see things differently than you did A MONTH ago? Has your attitude changed? Do you understand how and why you accumulated excess weight? How do you feel about making changes to your diet, physical activity, and lifestyle?

JF: I see a lot of things differently. Now I'm equipped with a lot of new information for what is good for my body.

All of my excess weight, if I had to sum it up, is because of excuses. I travel a lot and don't spend much time at home, but there is no reason I can't use what I know now while on the road.

You: _____

_____

What's the best thing you learned in the last four weeks?

JF: A lot of what I have learned has made me incredibly sad. But I guess if all the information I have been getting was happy "keep eating that" news, this entire process would have been easy. I have had to have "the talk" with some favorite foods and tell them that I am going to start to see other foods. Some of the foods didn't like that I was letting them go; some even threatened to hurt me if I left, but breaking up is hard to do …. Sorry, Pringles Potato Crisps, Sour Cream & Onion.

You: _____

_____

Assessing How You've Done

As a registered dietitian nutritionist, it's my responsibility to help you be successful. I make *The Food Is My Friend Diet* engaging, interactive, and fun. Hopefully, you got to know yourself better. Maybe it was easy. Maybe it was harder than you thought. Consider it a turning point. This is an opportunity to grow and look at yourself in a *new* way. It's a chance for hope, optimism, and a healthier you.

It's time to weigh in.

*Weight:*_____Weight (Jackie): 188.5 pounds

Are you happy with the results? Could you have done better? Is there anything stopping you?

JF: I am getting happy with the results. I am also in a lot of pain and very sore because of all the new activity in my life, but it is worth it. I could, of course, have done better. However, what I have learned is that despite having setbacks I cannot and should not quit. A bad day is only a diversion, and I don't need to throw away a plan because someone forced a red velvet cupcake down my throat (it could happen!). My only real obstacle is me, and I have given myself a good talking to about sticking with my plan to keep dropping the pounds.

You: _____

_____

Yes ... You're Losing Weight!

If you lost weight, *excellent*. Repeat the four weeks and lose some *more* weight. Every time you identify a problem or hurdle, come up with a solution. Set a goal and *go for it*. Keep eating healthy. Keep getting physical activity. If you haven't been eating healthy, it won't be that easy to switch over to a new lifestyle. *Take baby steps.*

Two to eight pounds in four weeks is possible. For some people, losing 8 pounds in a year is an achievement. Weight loss could be slower if you don't get some kind of physical activity most days of the week.

If you lost four pounds, jump for joy. That could amount to 52 pounds in a year. *That's fantastic.* It's encouraging to lose weight quickly. However, that doesn't mean that you're changing your habits and behaviors. You need the test of time. Losing weight quickly could result in muscle loss. You want *fat loss*. Go slow and steady. Be patient. It would be unrealistic to lose 5 or 10 pounds in a week and keep it off.

No Progress on the Scale?

Is your weight the same? Repeat the four weeks. Four weeks isn't long compared to a lifetime, so even just maintaining the same weight can be an accomplishment. Losing weight takes a little more effort than simply wanting to lose weight.

If you didn't lose any weight, you may feel discouraged. The energy going in balanced the energy going out. I understand how frustrating it can be to not see the scale go down. Take a look at what you did. Were you too busy to exercise? Did you eat when you weren't hungry? Did you eat when your stomach whimpered instead of growled? Did you eat out too much? Was there a lot of special-occasion eating? Is someone sabotaging your efforts? Are there still too many high-calorie goodies around? Are you lacking self-discipline? Whatever happened, don't worry about it. *Keep trying.*

If you don't think that you eat much and you didn't lose weight, start keeping a food journal again. Learn from it. In reality, maybe you ate more than you needed. Very few people can eat whatever they want and lose weight. Don't let occasional binges make you give up.

If you don't obsess over it, weigh yourself every day. Use the scale as a tool. If the scale isn't budging, it's telling you that you're eating too many calories to lose weight. If you can pinch an inch, you're eating more calories than you need. It's okay to eat fewer calories. The reward of seeing the scale go down will be worth the effort. Keep in mind that weight can fluctuate depending on water retention, the time of day, and clothes. If you eat two eggs and two pieces of toast for breakfast, start eating one egg and one piece of toast. You may be *used* to eating that much but you may not *need* that much. You might find the lesser amount to be "just right."

If your weight is stuck, assess your hunger. If hunger wasn't an issue, it would be a lot easier to lose weight. Step outside your comfort zone. You may need to feel more hunger than what is comfortable to you. When you eat, don't eat until you feel full. Crank up the physical activity to jump-start your metabolism. Your body likes things the way it is and it's trying to keep it the same. You're in charge of what you eat. Show your body who's the boss.

As you get older, you may be eating less and still not losing weight. Your metabolism is probably taking a dive. You need to eat even fewer calories to lose weight, and you want to avoid *sarcopenia*. This sounds like a horrible disease. In a way, it is. It's the loss of muscle mass. *Get busy. Move your body.* Unfortunately, older people can no longer eat like teenagers. Knees may hurt, making physical activity more difficult. *Do your best.*

Even Heavier Now?

If you've gained weight, pick up the pieces and start over again. Don't wait until you've added five more pounds before you start making changes. Things don't always go the way you want them to go. Bounce back. Keep making improvements. *You can do it!* It's all about getting your head in the game. Consistency, moderation, and persistence. Maybe part of you is resisting, and you need to hit rock bottom a few times before you've had enough. Then get serious. If you feel angry that you can't have a piece of cheesecake, go get one. Get it out of your system. *No foods are restricted, just the amount.*

If you're not ready, you're not ready. If someone gave you $1,000 a day to lose weight, it might not be enough. When you're ready, even $20 a day would be a nice reward. Decide if you will be ready "someday" or if you are "now."

Some medications make people gain weight. See if your medications caused an increase in appetite or water retention. Maybe there's another type of drug for you.

Are there still triggers that set off excess eating? Be aware of foods or situations that result in a lack of control. *Be proactive.* Be ready to stop yourself from eating *before* you're going to binge. Don't leave anything to chance. Plan your meals and snacks. Know what and how much you're going to eat. Try a little harder every day.

Continue to Use This Book as a Loyal Friend, Wise Counselor ◌

*"Some books are to be tasted, others to be swallowed,
and some few to be chewed and digested;
that is, some books are to be read only in parts,
others to be read, but not curiously,
and some few to be read wholly, and with diligence and attention."*

~ Sir Francis Bacon, English author (1561-1626)

Don't eat this book to increase your intake of fiber, but get the most out of it that you can. Keep reading the chapters until you understand everything and can apply it.

Need a Pep Talk?

Are you the chronic dieter who can't lose weight? Or if you lose weight, you regain it?

Do you care? Is it really important to you to eat less? *You have to care.* Keep thinking of reasons why you want to lose weight. If you're used to having a sweet treat in the afternoon or grabbing a snack before you go to sleep, the urge to eat will hit you hard. This is the time that you have to get tough. Deep down you know that you aren't really hungry but you feel like eating anyway. *Stay strong.* In the morning, you will feel triumphant. You survived, and it wasn't that bad. If a celery stick doesn't appeal to you, maybe you aren't that hungry. As time goes on, it will get easier to resist the urges. Soon your new healthier habits will take over.

Give yourself a pep talk. Say this out loud: *"I want to eat but I'm not hungry. I really want to lose weight. My stomach is too big. I can do this. I am not going to eat!"* It's not business as usual anymore. Take it one nibble, snack, and meal at a time. If other people can lose weight, so can you. Give yourself tough love. When you feel "just right," shout, *"I'm done eating. No more!"*

What if you reach a plateau? Many people reach a certain weight and can't lose any more. If this happens to you, take it easy. When you were at a higher weight, you were eating a lot more calories. Maintain for a while. Then eat fewer carbs, less protein and fewer sweets. What calories can you sacrifice? Watch the alcohol. You need fewer and fewer calories at a lower weight. You can't go back to eating the same amount of calories that you were eating at your highest weight. Try increasing physical activity.

Keep Active ☜

Physical activity seems to be a critical factor in losing and maintaining. Find pleasure in a variety of physical activities. It shouldn't be a form of punishment. Walking, dancing, and cleaning do not cost money. Physical activity will maintain muscle mass and strength. Physical activity reduces jiggle. Set measurable goals. Walk 10 minutes three times a week on Monday, Wednesday, and Friday. Gradually increase the time and the days. Begin to establish a routine. Soon it becomes: *"It's Saturday. I can't wait to do weights."*

Beware of Feeling Deprived

People get used to eating a certain amount of food. They eat for the sake of eating. If they're "dieting," they may not want to eat less – especially if people around them are eating everything in sight. Eating less or being told to eat less makes some people feel deprived.

Even though you can eat smaller amounts of whatever you want, do you feel deprived?

JF: I don't feel deprived, just a little nostalgic. I sometimes cry when standing in front of a display case filled with baked goods. However, I have to remember a minute on the lips is a lifetime standing in front of the mirrors in a fitting room crying my eyes out.

You: _____

Practice Being Careful and Maintain Your Weight

After you reach your ideal weight, it may be difficult to maintain. In the beginning, you are disciplined. Life starts getting in the way, and you give yourself some slack. *"Oh, a few fries won't hurt." "I'll just have a little ice cream."* All the little bites add up, and slowly the weight comes back. *Be careful.*

Be Careful

Be careful of your thoughts
For your thoughts become your words
Be careful of your words
For your words become your actions
Be careful of your actions
For your actions become your habits
Be careful of your habits
For your habits become your character
Be careful of your character
For your character becomes your destiny.

~ Author Unknown

Apply this poem to losing weight. One day you think that a donut would taste good (thoughts). You drive by the donut shop and say, "I feel like getting a donut" (words). You stop and buy a couple of donuts (actions). They taste good to you so you pick up a couple of donuts every day on your way to work (habits). After a few months, you start gaining weight. You continue gaining weight throughout the year (character). Eventually, you have excess amounts of weight, along with high blood pressure and elevated cholesterol (destiny). It all started with a thought.

You can also put a positive twist to the poem. You have been thinking about working out and going to the gym (thoughts). You ask some friends if they want to join a gym with you (words). You get a gym membership (actions). You go to the gym three times a week (habits). You start building muscle mass and losing weight (character). Your blood pressure improves, and you have more energy (destiny). *It all started with a thought.*

Don't put yourself down or let others put you down. Change your way of thinking. Do the old switcheroo.

Instead of Eating When:	Say:
Angry	*I'm too angry to eat.*
Sad and lonely	*I don't feel like eating.*
Stressed	*Rewarding myself with food doesn't work for me.*
Proud of yourself	*I feel like being with friends, not eating.*
Happy	*I don't need to eat.*
Bored	*I'll find something to do.*

Stay hungry for a change. Often people let the passion die and go back to their old habits. It's easier and much more fun to gain weight than lose it, but you can't go back to the good old days. Has this ever happened to you? You're not that hungry. You get tempted to eat something with lots of calories. You feel a little down. You go ahead and eat to feel better. Then you feel frustrated for eating. *Break the chain of events. Care.* If you truly want to lose the weight and keep it off, you will.

Many clients have told me that they have lost 20-50 pounds. The trick is keeping it off. Don't frequent the "Lost and Found" Department. If you lost weight and regained it, how will this time be different?

JF: This time is different because I am not aiming at losing a massive amount of weight just to be able to say I dropped 30 pounds in three weeks. I have a more realistic view of health and weight loss. I have lost up to 25 pounds in the past and put some of it back on little by little. I have learned that maintenance requires the same amount of discipline as losing.

You: _____

_____

A Weight That's Out of This World ☙

If you absolutely can't lose weight and you refuse to accept extra weight, there is a Plan B. *Live on the moon.* If you weigh 170 pounds on Earth, on the moon you will only weigh 28 pounds. *Cool!* Thinking about going to Jupiter? You'd weigh 401 pounds there!

Tips for Eating Healthy and Managing Your Weight

Here are some ideas to help you succeed long-term in your weight-loss journey. When you need an overall refresher, come back and review these tips.

- **Choose a variety of nutrient-rich foods.** Eat 4-4½ cups of fruits and vegetables and three sources of low-fat or fat-free milk products every day. Choose whole grains, lean sources of protein, and healthy fats. Limit salt.
- **Unwind with exercise.** Get at least 30-60 minutes of physical activity *every day.* The more you exercise, the more calories you burn. You know what they say ... *"Seven days without physical activity makes one weak."* Exercise is nature's medicine.
- **Only eat if you're hungry!! Stop when you feel "just right."** You could pack away a little more to feel "full," but don't. Keep

the temptations out of sight. Avoid watching television, reading, or sitting in front of your computer while eating. *Just eat.*

♦ **Avoid emotional eating.** Eat comfort foods with little or no calories. Find simple pleasures in life to lift your spirits.

♦ **Bad eating habits are learned behaviors. Watch the empty calories.** Limit calories from alcohol, solid fats, and added sugars (SoFAS). In other words, get off the SOFA. (That's more dietitian humor.)

♦ **When you want to eat and you aren't hungry, fill up on hot or cold beverages with little or no calories.**

♦ **If you feel like you're starving, eat or drink 50-100 calories of carbohydrate to boost your blood sugar level.**

♦ **Avoid high-fat and fried foods.** They contain too many calories and not enough nutrients.

♦ **The more you weigh, the more you eat.** Substitute low-calorie fruits and vegetables with lots of fiber for high-calorie foods to get the full feeling.

♦ **Stop and take a 10-15 minute break from eating. Then go back and see if you're still hungry.**

♦ **Slow down. Gobbling is for turkeys.** You could end up eating too much.

♦ **Make an eating schedule.** Wait until 3 p.m. to eat a snack, instead of random munching.

♦ **Decide how much of your meal you're going to eat at the restaurant.** Before the meal is over, get a container for the leftovers.

♦ **Exercise more than you normally would.** Think about how much physical activity construction workers get in a day. Think about how much physical activity you get sitting in front of a desk in a day.

♦ **It's okay to feel hunger.** You can go a long time without food. Say, "No, thank you. I ate earlier."

♦ **Don't feel the need to finish what's on your plate.** Remember, restaurant portions can be gigantic!

♦ **Take one or two bites to try a food.** Go for bite-size desserts.

♦ **If it keeps you on track, keep using a food journal.** Use it to identify emotions or activities that trigger overeating.

- **Get busy.** Being busy takes your mind off food.
- **Focus on what you're eating.** Look at your food. Smell it. Taste it. Chew it slowly. Swallow it. Pause. Savor the flavor.
- **Speed up your metabolism. Build muscle mass.**
- **Cook more at home.** Modify recipes.
- **If you binge on snacks, don't put yourself down.** Work it off and start over ASAP.
- **Be optimistic. Let things go.** Be happy. Stay positive. Do what makes you happy. Compliment yourself every day. Improve the world. View the world sunny side up.
- **Stay hydrated.** You'll have more energy.
- **If you can't do it alone, ask for support from family, friends, or co-workers.** Tell them what you want and what you need. Support one another. But don't compare yourself to others.
- **Weigh yourself once a week, more if needed.** If your weight goes up, eat less and exercise more *immediately.*
- **Base your food choices on science, not science fiction.** Get help from an expert. Ask a registered dietitian nutritionist.
- **When you feel like giving up, try harder.**

Make a Lifetime Commitment to Your Health

For thousands of years, people have used food to stay healthy. Look at this ancient Ayurvedic proverb for the journey of a long life. It's never too late to eat healthy and get physical activity.

> *"When diet is wrong, medicine is of no use.*
> *When diet is correct, medicine is of no need."*

Pledge: I want this to be a lifelong commitment. I will continue eating healthy foods (follow MyPlate guidelines) and get daily physical activity (may involve sweat).

Signed: *Jackie Fabulous*

Signed:_____

Will you be a role model to your family, friends, co-workers and the community to eat healthy and get physical activity? (Say "yes.")

JF: Hell, yes!

You: _____

_____

Many Americans are overweight and undernourished. People are eating too many foods with sodium, saturated fat, trans fatty acids, refined grains, and added sugars. Many people are not getting enough calcium, potassium, magnesium, fiber, and vitamins A, C, D, and E. We can meet these nutrient requirements if we eat more nutrient-rich foods, such as dark greens, red/orange vegetables, beans and peas, nuts, fruits, whole grains, oils, and low-fat or fat-free milk products. Follow the MyPlate meal patterns. Eat the right amounts of a variety of foods to maintain a healthy weight. Continue eating fewer calories and move your body more. _Obesity is the number one preventable disease._

There is a proliferation of diet books on the market every year. Yet most Americans are still overweight or obese. Forget about fad diets. Most of the diet books are not helpful and contain nutrition misinformation. Don't believe empty promises and miracles. Here's a fact: If you eat 1,500 calories worth of candy bars every day for a week and nothing else, you will lose weight because of the total amount of calories. HOWEVER, The Candy Bar Diet is not recommended, BECAUSE IT IS NOT HEALTHY.

Worst case scenario: If you have trouble losing weight, what would be the last straw? What horrible thing would have to happen to you before you made changes? (Can't walk? Can't get out of bed? Heart surgery? Blind from diabetes?)

JF: Probably a pool party that I had to attend. Public nudity is a great motivator.

You: _____

_____

Don't wait another ounce.

Reliable nutrition knowledge is important but it isn't enough to make some people change. Many people change their habits for emotional reasons, not facts. Knowing that eating fruit reduces the risk of cancer may not be enough motivation. Seeing a friend lose their hair from chemo may be the deciding factor. I give you the oars. You have to get in the boat and start rowing.

When emotions take over, many people are unable to listen to their hunger cues. People have learned to use food to satisfy their emotional hunger. Are you still using food for comfort, to soothe yourself, to escape, or as a distraction in the darkest of times? Are you using food to celebrate, to relax, or to seek pleasure in good times? How is your emotional health?

JF: I talk out my feelings now and exercise to control my cravings. I still love to celebrate good times with treats like wine, but now I will only have a glass instead of a bottle.

You: _____

_____

Where do you see yourself in a year? What do you want to change?

JF: I will be at my goal weight and sexy in a year. I don't want to change too much about me; just to be able to walk around during the summer half-naked is my wish.

You: _____

_____

What are your food and physical activity goals for the next five years? Come up with a plan to optimize your health. Where do you see yourself in five years?

JF: I will have a black belt in karate in five years. Mainly, my goal is health overall.

You: _____

_____

Repeat *The Food Is My Friend Diet,* reading one chapter a week. If you prefer, focus on one chapter a month. Take your time. Most people aren't eating enough healthy foods. They could … but they don't.

Most people are not getting enough physical activity. They could ... but they don't. It may take a while to routinely eat vegetables and go for a walk. *Never give up.* Turn your "I can'ts" into "I cans." You can and you will. LET'S SEE SOME ATTITUDE! *Stay with it.* Get more out of life than food. Because you know what?

You are your best friend. Believe in yourself. Do it for you.

I have enjoyed our time together and hope you have, too – even if it's been a bit difficult at times. I will be with you in spirit and will be thinking of you. Have a long and happy life.

End of 30 Days

Repeat the process of working your way through this book as many times as needed. Keep learning and changing. Build on previous successes. Your reward is losing weight. Instead of using your emotions to put on the pounds, use your emotions to stay motivated and keep your inner glow alive. Expect to succeed. Why do you want to lose the pounds? Keep the reason in your heart and watch the weight fall off. *The best is yet to come.*

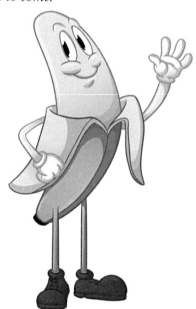

$\mathcal{D}$ay 30 CHECK-IN ☑

What did you accomplish yesterday?

JF: I finished a major project of learning who I am in food and fitness.

Now the journey continues ….

You: _____

_____

What is your goal for today? (Pick some ideas from "Tips for Eating Healthy and Managing Your Weight.")

JF: My goal today is to go grocery shopping and to fill my cart with foods that will truly feed me, not just fill it up with the crap I am used to eating. I might be a little obnoxious too while shopping and point out how bad someone's food choices are by asking, "Do you know what's really in that cereal?" I have always wanted to be the annoying health nut. Thanks to TFIMFD, now I can be.

You: _____

_____

The Food Is My Friend Diet
Measurements and Weight Record

Measurements

	Start	1 Month	2 Months	3 Months	4 Months	5 Months	6 Months
Chest							
Waist							
Hips							
Thighs							

Weight

Start	

Week 1		Week 11		Week 21	
Week 2		Week 12		Week 22	
Week 3		Week 13		Week 23	
Week 4		Week 14		Week 24	
Week 5		Week 15		Week 25	
Week 6		Week 16		Week 26	
Week 7		Week 17		Week 27	
Week 8		Week 18		Week 28	
Week 9		Week 19		Week 29	
Week 10		Week 20		Week 30	

Index

The Food Is My Friend Diet
ORDER FORM

Shipping

Name _____

Organization _____

Address _____

_____

City _____

State/Prov _____ Zip/Postal Code _____

Country _____

Phone _____ Fax _____

Email _____

Number of Copies _____ x $21.95 US ($24.95 Can) _____

Add 9.5% sales tax for CA orders _____

*Shipping & Handling
☐ 1 Book $6.00
☐ 2-5 Books $12.00
☐ 6 or more contact Gales Publishing

Shipping & Handling* _____

TOTAL _____
Thank you for your order!

Payment
☐ Credit Card   ☐ Check (to Gales Publishing)
☐ Visa   ☐ MasterCard   ☐ Discover   ☐ PayPal
(galespublishing@gmail.com)

Name on Card: _____

Card # _____ Exp Date _____

Orders

Mail:
Gales Publishing
P.O. Box 11721
Burbank, CA 91510

Phone: (818) 843-6628
Fax: (818) 846-1822
Email: GalesPublishing@gmail.com
Website: www.RuthFrechman.com

Please contact for: ☐ Skype counseling ☐ Speaking/Seminars